Respiratory Medicine

Series Editor: Sharon I.S. Rounds

For further volumes:
http://www.springer.com/series/7665

Keith C. Meyer • Allan R. Glanville
Editors

Bronchiolitis Obliterans Syndrome in Lung Transplantation

Humana Press

Editors
Keith C. Meyer, MD, MS, FACP, FCCP
Department of Internal Medicine
Section of Allergy
Pulmonary and Critical Care Medicine
University of Wisconsin School
of Medicine and Public Health
Madison, WI, USA

Allan R. Glanville, MBBS, MD, FRACP
Lung Transplant Unit
St. Vincent's Hospital
Sydney, NSW, Australia

ISBN 978-1-4614-7635-1 ISBN 978-1-4614-7636-8 (eBook)
DOI 10.1007/978-1-4614-7636-8
Springer New York Heidelberg Dordrecht London

Library of Congress Control Number: 2013942309

Printed on acid-free paper

Springer is part of Springer Science+Business Media (www.springer.com)

Keith Meyer and Allan Glanville dedicate this book to their families, mentors, and patients.

Keith Meyer especially dedicates this book to his parents-in-law, Wanda and Robert Auerbach, who have provided invaluable and loving support and guidance as he struggled to pursue a career in science and medicine.

Allan Glanville, in particular, dedicates this book to the many patients who have educated him regarding bravery, trust, and fellowship during their combined journey in this amazing field of lung transplantation.

Preface

It has been 50 years since the first successful human lung transplant was reported in 1963 by Hardy and colleagues. However, the success of this first transplant was transient, and outcomes remained poor until the early 1980s, when cyclosporine A (CsA) was first used for clinical immunosuppression. This was associated temporally with improved techniques for donor lung preservation, better surgical techniques, and advances in postoperative management. Most importantly, after an initial experience with dual immunosuppression (CsA and corticosteroids), it was found that a triple drug regimen of CsA, azathioprine, and corticosteroids given post-transplant could prevent acute rejection quite effectively. In the 1990s another calcineurin inhibitor (tacrolimus) and antimetabolite (mycophenolate) became available as alternates to CsA and azathioprine, respectively. Along with improved post-transplantation triple-drug immunosuppression, prophylactic regimens were devised over the past 2 decades to prevent opportunistic infection with viruses (cytomegalovirus and herpes simplex) and fungi (*Candida*, *Aspergillus*, and *Pneumocystis*).

Nonetheless, despite numerous developments in clinical lung transplantation and substantially improved survival statistics from a median survival of approximately 3.9 years in the early 1990s to 5.5 years in the early 2000s, delayed loss of allograft function due to the onset of obliterative bronchiolitis (OB) remains the prime cause of debilitation and recipient death for patients who successfully recover from the transplant and achieve good graft function during the initial recovery period. Because a confident diagnosis of chronic allograft rejection due to OB is difficult to make without a surgical lung biopsy, with its attendant risks of significant morbidity and mortality, a persistent decline of FEV_1 on spirometric testing ($\geq$20 % from baseline) was adopted as a clinical surrogate that is considered highly specific for the development of the syndrome of constrictive bronchiolitis and small airway obliteration that has become known as the bronchiolitis obliterans syndrome (BOS). BOS is generally considered to occur as a consequence of chronic allograft rejection. Attempts to prevent BOS or arrest its progression when it occurs in lung transplant recipients have been ineffective. The identification of risk factors that can be modified, the discovery of interventions that can prevent it from occurring, the development of sensitive and specific tests to facilitate early detection, and the advent of effective therapies to reverse it or prevent its progression would greatly improve survival and quality of life for lung transplant recipients. Recipients without BOS in particular can survive more than 2 decades post-transplant if significant complications do not occur.

This book is intended to provide readers with a comprehensive understanding of the definition and changing perceptions of the nature of BOS as a clinical and pathologic entity, immune and nonimmune mechanisms that have been identified as risk factors for the development of BOS, and interventions that may prove to be clinically useful for the prevention or treatment of BOS. Chapter 1 reviews observations that lead to the recognition of BOS as a clinical entity, risk factors that have been associated with its appearance, and evolving nomenclature and recognition of chronic lung allograft dysfunction (CLAD) phenotypes. Chapters 2, 3, 4, and 5 examine clinical aspects of BOS and other forms of CLAD. Drs. Lagstein and Myers review the histopathology of obliterative bronchiolitis and related entities that can cause allograft dysfunction in Chap. 2. Drs. Snell, Levvey, and Westall comprehensively review the multitude of abnormalities that can cause CLAD (which must be considered in the differential diagnosis of BOS) in Chap. 3. Dr. Kanne provides a review of the diagnostic capabilities and limitations of thoracic imaging when evaluating patients with suspected CLAD in Chap. 4. Finally, Drs. Brown and Nathan provide a comprehensive discussion of approaches that are currently used to screen for declining lung function and to make a confident diagnosis of BOS when a decline in allograft function is detected.

Chapters 6, 7, 8, 9, 10, and 11 examine the role of allo- and autoimmune responses, infection, and gastroesophageal reflux (GER) in the pathogenesis of BOS. Dr. Martinu thoroughly examines the role of T cell-mediated alloimmunity in OB pathogenesis in Chap. 6. In addition to adaptive immune T-cell response, there is growing recognition that B cells and antibody-mediated immune responses can play a key role in BOS, and Mr. Ainge-Allen and Dr. Glanville examine the expanding knowledge of antibody-mediated rejection (AMR) in the context of lung transplantation and present current recommendations for the diagnosis and treatment of AMR in Chap. 7. There is also increasing awareness that innate immune mechanisms, in concert with adaptive immune responses, play key roles in BOS, and Drs. Todd and Palmer review our current and evolving knowledge of innate immunity and BOS pathogenesis in Chap. 8. In addition to alloimmune responses to lung allograft implantation in human lung transplantation, there is increasing evidence that autoimmunity may develop and play a significant role in BOS pathogenesis, and such autoimmune sensitization may even exist prior to transplant. Drs. Braun, Meyer, and Burlingham review new and evolving knowledge of autoimmune responses that are associated with chronic rejection and BOS, the role of interleukin-17 responses, and the utility of animal models of BOS in Chap. 10. Finally, Chaps. 11 and 12 cover two major risk factors that have been associated with BOS. Dr. Avery provides a comprehensive discussion of the role of various infections in BOS pathogenesis in Chap. 11, and Drs. D'Ovidio and Aramini explore the role of GER with pulmonary aspiration of refluxate in BOS pathogenesis in Chap. 12 and provide current approaches to the diagnosis and treatment of significant GER in lung transplant candidates and recipients.

Approaches to the diagnosis and management of BOS in infants and small children can vary significantly from what is done for older children and adults, and Drs. Robinson and Aurora give an overview of current approaches to detect and manage BOS in children in Chap. 13. Finally, Chaps. 14, 15, and 16 cover important aspects of BOS prevention and management. Dr. Bhorade provides a comprehensive overview of the role of immunosuppression in the prevention and treatment of BOS in Chap. 14, and Drs. Vos, Stijn Verleden, Ruttens, Vanaudenaerde, and Geert Verleden provide a nicely comprehensive review of the immunomodulatory properties of azithromycin and its role as an agent that can be used to effectively treat and possibly prevent BOS. Lastly, Dr. Hachem provides an up-to-date and comprehensive review of the status of other therapies, such as extracorporeal photopheresis or total lymphoid irradiation, that may provide benefit for patients who have developed BOS in Chap. 16.

We hope that those who read this book will benefit from its contents and that it may stimulate future research endeavors that seek to better understand the pathogenesis of BOS and identify strategies to prevent its occurrence, to detect its onset before significant allograft impairment has occurred to allow therapeutic interventions, and to treat BOS such that further loss of allograft function can be prevented and even possibly restored.

Madison, WI, USA — Keith C. Meyer, MD, MS, FACP, FCCP
Sydney, NSW, Australia — Allan R. Glanville, MBBS, MD, FRACP

Contents

Contributors

Henry W. Ainge-Allen, M.D., Ph.D. Lung Transplant Unit, St. Vincent's Hospital, Sydney, NSW, Australia

Beatrice Aramini, M.D., Ph.D. Dipartimento di Scienze Mediche e Chirurgiche Materno-Infantili e dell'Adulto, Azienda Ospedaliero-Universitaria Policlinico di Modena, Modena, Italy

Paul Aurora, M.B.B.S., M.R.C.P., Ph.D., Department of Paediatric Respiratory Medicine, Great Ormond Street Hospital for Children, London, UK

Robin K. Avery, M.D., Division of Infectious Disease (Transplant/Oncology), Johns Hopkins Hospital, Baltimore, MD, USA

Sangeeta M. Bhorade, M.D., University of Chicago Medical Center, Chicago, IL, USA

Rudolf K. Braun, Ph.D., Department of Pediatrics, University of Wisconsin Madison, Madison, WI, USA

A. Whitney Brown, M.D., Advanced Lung Disease and Lung Transplant Program, Inova Fairfax Hospital, Falls Church, VA, USA

William J. Burlingham, Ph.D., Department of Surgery, University of Wisconsin, Madison, WI, USA

Frank D'Ovidio, M.D., Ph.D., Department of Surgery, NewYork-Presbyterian Hospital, Columbia University Medical Centre, New York, NY, USA

Allan R. Glanville, M.B.B.S., M.D., F.R.A.C.P., Lung Transplant Unit, St. Vincent's Hospital, Sydney, NSW, Australia

Ramsey Hachem, M.D., Washington University School of Medicine/Barnes-Jewish Hospital Pulmonary and Critical Care, St. Louis, MO, USA

Jeffrey P. Kanne, M.D., Department of Radiology, University of Wisconsin School of Medicine and Public Health, Madison, WI, USA

Amir Lagstein, M.D., Department of Pathology, University of Michigan, Ann Arbor, MI, USA

Vibha N. Lama, M.D., M.S., Department of Internal Medicine, University of Michigan, Ann Arbor, MI, USA

Bronwyn J. Levvey, R.N., B.Ed. Stu., Grad. Dip. Clin. Epi, Faculty of Medicine, Nursing and Health Sciences, Monash University, Melbourne, VIC, Australia

Department of Allergy, Immunology and Respiratory Medicine, The Alfred Hospital, Melbourne, VIC, Australia

Tereza Martinu, M.D., Department of Medicine, Duke University Medical Center, Durham, NC, USA

Keith C. Meyer, M.D., M.S., Department of Internal Medicine, Section of Allergy, Pulmonary and Critical Care Medicine, University of Wisconsin School of Medicine and Public Health, Madison, WI, USA

Jeffrey Myers, M.D., Divisions of Anatomic Pathology and MLabs, Department of Pathology, University of Michigan, Ann Arbor, MI, USA

Steven D. Nathan, M.D., Advanced Lung Disease and Lung Transplant Program, Inova Fairfax Hospital, Falls Church, VA, USA

Scott M. Palmer, M.D., M.H.S., Division of Pulmonary Allergy, and Critical Care Medicine, Department of Internal Medicine, Duke University Medical Center, Durham, NC, USA

Paul D. Robinson, M.B.Ch.B., M.R.C.P.C.H., F.R.A.C.P., Ph.D., Department of Pediatric Respiratory Medicine, The Children's Hospital at Westmead, Sydney, NSW, Australia

Portex Respiratory Unit, UCL Institute of Child Health, London, UK

David Ruttens, M.D. Lung Transplantation Unit, University Hospital Gasthuisberg, Leuven, Belgium

Gregory I. Snell, M.B.B.S., F.R.A.C.P., M.D., Department of Allergy, Immunology and Respiratory Medicine, The Alfred Hospital, Melbourne, VIC, Australia

Jamie L. Todd, M.D., Division of Pulmonary, Allergy, and Critical Care Medicine, Department of Internal Medicine, Duke University Medical Center, Durham, NC, USA

Bart M. Vanaudenaerde, Ph.D., Lung Transplantation Unit, University Hospital Gasthuisberg, Leuven, Belgium

Geert M. Verleden, M.D., Ph.D., Lung Transplantation Unit, University Hospital Gasthuisberg, Leuven, Belgium

Stijn E. Verleden, M.Sc., Lung Transplantation Unit, University Hospital Gasthuisberg, Leuven, Belgium

Robin Vos, M.D., Ph.D., Lung Transplantation Unit, University Hospital Gasthuisberg, Leuven, Belgium

Anish Wadhwa, M.D., Pulmonary and Critical Care Medicine, University of Michigan Health System, Ann Arbor, MI, USA

Glen P. Westall, M.D., Ph.D., Department of Allergy, Immunology and Respiratory Medicine, The Alfred Hospital, Melbourne, VIC, Australia

Chapter 1
Bronchiolitis Obliterans Syndrome and Chronic Lung Allograft Dysfunction: Evolving Concepts and Nomenclature

Keith C. Meyer and Allan R. Glanville

Abstract Bronchiolitis obliterans syndrome (BOS) eventually occurs in the majority of lung transplant recipients who survive beyond 1 year, can greatly impair quality of life, and is, directly or indirectly, the major cause of delayed allograft dysfunction and recipient death. A number of associated events or conditions are strongly associated with the risk for developing BOS; these include acute rejection, gastro-esophageal reflux, infections, and autoimmune reactions that can occur in the setting of alloimmune responses to the lung allograft as recipients are given intense immunosuppression to prevent allograft rejection. The term chronic lung allograft dysfunction (CLAD) is being increasingly used to refer to recipients with late allograft dysfunction that meets the spirometric criteria for the diagnosis of BOS, but clinicians should recognize that such dysfunction can occur for a variety of reasons other than BOS. The recently identified entity of restrictive allograft syndrome, which is now recognized as a relatively distinct phenotype of CLAD, has features that differentiate it from classic obstructive BOS. A number of other entities that can also significantly affect allograft function must also be considered when significant allograft dysfunction is encountered following lung transplantation.

Keywords Lung transplantation • Bronchiolitis obliterans syndrome • Obliterative bronchiolitis • Lung allograft rejection • Chronic lung allograft dysfunction • Restrictive allograft syndrome • Neutrophilic reversible allograft dysfunction

---

K.C. Meyer, M.D., M.S. (✉)
Department of Internal Medicine, Section of Allergy, Pulmonary and Critical Care Medicine, University of Wisconsin School of Medicine and Public Health, K4/910 Clinical Science Center, 600 Highland Avenue, Madison, WI 53792-9988, USA
e-mail: Kcm@medicine.wisc.edu

A.R. Glanville, M.B.B.S., M.D., F.R.A.C.P. (✉)
Lung Transplant Unit, St. Vincent's Hospital, Victoria Street, Darlinghurst, Sydney, NSW 2010, Australia
e-mail: aglanville@stvincents.com.au

K.C. Meyer and A.R. Glanville (eds.), *Bronchiolitis Obliterans Syndrome in Lung Transplantation*, Respiratory Medicine 8, DOI 10.1007/978-1-4614-7636-8_1,

Introduction

Late lung allograft dysfunction with progressive loss of function and graft loss was originally described for heart–lung transplant recipients in 1984 [1]. Histopathological postmortem examination of these lungs revealed lesions of constrictive bronchiolitis with airway fibrosis and luminal obliteration that was designated as obliterative bronchiolitis (OB). Late decline in allograft function following recovery and stabilization of lung function after the initial lung implantation was increasingly encountered as more lung transplants were performed in the late 1980s, and the consensus document that suggested that the term bronchiolitis obliterans syndrome (BOS) could be used to designate the syndrome of persistent loss of function with decline in FEV_1 that could not be explained by other, potentially reversible complications such as acute rejection or infection was published in 1993 [2].

Clinical experience that evolved over the subsequent 2 decades of lung transplantation has confirmed that the pathologic finding that usually correlates with a persistent decline in post-transplant FEV_1 that is consistent with the clinical diagnosis of BOS is the presence of the lesion of OB. The threshold of a ≥20 % decline in FEV_1 (with a pattern of airflow obstruction) from an established baseline was chosen in previous consensus documents [2, 3] as an appropriate surrogate marker of OB due to the strong association of OB with late chronic allograft dysfunction. Major considerations that led to choosing FEV_1 as a surrogate marker were (1) the relative difficulty of obtaining adequate diagnostic tissue via transbronchial lung biopsy (TBLB) plus (2) the desire to avoid the substantially increased risks of performing more invasive diagnostic procedures (i.e., surgical lung biopsy), although more extensive sampling of lung tissue could facilitate a more confident diagnosis (and may be considered necessary in certain situations). This chapter will provide an overview of current concepts pertaining to BOS and the terminology used to describe delayed or chronic allograft dysfunction.

An Overview of BOS Pathogenesis and Associated Risk Factors

Post-transplant OB is characterized by progressive obliteration of small airways accompanied by a persistent decline in FEV_1, an obstructive spirometric pattern, an essentially clear chest radiograph, and the lack of an alternative diagnosis to explain a persistent decline in lung function [2]. This syndrome was presumed to be caused by chronic allograft rejection, and the term chronic lung allograft dysfunction (CLAD) was coined and used to refer to allograft dysfunction that met the criteria that were adopted to indicate a diagnosis of BOS. Previously published consensus statements have designated a persistent decline in FEV_1 to ≤80 % of baseline post-transplant FEV_1 (that is present for a minimum of 3 weeks in the absence of confounding conditions) as a surrogate marker of probable OB (Table 1.1), and a staging system was devised to qualify the level of FEV_1 decline, which correlates fairly well with severity of allograft dysfunction.

Table 1.1 Diagnosis and grading of bronchiolitis obliterans syndrome

	Spirometry (% of baseline)	
BOS grade	1993 Classification	2002 Classification
0	FEV_1 ≥80 % of baseline	FEV_1 >90 % of baseline and FEF_{25-75} >75 % of baseline
0p	Not applicable	FEV_1 81–90 % of baseline and/or FEF_{25-75} ≤75 % of baseline
1	FEV_1 66–80 % of baseline	FEV_1 66–80 % of baseline
2	FEV_1 51–65 % of baseline	FEV_1 51–65 % of baseline
3	FEV_1 ≤50 % of baseline	FEV_1 ≤50 % of baseline

By definition, 3 or more months were required to have elapsed from the time of transplantation in order for the diagnosis of BOS to be made [2, 3]. This qualification was made to help distinguish BOS from non-BOS acute and/or subacute complications of lung transplantation as well as to take into account the time needed to establish both a baseline FEV_1 and a confirmed decline in FEV_1 with FEV_1 measurements taken 3 weeks apart. Because of concern that the cutoff value for FEV_1 at 80 % of the best post-transplant value may be insensitive to early decline in allograft function due to early OB, stage BOS-0p (FEV_1=81–90 % of baseline and/or FEF_{25-75}≤75 % of baseline) was added to the staging system to signify "potential BOS" [3]. One problem with this scheme is the considerable variation in FEV_1 values that some recipients may have due to the timing and fluctuation in spirometric measurements caused by various post-transplant complications that can prevent a recipient from achieving a graft function plateau with reasonably stable post-transplant FEV_1 values that accurately represent the zenith of attainable function. Such fluctuation and the consequent inability to establish stable post-transplant lung function make it difficult, if not impossible, to identify an accurate baseline value. The identification of other surrogate markers (e.g., biomarkers) that accurately reflect pathological airway and/or parenchymal processes for which specific interventions should be considered is much needed.

A considerable number of risk factors have been associated with the development of BOS (Table 1.2). BOS is widely perceived as the physiological surrogate of an immunologically mediated phenomenon due to many observations that include its association with acute cellular rejection [4], the association with greater degrees of HLA mismatch with BOS risk [5], and evolving evidence of the involvement of autoimmune pathways [6] and the interplay of alloimmune and autoimmune processes that can lead to allograft rejection [7]. Furthermore, lung histopathology in patients with BOS shows striking similarities to the OB that can occur in allogeneic bone marrow or stem cell transplant recipients as well as constrictive bronchiolitis in patients with connective tissue diseases [8–10], and these airway changes are perceived as alloimmune or autoimmune disorders, respectively. Nonetheless,

Table 1.2 Risk factors associated with BOS

Alloimmune rejection events
• Acute cellular rejection
• Lymphocytic bronchiolitis
• Humoral rejection (e.g., anti-HLA antibodies)
Acute allograft injury
• Primary graft dysfunction[a]
Autoimmune sensitization to self-antigens
• Collagen V
• κ (kappa)-α (alpha) 1 tubulin
"Non-immune"[a]
• Persistent BAL neutrophilia
• Gastroesophageal reflux and [micro]aspiration
▪ Acid reflux
▪ Nonacid reflux
• Infection or colonization
▪ Virus
• Cytomegalovirus
• Non-CMV community-acquired virus infection
▪ Bacterial (e.g., *Pseudomonas*)
▪ Fungal (e.g., *Aspergillus*)
▪ Air pollution
Other (putative) risks
• Ischemic airway injury due to disrupted bronchial microcirculation
• Accelerated allograft aging due to cell/tissue senescence
• Inadequate recipient compliance with outpatient drug therapies

BAL bronchoalveolar lavage, *CMV* cytomegalovirus, *HLA* human leukocyte antigen

[a]These likely involve allograft injury combined with triggering of innate immune responses that may also trigger or potentiate alloimmune/adaptive immune responses

although BOS is frequently equated with the term chronic rejection, various interventions, including intensified immunosuppression, may have little or no effect on the progressive loss of allograft function that is usually observed in lung transplant recipients who develop BOS. However, some patients can have significant clinical responses to alternative immunomodulatory therapies such as total lymphoid irradiation [11], or extracorporeal photopheresis [12], although these responses generally consist of stabilization or a decrease in the tempo of lung function loss over time and are unlikely to improve lung function (see Chap. 16).

In addition to alloimmune and/or autoimmune phenomena associated with BOS, various "non-immune" mechanisms have been implicated as playing a role in BOS pathogenesis. Although often referred to as nonimmune, these events/phenomena likely trigger or potentiate innate immune responses, which may also trigger or intensify alloimmune or autoimmune responses. These mechanisms include injury caused by primary graft dysfunction (PGD), gastroesophageal reflux (GER), and infections caused by viruses, bacteria, or fungi [13–15].

PGD, which affects 10–25 % of all lung transplants and is a leading cause of early morbidity and mortality, represents a form of acute lung injury that is considered to occur largely as a consequence of the periods of ischemia and reperfusion as the donor lung is procured and then implanted in the recipient [16–19]. Although a number of studies have not consistently linked PGD to BOS [20–24], more recent studies support a link between PGD and the development of BOS [25–27]. Daud et al. [25] found a convincing association of PGD grade with increased risk of developing BOS Stage 1 using International Society for Heart and Lung Transplantation (ISHLT) consensus definitions for PGD, and a more recent analysis of outcomes by this group identified a direct relationship between PGD severity at 24, 48, and 72 h post-transplant and increased risk of BOS [28]. The most severe grade of PGD (grade 3) at all three time points was associated with the highest risk of developing BOS (RR was 3.31 for grade 3 PGD at 24 h).

The presence of significant GER (GER that is increased in frequency/severity over what is considered normal) increases the risk that refluxate can be aspirated into the lower respiratory tract and has been linked to both subacute and chronic lung allograft dysfunction [29–36]. Multiple studies have reported a high prevalence of an abnormal degree of GER among patients with advanced lung disease and patients referred for lung transplantation [37, 38]. Approximately 70 % of patients who undergo transplant evaluation have some evidence of significant GER [38], and acid reflux may worsen following transplantation [39]. Gastroparesis and/or esophageal dysmotility may also be present and increase the risk of reflux and microaspiration. A negative correlation was found between increasing severity of acid reflux (as measured by 24-h pH study) and post-transplant FEV_1 [36], and the presence of nonacid reflux (as measured by impedance testing) was reported to increase the risk for BOS nearly threefold [33]. Refluxed bile acids in BAL fluid have been found to be increased in cross-sectional studies of patients with BOS [40, 41], and GER associated with aspiration of bile acids (bile acids detected in BAL) has been linked to BOS [40], a significantly increased risk of BOS onset [41], and poor response to azithromycin therapy [42]. Recent studies in animal models of lung transplantation suggest that gastric aspiration might enhance allorecognition and promote lung allograft rejection [43, 44], and GER has been linked to collagen V sensitization and BOS in transplant recipients [45].

Infections caused by viruses, bacteria, and fungi have been linked to risk for developing BOS (see Chap. 11). A large number of studies have linked pulmonary CMV infection to the subsequent development of BOS and/or diminished post-transplant survival [46–52]. Prophylactic and preemptive strategies to prevent/treat CMV infection have significantly reduced the incidence of CMV disease in lung transplant recipients [53–56], and retrospective studies of perioperative ganciclovir prophylaxis suggest that preventing CMV disease may delay the onset of BOS [57–59]. However, a recently published prospective, single-center study reported an incidence of CMV pneumonitis of 21 % within 6 months of transplant (in a cohort of 231 recipients) despite short-course prophylaxis being given to high-risk recipients [52]. These investigators observed that CMV pneumonitis was associated with a significantly increased risk of BOS (HR 2.19) and diminished survival (HR 1.89).

Interestingly, a prospective, randomized 11-center trial that examined the effects of 3 vs. 12 months of post-transplant valganciclovir prophylaxis for D+R−, D+R+, and D−R+ recipients showed that the 12-months prophylaxis strategy significantly diminished the incidence of CMV infection (64 % vs. 10 %), CMV disease (32 % vs. 4 %), and disease severity without any significant difference in rates of acute rejection, opportunistic infection, CMV UL97 ganciclovir-resistance mutations, or adverse events [60]. However, it remains unclear whether such prolonged prophylaxis can reduce risk for BOS.

Infection with other β(beta)-herpes viruses may also cause serious complications. The non-CMV β-herpes viruses include Epstein-Barr virus (EBV), herpes simplex virus (HSV), varicella zoster virus (VZV), and human herpes viruses 6 (HHV-6) and 7 (HHV-7). A prospective cohort study of 385 lung transplant recipients linked repetitive detection of EBV DNA in peripheral blood with the development of BOS [61], and HHV-6 or HHV-7 infection has been associated with BOS [62, 63].

Infection with community-acquired respiratory viruses (CARV) can be asymptomatic, cause mild symptoms, cause significant respiratory tract disease, or lead to acute respiratory insufficiency and death. Recovery of CARV (influenza A and B, respiratory syncytial virus, parainfluenza viruses, rhinoviruses, enteroviruses, adenoviruses, human metapneumovirus, human coronavirus, and human bocavirus) during infections suspicious for CARV in lung transplant recipients can range from 34 to 66 % [64–66], and retrospective as well as recent prospective investigations have linked CARV infections with BOS risk [64, 67–73].

Post-transplant bacterial infection is exceedingly common in recipients with prior septic lung disease (CF and non-CF bronchiectasis) and is a leading cause of death in recipients with established BOS. Botha et al. [74] reported that de novo allograft colonization with *Pseudomonas aeruginosa* was strongly associated with developing BOS within 2 years of transplant (23.4 % colonized vs. 7.7 % non-colonized), Vos et al. [75] reported that persistent *Pseudomonas* colonization was an even greater risk for BOS than de novo colonization, and Gottlieb et al. [76] found that persistent allograft *Pseudomonas* colonization in a cohort of 59 patients with CF significantly increased the prevalence of BOS. Additionally, Vos et al. [77] reported that BAL bile acid levels, neutrophils, and IL-8 levels correlated significantly with *Pseudomonas* colonization and suggested that the presence of abnormal GER and microaspiration can lead to persistent colonization with *Pseudomonas*.

Invasive fungal infections can be an important cause of morbidity and mortality in lung transplant recipients. Valentine et al. [78] reported that the diagnosis of fungal pneumonia or pneumonitis in a cohort of 160 recipients was an independent predictor of BOS with a hazard ratio of 2.1 (95 % CI 1.1–4.0) for early (0–100 days post-transplant) and 1.5 (95 % CI 1.1–1.9) for late (≥1 year) fungal pneumonia on multivariate analysis. Another study of 201 recipients reported that *Aspergillus* colonization was independently associated (multivariate Cox regression analysis) with the subsequent development of BOS (HR = 1.81; 95 % CI 1.03–3.19) and BOS-associated mortality (HR = 2.57; 95 % CI 1.19–5.55). Additionally, recipients with new or persistent *Aspergillus* colonization after developing BOS had increased risk of progression to Stage 3 BOS or death [79].

Recent observations also suggest that environmental exposures can lead to airway injury and obliteration in non-transplant patients [80–82], and higher ambient levels of pollutants have recently been linked to BOS in lung transplant recipients [83]. Additionally, airway ischemia caused by disruption of the bronchial circulation has also been suggested as a potential cause of BOS [84]. Because established OB displays variable evidence of inflammation combined with evidence of heightened innate immune responses, alloimmune reactions, autoimmunity, and fibroproliferation with airway obliteration that leads to allograft airway remodeling and loss of function, OB likely represents a final common endpoint for allograft bronchiolar injury that can be precipitated and/or driven by a variety of insults and mechanisms.

Evolving Therapies That May Stabilize or Improve Delayed/Chronic Allograft Dysfunction

Over the past decade it has become increasingly recognized that many recipients with declining lung function consistent with FEV_1 criteria for BOS can respond to certain interventions (see Chaps. 12, 14, 15, and 16) (Table 1.3). Macrolides and neo-macrolides such as the azalide, azithromycin, possess anti-inflammatory effects and inhibit IL-8 production and neutrophil recruitment, suppress bronchial inflammation, and prevent or modulate airway damage for a number of respiratory disorders [85]. Observations from many centers indicate that a substantial number of patients who develop clinical BOS respond to azithromycin and may have their lung function stabilized or significantly improved (see Chap. 15), such that some patients may no longer meet FEV_1 criteria for BOS after responding to the drug [86, 87]. Azithromycin appears to be capable of diminishing the risk of graft loss and recipient death when given to patients with established BOS [88, 89]. Additionally, the recently published, randomized prospective, placebo-controlled clinical trial conducted by Vos et al. [90] suggested that prophylactic administration of azithromycin initiated shortly after transplantation can significantly decrease the risk of developing BOS, although a significant impact on survival was not shown over the relatively brief, 2-year evaluation period.

As mentioned above, abnormal GER is highly prevalent in patients with advanced lung disease and in lung transplant recipients [37, 91], and the prevalence may increase post-transplant [39, 40]. Notably, abnormal acid GER has been strongly linked to risk for BOS (see Chap. 12). However, pharmacologic therapy with proton-pump inhibitors (PPI), although such therapy can increase the pH of gastric secretions and relieve symptoms, may have little effect on GER [41]. Indeed, PPI therapy may have negligible effect on nonacid reflux, which may contain bile acids that can be very injurious to the lung [40, 92]. Because pharmacologic suppression of gastric acid secretion may not significantly suppress abnormal GER (especially weakly acid or nonacid reflux) and microaspiration, gastric fundoplication has been investigated to a considerable degree as a means of preventing lung transplant complications and as a treatment for BOS when reflux appears to be present [93–95].

Table 1.3 Emerging phenotypes of CLAD: key features[a]

Entity	Classic BOS	RAS	NRAD
Time of onset	• Late (usually 2–3 years post-transplant, but may occur earlier)	• Tends to occur later but may occur at any time	• Usually occurs early (e.g., 3–6 months post-transplant)
Physiology	• Obstructive (FEV_1 ≤80 % of stable baseline value)	• Restrictive (e.g., FEV_1 ≤80 % and TLC ≤90 % of stable baseline values)	• Obstructive (FEV_1 ≤80 % of stable baseline value)
HRCT imaging	• Air trapping often present	• Parenchymal infiltrates usually present (DAD and/or fibrosis often present)	• Changes of bronchiolitis ("tree-in-bud," thickened airway walls, peribronchiolar infiltrates often present)
	• Infiltrates usually not present • ±Bronchiectasis	• ±Bronchiectasis • ±Air trapping	• ±Air trapping
Histopathology	• OB (difficult to diagnose via transbronchial biopsy)	• Fibrosis (thickened septae and pleurae) • DAD often present • OB may be present	• Cellular bronchiolitis
Clinical course	• Typically progressive but may stabilize	• Tends to be relentlessly progressive (especially if early DAD on TBB)	• High likelihood of significant response to azithromycin (may no longer meet FEV_1 criteria for BOS if recipient responds to azithromycin)
	• Recipients may have coexistent chronic bacterial infection	• Significantly worse prognosis than BOS	
Other	• Usually responds poorly to pharmacologic therapies • Can have outcome similar to primary transplant following lung retransplantation	• Increased risk of RAS if new onset DAD detected >90 days post-transplant	• BAL neutrophilia (e.g., ≥15 % on differential cell count) correlates with response to azithromycin therapy

BAL bronchoalveolar lavage, *BOS* bronchiolitis obliterans syndrome, *CLAD* chronic lung allograft dysfunction, *DAD* diffuse alveolar damage, *FEV_1* forced expiratory volume in 1 s, *NRAD* neutrophilic reversible allograft dysfunction, *OB* obliterative bronchiolitis, *RAS* restrictive allograft syndrome

[a]Infection, other pathologies (e.g., acute cellular rejection, lymphocytic bronchiolitis, antibody-mediated rejection), and/or other causes of allograft dysfunction (e.g., significant gastroesophageal reflux, pleural disorders, anastomotic dysfunction, obesity, thromboembolic disease, recurrent primary lung disease, etc.) must be ruled out

One case series suggests that it may prevent the appearance of BOS or prevent its progression if abnormal GER is diagnosed in patients who have developed BOS [35]. Additionally, as with the improvement in FEV_1 that has been observed with azithromycin therapy, fundoplication has been reported to lead to improved lung function such that patients can revert to BOS Stage 0 [34].

In summary, it has become clear that lung function decline that is consistent with a diagnosis of BOS can stabilize in some patients and not lead to sustained, progressive deterioration in allograft function and graft loss. Allograft functional decline that is consistent with the onset of BOS may respond to azithromycin therapy or anti-reflux surgery such that spirometric criteria for BOS are no longer met due to improved FEV_1 and clinical status. However, treatment of BOS with intensified immunosuppression or other modalities remains relatively ineffective to date, and more research into the basic pathogenetic mechanisms, preventive strategies, and treatment interventions is greatly needed.

Nomenclature and Phenotypes of Delayed-Onset Lung Allograft Dysfunction

It seems logical to use the term CLAD to indicate a late or delayed, significant decline in lung function that can be due to evolving OB as well as other causes of allograft dysfunction in the chronic setting. However, it should be recognized that CLAD (which is increasingly used to indicate a decline in FEV_1 that appears to meet criteria for BOS) may not necessarily be caused by "chronic rejection" that is mediated by classical alloimmune responses (see Chap. 3). Additionally, a number of processes may be operant simultaneously and contribute to declining allograft function. For example, the presence of significant anastomotic dysfunction combined with OB. The ability to identify characteristics that identify subsets of lung transplant recipients who have allograft function decline that meets criteria for BOS but may have specific disease mechanisms, specific triggering events and pathways, or characteristics that predict beneficial response to a specific treatment intervention can aid efforts to provide specific treatments and make key management decisions concerning specific therapies to treat BOS.

A cause of CLAD has been recently described that has characteristics that distinguish it from typical BOS/OB (Table 1.4). Sato et al. [96] identified 156/468 recipients transplanted from 1996 to 2009 who developed a clinical picture consistent with CLAD (defined as an irreversible decline in FEV_1 to <80 % of baseline), and 47 (30 %) of those diagnosed with CLAD displayed evidence of restriction (irreversible decline in total lung capacity [TLC] to <90 % of baseline) associated with thoracic imaging (HRCT) changes consistent with interstitial lung disease (ILD) and peripheral parenchymal lung fibrosis. This constellation of findings was termed restrictive allograft syndrome (RAS). Survival was worse for patients with (RAS) vs. patients with typical BOS (541 vs. 1,421 days; $p=0.0003$). Two other groups have also described a subset of BOS patients with features of restriction via

Table 1.4 Management of BOS

• Identify and treat potentially reversible non-BOS causes of impaired graft function
• Administration of neo-macrolides (e.g., azithromycin)
• Adjust maintenance immunosuppression
° Optimize regimen
° Switch to tacrolimus if FEV_1 decline occurred on CsA-based regimen
° Avoid sustained, high-dose corticosteroids
• Evaluate for abnormal GER (acid and nonacid)
° Consider fundoplication if significant GER is identified
• Screen for appearance of de novo anti-HLA antigen
° Consider IVIG, plasma exchange, and/or rituximab if detected
• Therapies for progressive BOS refractory to other interventions
° Total lymphoid irradiation
° Extracorporeal photopheresis
° Retransplantation

CsA cyclosporine A, *GER* gastroesophageal reflux, *IVIG* intravenous immunoglobulin

pulmonary function testing. Verleden et al. [97] diagnosed CLAD in 71 of 294 recipients and found that 20 (28.2 %) patients had restrictive changes on pulmonary function testing; 17 of these 20 recipients had persistent parenchymal infiltrates on HRCT, and multivariate analysis showed that a restrictive pattern on pulmonary function testing (decline in TLC in 15, decline in FEV_1 and FVC in 5 with restrictive FEV_1/FVC ratio) was associated with worse survival. Woodrow et al. [98] also identified a substantial number of recipients with CLAD who met the FEV_1 criterion for BOS and had evidence of restriction (47 of 62, 44 %) via spirometric testing (TLC data were not reported) showing forced vital capacity decline from baseline ≥20 %; however, the prevalence of parenchymal infiltrates on HRCT was similar for the restrictive vs. obstructive groups that met BOS criteria, and survival did not differ between the groups.

A more recent analysis of recipient cohorts who developed BOS by Sato et al. [99] has shown that the detection of diffuse alveolar damage (DAD) on lung biopsy specimens may have important implications for both obstructive BOS and RAS. They reported that DAD was seen at least once on TBLB in 320/720 (44 %) recipients, and early DAD (≤3 months post-transplant) was associated with a significantly increased mortality risk. They also found that bilateral lung recipients with adequate pulmonary function testing to distinguish RAS from BOS had earlier onset of BOS if early DAD was detected. Additionally, late new-onset DAD (>90 days post-transplant) was a significant risk factor for developing RAS. A review of temporal changes on lung biopsy in recipients with RAS showed that DAD tended to be followed by development of pleuroparenchymal fibroelastosis [100]. Additional characterization of a subset of patients showed that ground-glass opacities on HRCT correlated with DAD episodes, and such episodes were accompanied by a decline in lung function with subsequent stabilization during interval periods that correlated with allograft fibrosis [101].

The existence of distinct phenotypes on the basis of length of time from transplant to BOS development and the tempo of disease progression have been suggested in the literature. Those recipients with early-onset BOS may represent a group of patients that is prone to rapid progression and poor prognosis [20, 25, 102, 103]. Median survival for recipients with acute-onset BOS has been noted to be 29 vs. 58 months for later, chronic-onset BOS [104]. Additionally, Burton et al. [105] found that progression of BOS from lower to higher grade increases the risk of mortality up to threefold, and a rapid decline in FEV_1 of >20 % has been associated with worse prognosis [106]. Brugiere et al. [107] found that recipients with early-onset BOS had lower mean FEV_1, need for supplemental oxygen, and poorer graft survival than those with later-onset BOS. These observations suggest that patients with early-onset BOS represent a subset of recipients that are at risk for a more rapid decline in lung function plus a higher incidence of graft failure and death as compared to patients with late-onset BOS. However, not all patients with rapidly declining lung function associated with BOS have relentless progression; some may stabilize despite an initial rapid BOS onset and FEV_1 decline [108].

The presence of significant bronchoalveolar lavage (BAL) neutrophilia that is often associated with high-resolution computed tomographic (HRCT) changes of probable cellular bronchiolitis in patients with FEV_1 decline that meets the criterion for BOS Stage >0 has been perceived as representing a variant of BOS. These individuals are likely to respond to azithromycin therapy [88, 109], and FEV_1 may improve such that the recipient no longer meets spirometric criteria for BOS. Indeed, this reversibility, should it occur in response to azithromycin, poses an issue in terms of classifying this entity as a phenotype or subtype of BOS if criteria for BOS Stage ≥1 or even BOS-0p are eventually no longer met due to a significant therapeutic response. This phenomenon has been termed neutrophilic reversible allograft dysfunction (NRAD) [15, 88], and it has been suggested to represent a specific phenotype of CLAD. In contrast to NRAD, patients who meet BOS criteria but do not respond to azithromycin have been proposed to represent a fibroproliferative BOS phenotype [88]. Nonetheless, distinct phenotypes of BOS that are based upon specific risk factors or other parameters have yet to be firmly established, and azithromycin-unresponsive individuals may have significant variation in their underlying histopathological changes from those who respond to azithromycin.

The data from Sato et al. [96] and Verleden et al. [97] indicate that recipients with RAS may comprise a relatively specific CLAD phenotype that is distinguishable from patients with the more common BOS pattern of airflow obstruction that is usually not associated with parenchymal infiltrates. These observations suggest that HRCT imaging and lung volume determinations (and perhaps FVC and the FEV_1/FVC ratio) can be useful to differentiate recipients with the RAS phenotype from those with a typical obstructive BOS pattern when spirometric criteria for the onset of BOS are met. However, OB lesions may be present in lung specimens from recipients who develop allograft dysfunction that is consistent with a RAS phenotype [96].

Nomenclature and Classification of Allograft Dysfunction Syndromes: A Suggested Approach

The differential diagnosis of acute lung allograft dysfunction includes surgical complications, PGD, or hyperacute rejection. Early allograft dysfunction that occurs outside of the immediate postoperative period is generally caused by acute cellular rejection, lymphocytic bronchiolitis, or infection, but other entities such as vascular or humoral rejection, pleural effusion or empyema, or venous thromboembolism must be considered.

Similarly, the differential diagnosis of late or delayed chronic allograft dysfunction must include a considerable number of potential complications as discussed in Chap. 3, and the recent observations discussed above suggest that imaging and the determination of lung volumes can differentiate graft dysfunction caused by RAS from classical obstructive BOS. Distinguishing between these entities may be important in decision making (e.g., considering early listing for retransplantation for RAS that is progressive and unresponsive to therapeutic interventions), as the prognosis associated with RAS appears to be significantly worse than that associated with obstructive BOS. Additionally, HRCT imaging combined with a BAL differential cell count can identify changes (cellular bronchiolitis on HRCT, BAL neutrophilia) that identify patients with a high likelihood of having NRAD, which can improve with neo-macrolide therapy. As our knowledge of these evolving syndromes with their differing phenotypic characteristics advances, therapies may be identified that provide benefit for a specific subset of CLAD but may not have efficacy for other phenotypes.

We suggest that delayed allograft dysfunction with a persistent decline in $FEV_1 \geq 10\ \%$ of baseline can be used as a threshold value to signify the likely onset of CLAD, and such an FEV_1 decline should trigger consideration of the various entities that could cause such a decline in graft function and appropriate diagnostic testing to determine the cause(s). Imaging should be performed, and HRCT with expiratory views may provide more useful information than a routine chest radiograph. Bronchoscopy with examination of bronchial anastomoses and performance of BAL and endoscopic lung biopsies is likely to provide useful information that can be combined with clinical presentation and physical examination, imaging, and pulmonary function studies to identify and/or rule out various potential causes of CLAD. If criteria for the diagnosis of BOS are met, the various risk factors associated with BOS should be considered and appropriate testing performed to determine the most likely etiology and identify treatments that are most likely to stabilize or possibly improve allograft function (e.g., anti-reflux surgery for significant GER). This evolving classification scheme (Fig. 1.1) needs to be validated, but its adoption would allow a more precise definition of terms used to describe delayed-onset allograft dysfunction and also convey the complexity of CLAD, set a lower threshold to investigate FEV_1 decline in the chronic setting (which may allow earlier diagnosis and interventions to

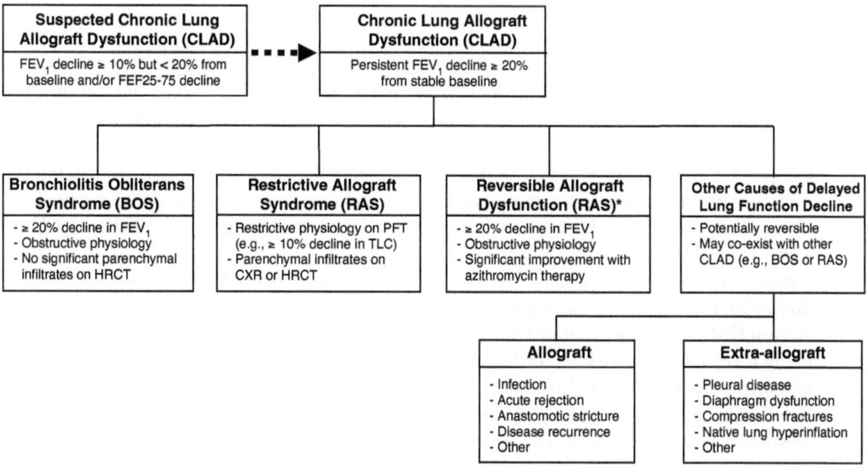

Fig. 1.1 Suggested definitions and characteristics of CLAD and its subcategories. *Decline in FEV_1 may be due to (probable cellular) bronchiolitis that can respond to azithromycin therapy such that FEV_1 significantly improves or normalizes: predictors of an increased likelihood of improvement with azithromycin include BAL neutrophilia (≥15 % neutrophils) and HRCT changes consistent with bronchiolitis (tree-in-bud opacities, peribronchiolar infiltrates, ±air trapping). *CXR* routine chest radiograph, FEF_{25-75} forced expiratory flow rate from 75 to 25 % of forced vital capacity, FEV_1 forced expiratory volume in 1 s, *FVC* forced vital capacity, *HRCT* high-resolution computed tomogram, *PFT* pulmonary function testing, *TLC* total lung capacity

preserve allograft function), and promote the evolving concept that distinct phenotypes of CLAD can be identified that may have varying prognoses and responses to therapeutic interventions.

Conclusion

Our perception of chronic allograft dysfunction is changing. While the terms OB, BOS, CLAD, and chronic rejection have been frequently used as synonymous and pertaining to allograft function due to OB, we now recognize that what we have termed BOS up to the present is actually a heterogeneous entity (e.g., RAS vs. BOS) and that (1) the term CLAD may be a better term to use for delayed allograft dysfunction, (2) CLAD can be caused by a variety of entities that have an impact on allograft function, (3) BOS is one of a number of relatively distinct CLAD entities, and (4) BOS phenotypes may better be identified according to time of onset post-transplant, rapidity of progression, underlying etiology (e.g., associated with GER, azithromycin-responsive), and response to therapies (e.g., azithromycin or anti-reflux surgery). We suggest that a new classification system with precise definitions should be created for delayed allograft dysfunction (i.e., CLAD).

References

1. Burke CM, Theodore J, Dawkins KD, Yousem SA, Blank N, Billingham ME, et al. Post-transplant obliterative bronchiolitis and other late lung sequelae in human heart-lung transplant recipients. Chest. 1984;86:824–9.
2. Cooper JD, Billingham M, Egan T, Hertz MI, Higenbottam T, Lynch J, et al. A working formulation for the standardization of nomenclature and for clinical staging of chronic dysfunction in lung allografts. International Society for Heart and Lung Transplantation. J Heart Lung Transplant. 1993;12:713–6.
3. Estenne M, Maurer JR, Boehler A, Egan JJ, Frost A, Hertz M, et al. Bronchiolitis obliterans syndrome 2001: an update of the diagnostic criteria. J Heart Lung Transplant. 2002;21:297–310.
4. Burton CM, Iversen M, Carlsen J, Mortensen J, Andersen CB, Steinbrüchel D, et al. Acute cellular rejection is a risk factor for bronchiolitis obliterans syndrome independent of post-transplant baseline FEV1. J Heart Lung Transplant. 2009;28:888–93.
5. Schulman LL, Weinberg AD, McGregor C, Galantowicz ME, Suciu-Foca NM, Itescu S. Mismatches at the HLA-dr and HLA-b loci are risk factors for acute rejection after lung transplantation. Am J Respir Crit Care Med. 1998;157:1833–7.
6. Burlingham WJ, Love RB, Jankowska-Gan E, Haynes LD, Xu Q, Bobadilla JL, et al. IL-17-dependent cellular immunity to collagen type V predisposes to obliterative bronchiolitis in human lung transplants. J Clin Invest. 2007;117:3498–506.
7. Saini D, Weber J, Ramachandran S, Phelan D, Tiriveedhi V, Liu M, et al. Alloimmunity-induced autoimmunity as a potential mechanism in the pathogenesis of chronic rejection of human lung allografts. J Heart Lung Transplant. 2011;30(6):624–31.
8. Barbareschi M, Cavazza A, Leslie KO. Bronchiolar disorders. In: Wick MR, Leslie KO, editors. Practical pulmonary pathology. 2nd ed. Philadelphia: Elsevier; 2011.
9. King T. Bronchiolitis. In: Schwarz M, King T, editors. Interstitial lung disease. 5th ed. Shelton, CT: People's Medical Publishing House; 2011.
10. Kitko CL, White ES, Baird K. Fibrotic and sclerotic manifestations of chronic graft-versus-host disease. Biol Blood Marrow Transplant. 2012;18(1 Suppl):S46–52.
11. Fisher AJ, Rutherford RM, Bozzino J, Parry G, Dark JH, Corris PA. The safety and efficacy of total lymphoid irradiation in progressive bronchiolitis obliterans syndrome after lung transplantation. Am J Transplant. 2005;5:537–43.
12. Morrell MR, Despotis GJ, Lublin DM, Patterson GA, Trulock EP, Hachem RR. The efficacy of photopheresis for bronchiolitis obliterans syndrome after lung transplantation. J Heart Lung Transplant. 2010;29:424–31.
13. Belperio JA, Weigt S, Fishbein MC, Lynch III JP. Chronic lung allograft rejection: mechanisms and therapy. Proc Am Thorac Soc. 2009;6:108–21.
14. Weigt SS, Wallace WD, Derhovanessian A, Saggar R, Saggar R, Lynch JP, et al. Chronic allograft rejection: epidemiology, diagnosis, pathogenesis, and treatment. Semin Respir Crit Care Med. 2010;31:189–207.
15. Verleden GM, Vos R, de Vleeschauwer SI, Willems-Widyastuti A, Verleden SE, Dupont LJ, et al. Obliterative bronchiolitis following lung transplantation: from old to new concepts? Transpl Int. 2009;22:771–9.
16. Christie JD, Carby M, Bag R, Corris P, Hertz M, Weill D. Report of the ISHLT Working Group on Primary Lung Graft Dysfunction part II: definition. A consensus statement of the International Society for Heart and Lung Transplantation. J Heart Lung Transplant. 2005;24:1454–9.
17. King RC, Binns OA, Rodriguez F, Kanithanon RC, Daniel TM, Spotnitz WD, et al. Reperfusion injury significantly impacts clinical outcome after pulmonary transplantation. Ann Thorac Surg. 2000;69:1681–5.
18. Arcasoy SM, Fisher A, Hachem RR, Scavuzzo M, Ware LB, ISHLT Working Group on Primary Lung Graft Dysfunction. Report of the ISHLT Working Group on Primary Lung Graft Dysfunction part v: predictors and outcomes. J Heart Lung Transplant. 2005;24:1483–8.

19. Christie JD, Kotloff RM, Ahya VN, Tino G, Pochettino A, Gaughan C, et al. The effect of primary graft dysfunction on survival after lung transplantation. Am J Respir Crit Care Med. 2005;171(11):1312–6.
20. Fisher AJ, Wardle J, Dark JH, Corris PA. Non-immune acute graft injury after lung transplantation and the risk of subsequent bronchiolitis obliterans syndrome (BOS). J Heart Lung Transplant. 2002;21:1206–12.
21. Fiser SM, Tribble CG, Long SM, Kaza AK, Kern JA, Jones DR, et al. Ischemia-reperfusion injury after lung transplantation increases risk of late bronchiolitis obliterans syndrome. Ann Thorac Surg. 2002;73:1041–7.
22. Girgis RE, Tu I, Berry GJ, Reichenspurner H, Valentine VG, Conte JV, et al. Risk factors for the development of obliterative bronchiolitis after lung transplantation. J Heart Lung Transplant. 1996;15:1200–8.
23. Hachem RR, Khalifah AP, Chakinala MM, Yusen RD, Aloush AA, Mohanakumar T, et al. The significance of a single episode of minimal acute rejection after lung transplantation. Transplantation. 2005;80:1406–13.
24. Burton CM, Iversen M, Milman N, Zemtsovski M, Carlsen J, Steinbrüchel D, et al. Outcome of lung transplanted patients with primary graft dysfunction. Eur J Cardiothorac Surg. 2007;31(1):75–82.
25. Daud SA, Yusen RD, Meyers BF, Chakinala MM, Walter MJ, Aloush AA, et al. Impact of immediate primary lung allograft dysfunction on bronchiolitis obliterans syndrome. Am J Respir Crit Care Med. 2007;175:507–13.
26. Bharat A, Narayanan K, Street T, Fields RC, Steward N, Aloush A, et al. Early posttransplant inflammation promotes the development of alloimmunity and chronic human lung allograft rejection. Transplantation. 2007;83:150–8.
27. Bharat A, Kuo E, Steward N, Aloush A, Hachem R, Trulock EP, et al. Immunological link between primary graft dysfunction and chronic lung allograft rejection. Ann Thorac Surg. 2008;86:189–95.
28. Huang HJ, Yusen RD, Meyers BF, Walter MJ, Mohanakumar T, Patterson GA, et al. Late primary graft dysfunction after lung transplantation and bronchiolitis obliterans syndrome. Am J Transplant. 2008;8(11):2454–62.
29. Reid KR, McKenzie FN, Menkis AH, Novick RJ, Pflugfelder PW, Kostuk WJ, et al. Importance of chronic aspiration in recipients of heart-lung transplants. Lancet. 1990;336:206–8.
30. Au J, Hawkins T, Venables C, Morritt G, Scott CD, Gascoigne AD, et al. Upper gastrointestinal dysmotility in heart-lung transplant recipients. Ann Thorac Surg. 1993;55:94–7.
31. Palmer SM, Miralles AP, Howell DN, Brazer SR, Tapson VF, Davis RD. Gastroesophageal reflux as a reversible cause of allograft dysfunction after lung transplantation. Chest. 2000;118:1214–7.
32. Halsey KD, Wald A, Meyer KC, Torrealba JR, Gaumnitz EA. Non-acidic supraesophageal reflux associated with diffuse alveolar damage and allograft dysfunction after lung transplantation: a case report. J Heart Lung Transplant. 2008;27:564–7.
33. King BJ, Iyer H, Leidi AA, Carby MR. Gastroesophageal reflux in bronchiolitis obliterans syndrome: a new perspective. J Heart Lung Transplant. 2009;28:870–5.
34. Davis Jr RD, Lau CL, Eubanks S, Messier RH, Hadjiliadis D, Steele MP, et al. Improved lung allograft function after fundoplication in patients with gastroesophageal reflux disease undergoing lung transplantation. J Thorac Cardiovasc Surg. 2003;125:533–42.
35. Cantu III E, Appel III JZ, Hartwig MG, Woreta H, Green C, Messier R, et al. J. Maxwell Chamberlain Memorial Paper. Early fundoplication prevents chronic allograft dysfunction in patients with gastroesophageal reflux disease. Ann Thorac Surg. 2004;78:1142–51.
36. Hadjiliadis D, Duane Davis R, Steele MP, Messier RH, Lau CL, Eubanks SS, et al. Gastroesophageal reflux disease in lung transplant recipients. Clin Transplant. 2003;17: 363–8.
37. D'Ovidio F, Singer LG, Hadjiliadis D, Pierre A, Waddell TK, de Perrot M, et al. Prevalence of gastroesophageal reflux in end-stage lung disease candidates for lung transplant. Ann Thorac Surg. 2005;80:1254–60.

38. Sweet MP, Patti MG, Hoopes C, Hays SR, Golden JA. Gastro-oesophageal reflux and aspiration in patients with advanced lung disease. Thorax. 2009;64:167–73.
39. Young LR, Hadjiliadis D, Davis RD, Palmer SM. Lung transplantation exacerbates gastroesophageal reflux disease. Chest. 2003;124:1689–93.
40. D'Ovidio F, Mura M, Tsang M, Waddell TK, Hutcheon MA, Singer LG, et al. Bile acid aspiration and the development of bronchiolitis obliterans after lung transplantation. J Thorac Cardiovasc Surg. 2005;129:1144–52.
41. Blondeau K, Mertens V, Vanaudenaerde BA, Verleden GM, Van Raemdonck DE, Sifrim D, et al. Gastro-esophageal reflux and gastric aspiration in lung transplant patients with or without chronic rejection. Eur Respir J. 2008;31:707–13.
42. Mertens V, Blondeau K, Van Oudenhove L, Vanaudenaerde B, Vos R, Farre R, et al. Bile acids aspiration reduces survival in lung transplant recipients with BOS despite azithromycin. Am J Transplant. 2011;11:329–35.
43. Meltzer AJ, Weiss MJ, Veillette GR, Sahara H, Ng CY, Cochrane ME, et al. Repetitive gastric aspiration leads to augmented indirect allorecognition after lung transplantation in miniature swine. Transplantation. 2008;86:1824–9.
44. Li B, Hartwig MG, Appel JZ, Bush EL, Balsara KR, Holzknecht ZE, et al. Chronic aspiration of gastric fluid induces the development of obliterative bronchiolitis in rat lung transplants. Am J Transplant. 2008;8:1614–21.
45. Bobadilla JL, Jankowska-Gan E, Xu Q, Haynes LD, Munoz del Rio A, Meyer K, et al. Reflux-induced collagen type v sensitization: potential mediator of bronchiolitis obliterans syndrome. Chest. 2010;138:363–70.
46. Reichenspurner H, Girgis RE, Robbins RC, Yun KL, Nitschke M, Berry GJ, et al. Stanford experience with obliterative bronchiolitis after lung and heart-lung transplantation. Ann Thorac Surg. 1996;62:1467–72.
47. Kroshus TJ, Kshettry VR, Savik K, John R, Hertz MI, Bolman III RM. Risk factors for the development of bronchiolitis obliterans syndrome after lung transplantation. J Thorac Cardiovasc Surg. 1997;114:195–202.
48. Heng D, Sharples LD, McNeil K, Stewart S, Wreghitt T, Wallwork J. Bronchiolitis obliterans syndrome: incidence, natural history, prognosis, and risk factors. J Heart Lung Transplant. 1998;17:1255–63.
49. Keller CA, Cagle PT, Brown RW, Noon G, Frost AE. Bronchiolitis obliterans in recipients of single, double, and heart-lung transplantation. Chest. 1995;107:973–80.
50. Keenan RJ, Lega ME, Dummer JS, Paradis IL, Dauber JH, Rabinowich H, et al. Cytomegalovirus serologic status and postoperative infection correlated with risk of developing chronic rejection after pulmonary transplantation. Transplantation. 1991;51:433–8.
51. Smith MA, Sundaresan S, Mohanakumar T, Trulock EP, Lynch JP, Phelan DL, et al. Effect of development of antibodies to HLA and cytomegalovirus mismatch on lung transplantation survival and development of bronchiolitis syndrome. J Thorac Cardiovasc Surg. 1998;116:812–20.
52. Snyder LD, Finlen-Copeland A, Turbyfill WJ, Howell D, Willner DA, Palmer SM. Cytomegalovirus pneumonitis is a risk for bronchiolitis obliterans syndrome in lung transplantation. Am J Respir Crit Care Med. 2010;181:1391–6.
53. Weill D, Lock BJ, Wewers DL, Young KR, Zorn GL, Early L, et al. Combination prophylaxis with ganciclovir and cytomegalovirus (CMV) immune globulin after lung transplantation: effective CMV prevention following daclizumab induction. Am J Transplant. 2003;3:492–6.
54. Palmer SM, Grinnan DC, Diane Reams B, Steele MP, Messier RH, Duane Davis R. Delay of CMV infection in high-risk CMV mismatch lung transplant recipients due to prophylaxis with oral ganciclovir. Clin Transplant. 2004;18:179–85.
55. Zamora MR, Nicolls MR, Hodges TN, Marquesen J, Astor T, Grazia T, et al. Following universal prophylaxis with intravenous ganciclovir and cytomegalovirus immune globulin, valganciclovir is safe and effective for prevention of CMV infection following lung transplantation. Am J Transplant. 2004;4:1635–42.

56. Humar A, Kumar D, Preiksaitis J, Boivin G, Siegal D, Fenton J, et al. A trial valganciclovir prophylaxis for cytomegalovirus prevention in lung transplant recipients. Am J Transplant. 2005;5:1462–8.
57. Chmiel C, Speich R, Hofer M, Michel D, Mertens T, Weder W, et al. Ganciclovir/valganciclovir prophylaxis decreases cytomegalovirus; related events and bronchiolitis obliterans syndrome after lung transplantation. Clin Infect Dis. 2008;46:831–9.
58. Valentine VG, Weill D, Gupta MR, Raper B, Laplace SG, Lombard GA, et al. Ganciclovir for cytomegalovirus: a call for indefinite prophylaxis in lung transplantation. J Heart Lung Transplant. 2008;27:875–81.
59. Ruttmann E, Geltner C, Bucher B, Ulmer H, Höfer D, Hangler HB, et al. Combined CMV prophylaxis improves outcome and reduces the risk for bronchiolitis obliterans syndrome (BOS) after lung transplantation. Transplantation. 2006;27:1415–20.
60. Palmer SM, Limaye AP, Banks M, Gallup D, Chapman J, Lawrence EC, et al. Extended valganciclovir prophylaxis to prevent cytomegalovirus after lung transplantation: a randomized controlled trial. Ann Intern Med. 2010;152:761–9.
61. Engelmann I, Welte T, Fühner T, Simon AR, Mattner F, Hoy L, et al. Detection of Epstein-Barr virus DNA in peripheral blood is associated with the development of bronchiolitis obliterans syndrome after lung transplantation. J Clin Virol. 2009;45:47–53.
62. Ross DJ, Chan RC, Kubak B, Laks H, Nichols WS. Bronchiolitis obliterans with organizing pneumonia: possible association with human herpesvirus-7 infection after lung transplantation. Transplant Proc. 2001;33:2603–6.
63. Neurohr C, Huppmann P, Leuchte H, Schwaiblmair M, Bittmann I, Jaeger G, et al. Human herpesvirus 6 in bronchoalveolar lavage fluid after lung transplantation: a risk factor for bronchiolitis obliterans syndrome? Am J Transplant. 2005;5:2982–91.
64. Kumar D, Erdman D, Keshavjee S, Peret T, Tellier R, Hadjiliadis D, et al. Clinical impact of community-acquired respiratory viruses on bronchiolitis obliterans after lung transplant. Am J Transplant. 2005;5:2031–6.
65. Garbino J, Gerbase MW, Wunderli W, Deffernez C, Thomas Y, Rochat T, et al. Lower respiratory viral illnesses: improved diagnosis by molecular methods and clinical impact. Am J Respir Crit Care Med. 2004;170:1197–203.
66. Milstone AP, Brumble LM, Barnes J, Estes W, Loyd JE, Pierson III RN, et al. A single-season prospective study of respiratory viral infections in lung transplant recipients. Eur Respir J. 2006;28:131–7.
67. Bridges ND, Spray TL, Collins MH, Bowles NE, Towbin JA. Adenovirus infection in the lung results in graft failure after lung transplantation. J Thorac Cardiovasc Surg. 1998;116:617–23.
68. Khalifah AP, Hachem RR, Chakinala MM, Schechtman KB, Patterson GA, Schuster DP, et al. Respiratory viral infections are a distinct risk for bronchiolitis obliterans syndrome and death. Am J Respir Crit Care Med. 2004;170:181–7.
69. Billings JL, Hertz MI, Savik K, Wendt CH. Respiratory viruses and chronic rejection in lung transplant recipients. J Heart Lung Transplant. 2002;21:559–66.
70. Vilchez RA, Dauber J, McCurry K, Iacono A, Kusne S. Parainfluenza virus infection in adult lung transplant recipients: an emergent clinical syndrome with implications on allograft function. Am J Transplant. 2003;3:116–20.
71. Palmer Jr SM, Henshaw NG, Howell DN, Miller SE, Davis RD, Tapson VF. Community respiratory viral infection in adult lung transplant recipients. Chest. 1998;113:944–50.
72. Gottlieb J, Schulz TF, Welte T, Fuehner T, Dierich M, Simon AR, et al. Community-acquired respiratory viral infections in lung transplant recipients: a single season cohort study. Transplantation. 2009;87:1530–7.
73. Kumar D, Husain S, Chen MH, Moussa G, Himsworth D, Manuel O, et al. A prospective molecular surveillance study evaluating the clinical impact of community-acquired respiratory viruses in lung transplant recipients. Transplantation. 2010;89:1028–33.
74. Botha P, Archer L, Anderson RL, Lordan J, Dark JH, Corris PA, et al. Pseudomonas aeruginosa colonization of the allograft after lung transplantation and the risk of bronchiolitis obliterans syndrome. Transplantation. 2008;85:771–4.

75. Vos R, Vanaudernaerde BM, De Vleeschauwer SI, Van Raemdonck DE, Dupont LJ, Verleden GM. De novo or persistent pseudomonal airway colonization after lung transplantation: importance for bronchiolitis obliterans syndrome? Transplantation. 2008;86:624–5.
76. Gottlieb J, Mattner F, Weissbrodt H, Dierich M, Fuehner T, Strueber M, et al. Impact of graft colonization with gram-negative bacteria after lung transplantation on the development of bronchiolitis obliterans syndrome in recipients with cystic fibrosis. Respir Med. 2009;103:743–9.
77. Vos R, Blondeau K, Vanaudenaerde BM, Mertens V, Van Raemdonck DE, Sifrim D, et al. Airway colonization and gastric aspiration after lung transplantation: do birds of a feather block together? J Heart Lung Transplant. 2008;27:843–9.
78. Valentine VG, Gupta MR, Walker Jr JE, Seoane L, Bonvillain RW, Lombard GA, et al. Effect of etiology and timing of respiratory tract infections on development of bronchiolitis obliterans syndrome. J Heart Lung Transplant. 2009;28:163–9.
79. Weigt SS, Elashoff RM, Huang C, Ardehali A, Gregson AL, Kubak B, et al. Aspergillus colonization of the lung allograft is a risk factor for bronchiolitis obliterans syndrome. Am J Transplant. 2009;9:1903–11.
80. Lockey JE, Hilbert TJ, Levin LP, Ryan PH, White KL, Borton EK, et al. Airway obstruction related to diacetyl exposure at microwave popcorn production facilities. Eur Respir J. 2009;34(1):63–71.
81. Rowell M, Kehe K, Balszuweit F, Thiermann H. The chronic effects of sulfur mustard exposure. Toxicology. 2009;263(1):9–11.
82. King MS, Eisenberg R, Newman JH, Tolle JJ, Harrell Jr FE, Nian H, et al. Constrictive bronchiolitis in soldiers returning from Iraq and Afghanistan. N Engl J Med. 2011;365(3): 222–30.
83. Nawrot TS, Vos R, Jacobs L, Verleden SE, Wauters S, Mertens V, et al. The impact of traffic air pollution on bronchiolitis obliterans syndrome and mortality after lung transplantation. Thorax. 2011;66:748–54.
84. Dhillon GS, Zamora MR, Roos JE, Sheahan D, Sista RR, Van der Starre P, et al. Lung transplant airway hypoxia: a diathesis to fibrosis? Am J Respir Crit Care Med. 2010;182(2): 230–6.
85. Kanoh S, Rubin BK. Mechanisms of action and clinical application of macrolides as immunomodulatory medications. Clin Microbiol Rev. 2010;23:590–615.
86. Vos R, Vanaudenaerde BM, Verleden SE, Ruttens D, Vaneylen A, Van Raemdonck DE, et al. Anti-inflammatory and immunomodulatory properties of azithromycin involved in treatment and prevention of chronic lung allograft rejection. Transplantation. 2012;94(2):101–9.
87. Verleden GM, Vanaudenaerde BM, Dupont LJ, Van Raemdonck DE. Azithromycin reduces airway neutrophilia and interleukin-8 in patients with bronchiolitis obliterans syndrome. Am J Respir Crit Care Med. 2006;174:566–70.
88. Vos R, Vanaudenaerde BM, Ottevaere A, Verleden SE, De Vleeschauwer SI, Willems-Widyastuti A, et al. Long-term azithromycin therapy for bronchiolitis obliterans syndrome: divide and conquer? J Heart Lung Transplant. 2010;29:1358–68.
89. Jain R, Hachem RR, Morrell MR, Trulock EP, Chakinala MM, Yusen RD, et al. Azithromycin is associated with increased survival in lung transplant recipients with bronchiolitis obliterans syndrome. J Heart Lung Transplant. 2010;29:531–7.
90. Vos R, Vanaudenaerde BM, Verleden SE, De Vleeschauwer SI, Willems-Widyastuti A, Van Raemdonck DE, et al. A randomized placebo-controlled trial of azithromycin to prevent bronchiolitis obliterans syndrome after lung transplantation. Eur Respir J. 2011;37:164–72.
91. Murthy SC, Nowicki ER, Mason DP, Budev MM, Nunez AI, Thuita L, et al. Pretransplant gastroesophageal reflux compromises early outcomes after lung transplantation. J Thorac Cardiovasc Surg. 2011;142(1):47–52e3.
92. D'Ovidio F, Mura M, Ridsdale R, Takahashi H, Waddell TK, Hutcheon M, et al. The effect of reflux and bile acid aspiration on the lung allograft and its surfactant and innate immunity molecules SP-A and SP-D. Am J Transplant. 2006;6:1930–8.

93. Linden PA, Gilbert RJ, Yeap BY, Boyle K, Deykin A, Jaklitsch MT, et al. Laparoscopic fundoplication in patients with end-stage lung disease awaiting transplantation. J Thorac Cardiovasc Surg. 2006;131:438–46.
94. Gasper WJ, Sweet MP, Hoopes C, Leard LE, Kleinhenz ME, Hays SR, et al. Antireflux surgery for patients with end-stage lung disease before and after lung transplantation. Surg Endosc. 2008;22:495–500.
95. Hoppo T, Jarido V, Pennathur A, Morrell M, Crespo M, Shigemura N, et al. Antireflux surgery preserves lung function in patients with gastroesophageal reflux disease and end-stage lung disease before and after lung transplantation. Arch Surg. 2011;146:1041–7.
96. Sato M, Waddell TK, Wagnetz U, Roberts HC, Hwang DM, Haroon A, et al. Restrictive allograft syndrome (RAS): a novel form of chronic lung allograft dysfunction. J Heart Lung Transplant. 2011;30:735–42.
97. Verleden GM, Vos R, Verleden SE, De Wever W, De Vleeschauwer SI, Willems-Widyastuti A, et al. Survival determinants in lung transplant patients with chronic allograft dysfunction. Transplantation. 2011;92:703–8.
98. Woodrow JP, Shlobin OA, Barnett SD, Burton N, Nathan SD. Comparison of bronchiolitis obliterans syndrome to other forms of chronic lung allograft dysfunction after lung transplantation. J Heart Lung Transplant. 2010;29:1159–64.
99. Sato M, Hwang DM, Ohmori-Matsuda K, Chaparro C, Waddell TK, Singer LG, et al. Revisiting the pathologic finding of diffuse alveolar damage after lung transplantation. J Heart Lung Transplant. 2012;31(4):354–63.
100. Ofek E, Sato M, Saito T, Wagnetz U, Roberts HC, Chaparro C, et al. Restrictive allograft syndrome post lung transplantation is characterized by pleuroparenchymal fibroelastosis. Mod Pathol. 2013;26(3):350–6.
101. Sato M, Hwang DM, Waddell TK, Singer LG, Keshavjee S. Progression pattern of restrictive allograft syndrome after lung transplantation. J Heart Lung Transplant. 2013;32(1):23–30.
102. Glanville AR, Aboyoun CL, Havryk A, Plit M, Rainer S, Malouf MA. Severity of lymphocytic bronchiolitis predicts long-term outcome after lung transplantation. Am J Respir Crit Care Med. 2008;177(9):1033–40.
103. Speich R, Schneider S, Hofer M, Irani S, Vogt P, Weder W, et al. Mycophenolate mofetil reduces alveolar inflammation, acute rejection and graft loss due to bronchiolitis obliterans syndrome after lung transplantation. Pulm Pharmacol Ther. 2010;23:445–9.
104. Jackson CH, Sharples LD, McNeil K, Stewart S, Wallwork J. Acute and chronic onset of bronchiolitis obliterans syndrome (BOS): are they different entities? J Heart Lung Transplant. 2002;21:658–66.
105. Burton CM, Carlsen J, Mortensen J, Andersen CB, Milman N, Iversen M. Long-term survival after lung transplantation depends on development and severity of bronchiolitis obliterans syndrome. J Heart Lung Transplant. 2007;26:681–6.
106. Lama VN, Murray S, Lonigro RJ, Toews GB, Chang A, Lau C, et al. Course of FEV(1) after onset of bronchiolitis obliterans syndrome in lung transplant recipients. Am J Respir Crit Care Med. 2007;175:1192–8.
107. Brugière O, Pessione F, Thabut G, Mal H, Jebrak G, Lesèche G, et al. Bronchiolitis obliterans syndrome after single-lung transplantation: impact of time to onset on functional pattern and survival. Chest. 2002;121(6):1883–9.
108. Borro JM, Bravo C, Solé A, Usetti P, Zurbano F, Lama R, et al. Conversion from cyclosporine to tacrolimus stabilizes the course of lung function in lung transplant recipients with bronchiolitis obliterans syndrome. Transplant Proc. 2007;39:2416–9.
109. Gottlieb J, Szangolies J, Koehnlein T, Golpon H, Simon A, Welte T. Long-term azithromycin for bronchiolitis obliterans syndrome after lung transplantation. Transplantation. 2008;85:36–41.

Chapter 2
Airway Pathology in Lung Transplants

Amir Lagstein and Jeffrey Myers

Abstract The histologic diagnosis of lung transplant rejection is based on the assessment of perivascular mononuclear cell inflammation, airway inflammation and fibrosis, and vasculopathic changes. This chapter describes the pathologic features of acute and chronic rejection of the small airways (i.e., lymphocytic and obliterative bronchiolitis). As transbronchial lung biopsy is the mainstay for the assessment of rejection, a brief discussion of some of the limitations of this technique is provided from the pathologist's perspective. Several important and common entities that can mimic airway rejection are described with practical guidance for distinguishing these potential confounders on transbronchial biopsy. The non-rejection findings that are discussed include the normal biopsy, nonspecific forms of chronic bronchiolitis, cytomegalovirus and pneumocystis pneumonia, bronchiolitis obliterans-organizing pneumonia, and aspiration pneumonia.

Keywords Lymphocytic bronchiolitis • Obliterative bronchiolitis • Bronchiolitis obliterans syndrome • Acute rejection • Chronic rejection

---

A. Lagstein, M.D. (✉)
Department of Pathology, University of Michigan, 1500 East Medical Center Drive, 2G332UH, Ann Arbor, MI 48109, USA
e-mail: alagstei@med.umich.edu

J. Myers, M.D.
Divisions of Anatomic Pathology and MLabs, Department of Pathology, University of Michigan, 1500 East Medical Center Drive, 2G332UH, Ann Arbor, MI 48109, USA
e-mail: myerjeff@umich.edu

K.C. Meyer and A.R. Glanville (eds.), *Bronchiolitis Obliterans Syndrome in Lung Transplantation*, Respiratory Medicine 8, DOI 10.1007/978-1-4614-7636-8_2,

Introduction

Lesions of the small airways are an important manifestation of both acute and chronic rejection of the pulmonary allograft, and two major forms are recognized. The first, lymphocytic bronchiolitis (LB), describes chronic mononuclear cell inflammation of the epithelium and submucosa of the distal small airways (i.e., at the level of and distal to the membranous bronchioles). The second, obliterative (or constrictive) bronchiolitis (OB), refers to partial or complete fibrous scarring of the distal airways and it is often, but not always, pauci-inflammatory. The term "obliterative bronchiolitis" is preferred over the term "bronchiolitis obliterans," so as not to confuse the former with the much more common bronchiolitis obliterans-organizing pneumonia (BOOP), also termed simply organizing pneumonia (OP), an unrelated disease process with different clinical, radiologic, and pathologic features.

OB is the histologic correlate of the clinically defined bronchiolitis obliterans syndrome (BOS) and remains the gold standard for its definitive diagnosis [1]. While OB is perhaps best known as the central feature of chronic lung rejection, it may also occur in a number of non-transplant settings. Patients with connective tissue diseases, especially rheumatoid arthritis, are perhaps the most commonly affected with OB outside of the transplant setting [2]. In addition, OB is an uncommon complication of various viral infections of the respiratory tract, particularly in children [3, 4], and is also a rare manifestation of medication toxicity (e.g., D-PENICILLAMINE) [5] and inhalational injury from various toxins such as ammonia [6], smoke [7], and cocaine [8]. Recently, OB has been described as an occupational lung disorder of microwave popcorn workers (possibly related to diacetyl exposure, a butter-flavoring agent) [9, 10]. OB is also a manifestation of graft-versus-host-disease in allogeneic bone marrow transplant recipients [11]. Interestingly, lesions histologically identical to LB have been observed in some of these conditions [11–13], providing a putative link between LB and OB. Indeed, LB is now widely accepted as not only a bona fide manifestation of acute rejection, but as an important risk factor for developing chronic airway rejection.

The occurrence of OB outside of the transplant setting has contributed to our understanding of the etiology and pathogenesis of this still enigmatic disorder [14–16]. However, post-transplant-related cases remain the most common and increasingly, the best understood examples of OB. As a consequence of the great success of modern immunosuppressive drugs, surgical techniques, and management of infections, with the attendant increase in allograft longevity, OB has emerged as the major long-term obstacle to both graft and patient survival in lung transplantation [17]. This challenge has led to greater emphasis on its early recognition, with the corresponding hope that early treatment can delay or prevent its development [18].

Lymphocytic and obliterative bronchiolitis are part of the formal histologic classification system of lung rejection, developed by the Lung Rejection Study Group of the International Society of Heart and Lung Transplantation (ISHLT).

The classification system is published as an ongoing series of working papers in order to maintain up-to-date and standardized nomenclature, and it has undergone two major revisions since the original working formulation was published in 1990 [19–21]. These changes reflect a combination of advances in the field of transplant rejection, experience with the application of the earlier grading schemes, and consensus expert opinion. The current ISHLT Working Formulation [21] recommends histologic assessment of rejection along four lines: Grade A for perivascular inflammation (acute cellular rejection [ACR]), Grade B for airway inflammation (lymphocytic bronchiolitis), Grade C for airway fibrosis (obliterative bronchiolitis), and Grade D for chronic vascular rejection (graft atherosclerosis). ACR is graded on the severity and density of perivascular and interstitial mononuclear cell inflammation in the following manner: A0, no perivascular infiltrates; A1, minimal acute rejection; A2, mild acute rejection; A3, moderate acute rejection; and A4, severe acute rejection. Lymphocytic bronchiolitis is graded as: B0, no airway inflammation; B1R, low-grade airway inflammation; and B2R, high-grade airway inflammation. Constrictive bronchiolitis and chronic vascular rejection are not graded but are designated as being either absent (C0 and D0) or present (C1 and D1). Because bronchoscopy with transbronchial biopsy (TBBx) is the mainstay for assessment of lung rejection, the classification system includes an "ungradeable" score for each parameter, designated by an X after the letter (e.g., AX), if it cannot be assessed in the sample. This reflects the limitations arising from the necessarily limited amount of tissue obtainable with TBBx, the patchiness of the histologic findings in graft rejection, and potential confounding factors, particularly concomitant infection. This classification system can also be applied to larger specimens, such as surgical lung biopsies, explanted allografts, and autopsy material, with the recognition that some findings, especially chronic vascular rejection (Grade D), are relatively uncommon and virtually never identified on TBBx. ACR and graft atherosclerosis will not be further discussed as they are beyond the scope of this chapter. The interested reader will find a good discussion of these topics elsewhere [21–23].

The focus of this chapter is the pathology of the small airways in acute and chronic rejection, with only brief discussion of the potential significance of large airway inflammation (bronchitis). In addition to rejection, the lung transplant patient is at greater risk for a variety of insults that manifest predominantly, both clinically and pathologically, as airway or airway-based abnormalities. Most importantly, this includes opportunistic infections. BOOP and aspiration pneumonia also occur more commonly in transplanted patients and are sometimes overlooked as potential causes of allograft dysfunction. We will also briefly review two entities that may be mistaken for rejection by the pathologist—the normal biopsy and nonspecific forms of chronic bronchiolitis. First however, given the central role that TBBx plays in the management of rejection, we will briefly review the limitations of TBBx, from the perspective of the pathologist.

The Limitations of Transbronchial Lung Biopsy/Adequacy (Fig. 2.1)

There continues to be a spirited debate within the transplant community regarding the utility of the surveillance TBBx (i.e., one that is performed in the asymptomatic patient according to a predetermined schedule) as compared to the clinically indicated TBBx (i.e., one that is performed after the development of signs or symptoms) [24, 25]. Like any procedure TBBx has intrinsic benefits and costs; it is not our intention to enter into the debate regarding the most appropriate role for TBBx. Our focus is instead on the histopathologic findings that facilitate accurate and timely diagnosis in lung transplant patients. Accurate interpretation of TBBx performed for rejection can be challenging for two main reasons. The first, which is common to currently available techniques for retrieving lung tissue with TBBx, stems from the small size and necessarily limited amount of tissue obtainable via the flexible bronchoscope. The second, which is unique to lung transplant patients, is the difficulty in separating bona fide rejection from other processes with a similar appearance. These potential confounders are discussed in greater detail in the latter sections of this chapter.

There is an inherent challenge in interpreting small pieces of tissue that may be crushed or torn. In addition, small pieces of tissue are more difficult to interpret due to problems stemming from oblique (or tangential) sectioning. This is unavoidable in TBBx. However, the problem of limited tissue is ameliorated, to a degree, by the goal for "adequacy" in rejection TBBx. The ISHLT recommends that adequate biopsy tissue sampling consists of at least five pieces of alveolated parenchyma, recognizing that the bronchoscopist may need to submit more pieces than this in order to increase the chances of including histologically assessable bronchioles within the submitted sample. Moreover, the bronchoscopist may need to submit more than five pieces as some, and sometimes all, of the submitted pieces are invariably comprised only of bronchial wall, exfoliated epithelium, and/or blood (see Fig. 2.1). As mentioned above, rejection is a histologically patchy phenomenon. While higher grades of acute rejection are, by definition, more diffuse processes, lower grades of rejection, including grade A2 (the traditional clinical threshold for pulse therapy), can still be very patchy. Moreover, increasing evidence suggests that episodes of even minimal acute rejection or low-grade LB are associated with higher subsequent rates of chronic rejection/BOS [26]. Therefore, obtaining adequate biopsies may be expected to increase the diagnostic yield of TBBx and allow clinicians to appropriately treat an acute rejection episode in patients who would have otherwise gone untreated.

The sensitivity of TBBx for the detection of rejection is less than 100 % even when technically adequate. The *yield* of TBBx should be distinguished from its *sensitivity*. The diagnostic *yield* of TBBx is the percentage of biopsies performed that are "positive" for rejection. Comparing experiences between centers is challenging, in part, because positivity is not uniformly defined. Some have defined as "positive" any biopsy with at least grade A1 rejection, while others define as

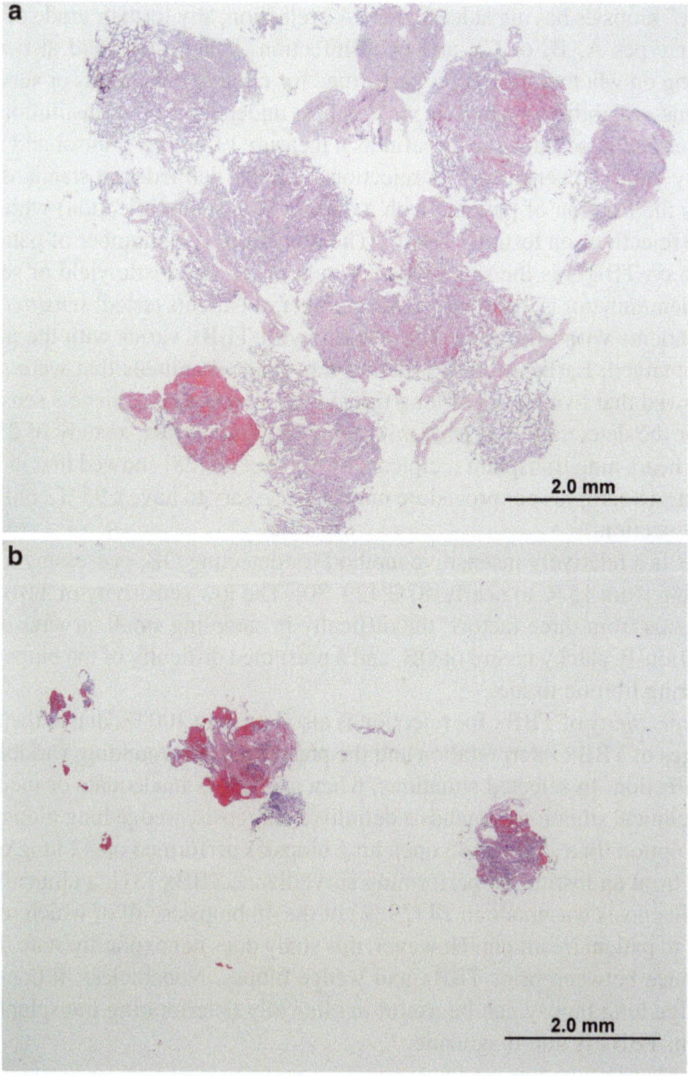

Fig. 2.1 Comparing an adequate (**a**) and a suboptimal (**b**) transbronchial biopsy (TBBx) at low magnification (hematoxylin and eosin, original magnification ×20). The TBBx in (**a**) is very generous and contains about eight substantial fragments of alveolated parenchyma. Both large and small airways are well represented (although difficult to discern at this magnification). By comparison, the TBBx in (**b**) is unsuitable for assessment of rejection. While it consists of about five fragments of tissue, only three are adequately alveolated. However, even these are small, torn, and show significant crush by the forceps. The other fragments are crushed bronchial wall, blood, and exfoliated epithelium, which are not useful for a meaningful histological assessment. The biopsy in (**a**) obviously provides much more information and is also easier to interpret

"positive" biopsies having at least grade A2 rejection, any form or grade of rejection (whether types A, B, or C), and even infection. Diagnostic *yield* also will vary depending on whether a TBBx is performed for clinical indications or surveillance. Given this variability, diagnostic *yield* is best understood as an institution-specific parameter and is perhaps most useful as a measure of quality control and improvement. By contrast, sensitivity of rejection TBBx is defined in a standard fashion, which is the fraction of patients with a disease (transplant rejection) who have the disease (rejection) on testing (TBBx). The numerator (i.e., number of patients with rejection on TBBx) is the same whether measuring diagnostic yield or sensitivity, but the denominator is different (*yield* = number of patients tested; *sensitivity* = number of patients with rejection). The sensitivity of TBBx varies with the number of pieces obtained. Earlier studies utilizing transplanted animals that were sacrificed [27] showed that five pieces of lung tissue were required to achieve a sensitivity of 92 % for the detection of at least mild rejection. In contrast, a study of 219 TBBx from 54 heart-lung transplant recipients by Scott et al. [28] showed that in the clinical setting 18 samples per procedure may be necessary to have a 95 % confidence of finding rejection.

TBBx is a relatively insensitive method for detecting OB, possessing a sensitivity ranging from 15 % to nearly 40 % [29, 30]. The low sensitivity of TBBx for OB likely stems from three factors: the difficulty in sampling small airways on TBBx, the notoriously patchy nature of OB, and a presumed difficulty of the biopsy forceps in acquiring fibrotic tissue.

The *specificity* of TBBx for rejection is also less than 100 %, due to the technical challenges of TBBx interpretation and the presence of confounding variables, especially infection. In selected situations, when a TBBx is inadequate or inconclusive and the clinical situation demands a definitive diagnosis, wedge lung biopsy may be a useful option. In a study of 48 open lung biopsies performed on 42 lung transplant patients from an institution performing surveillance TBBx [31], a clinically unsuspected diagnosis was made in 14 (29 %) of the 48 biopsies, all of which resulted in changes to patient treatment. However, this study does not explicitly state the rate of discordance between prior TBBx and wedge biopsy. Nonetheless, it does suggest that wedge lung biopsy can be useful in clinically deteriorating transplant patients for whom TBBx is non-diagnostic.

Lymphocytic Bronchiolitis (Figs. 2.2 and 2.3)

Lymphocytic bronchiolitis describes chronic mononuclear cell infiltrates involving the small airways. The current ISHLT Working Formulation subdivides LB into low-grade (B1R) and high-grade (B2R) forms. The "R" in the category designation stands for "revised," as it reflects a modification of the 1996 working formulation in collapsing the previous four tier grading system (minimal, mild, moderate, severe) into two (low grade and high grade). In addition, there is a category for no airway inflammation (B0) and an ungradeable category (BX) for those cases in which small

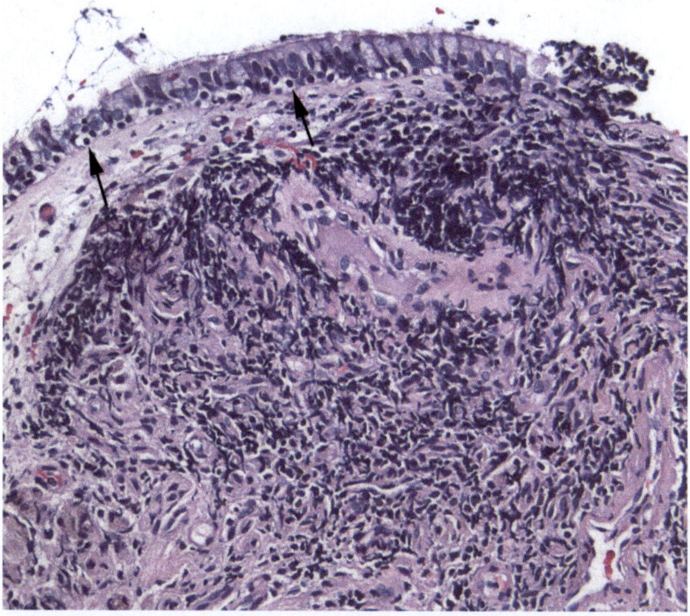

Fig. 2.2 Low-grade lymphocytic bronchiolitis, TBBx (hematoxylin and eosin, original magnification ×200). Mildly to moderately dense lymphocytic inflammation localized predominantly to the bronchiolar submucosa. Lymphocyte crush artifact is prominent, which is common in forceps biopsies. While there are scattered intra-epithelial lymphocytes (*arrows*), there is no evidence of epithelial cell injury

airways are not present, are not assessable (due to tangential sectioning for example), or for which the inflammation cannot be confidently ascribed to rejection. Indeed, potential confounders that mimic LB have delayed acceptance of utilizing LB as an independent or sole marker for establishing or grading acute rejection. These potential confounders are discussed in detail in the second portion of this chapter (see section on "Non-rejection Findings").

Low-grade LB is characterized by relatively sparse peribronchiolar lymphocytic inflammation, often in a circumferential or partially circumferential distribution. The lymphocytic infiltrates are localized to the submucosa, which is not expanded, and there should be no evidence of associated epithelial injury. Although the ISHLT definition of low-grade LB *restricts* the mononuclear infiltrates to the submucosa, scattered intra-epithelial lymphocytes can be observed in otherwise histologically straightforward cases of low-grade LB. For that reason a diagnosis of low-grade LB is appropriate when the infiltrates are not overly dense and localized *predominantly* to the submucosa.

High-grade LB, by contrast, is characterized by more frequent and increasingly dense peribronchiolar lymphoplasmacytic infiltrates. The lymphocytes may be larger

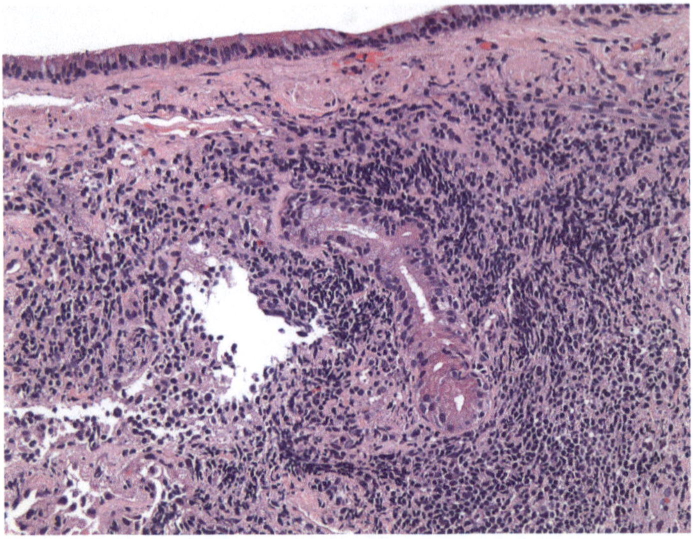

Fig. 2.3 High-grade lymphocytic bronchiolitis, TBBx (hematoxylin and eosin, original magnification ×100). Very dense lymphoplasmacytic inflammation involving the epithelium and submucosa of a bronchiole (*center*). The epithelium lining the adjacent larger airway (*top*) shows no mucosal inflammation. In other levels, the bronchiolar epithelium was necrotic and denuded

and possess an activated or plasmacytoid appearance. Plasma cells may be present in either low-grade or high-grade LB, but are more numerous in high-grade LB. In contrast to low-grade LB, the denser collections of mononuclear cells (lymphocytes and plasma cells) in high-grade LB tend to infiltrate the basement membrane and epithelium of the bronchioles. In such cases, there will usually be evidence of associated epithelial injury, ranging from epithelial cell apoptosis and necrosis to frank mucosal ulceration. Squamous metaplasia of bronchiolar epithelium may also be present and is testimony to attempts at epithelial regeneration. In addition to mononuclear cells, polymorphonuclear leukocytes, including eosinophils, may be seen with high-grade LB. Neutrophils are usually seen in cases with attendant epithelial necrosis or ulceration. If the luminal infiltrates are frankly purulent, or if there is evidence of distal airspace involvement with neutrophilic inflammation, then acute infection (bronchopneumonia) becomes a more likely explanation for the findings.

Obliterative (Constrictive) Bronchiolitis (Figs. 2.4 and 2.5)

OB is the histologic finding of complete or partial bronchiolar fibrosis, whereas BOS is clinically defined as a persistent decline in forced expiratory volume (FEV1) compared to an established post-transplant baseline. While OB is the presumed histologic correlate of BOS, the terms are not interchangeable because some transplant patients develop airflow limitation from other causes [1].

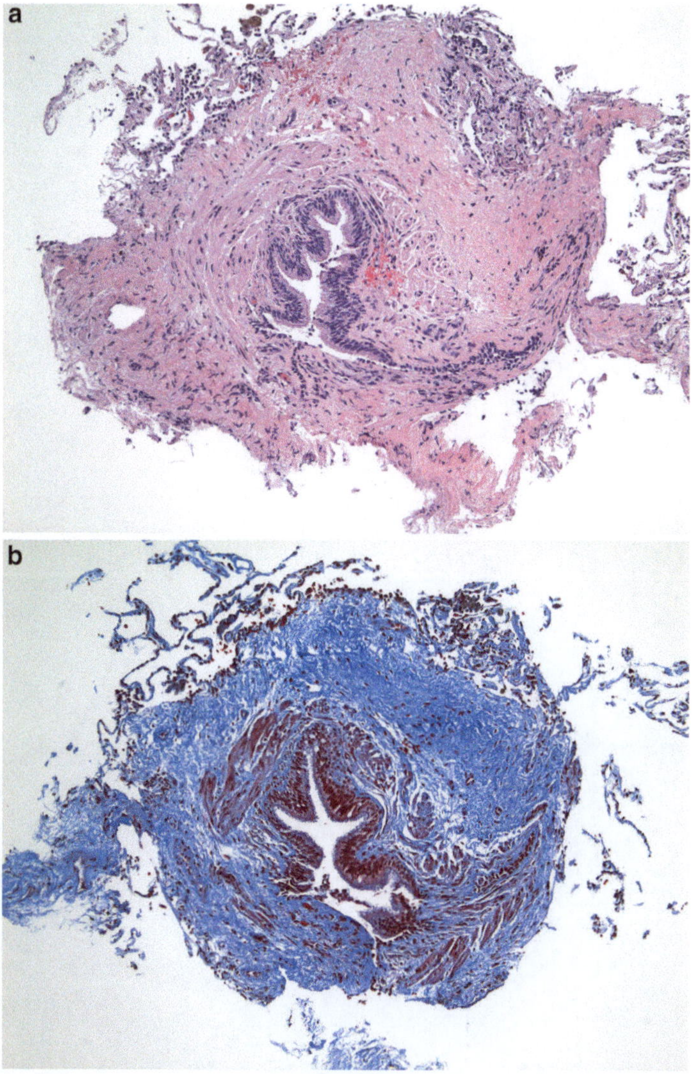

Fig. 2.4 Obliterative bronchiolitis, TBBx (original magnification ×40). (**a**) Hematoxylin and eosin-stained section showing collagen fibrosis of a small airway. There is far too much collagen in the wall and submucosa of this bronchiole, lending the wall an excessively thick appearance out of proportion to the caliber of the lumen. The patient showed spirometric evidence of the bronchiolitis obliterans syndrome (BOS). (**b**) Corresponding trichrome stain. The abnormal and excessive deposition of collagen (*blue*) within the submucosa and wall of the bronchiole is apparent

A great deal of basic science, animal model, and clinical research has begun to clarify the pathogenesis of OB and the risk factors predisposing to it [15, 16]. Both ACR and LB are well-established risk factors. Non-immunologic risk factors, including cytomegalovirus (CMV) and non-CMV infection, BOOP, donor age, and graft ischemia time (among others), have also been implicated as risk factors for developing OB/BOS.

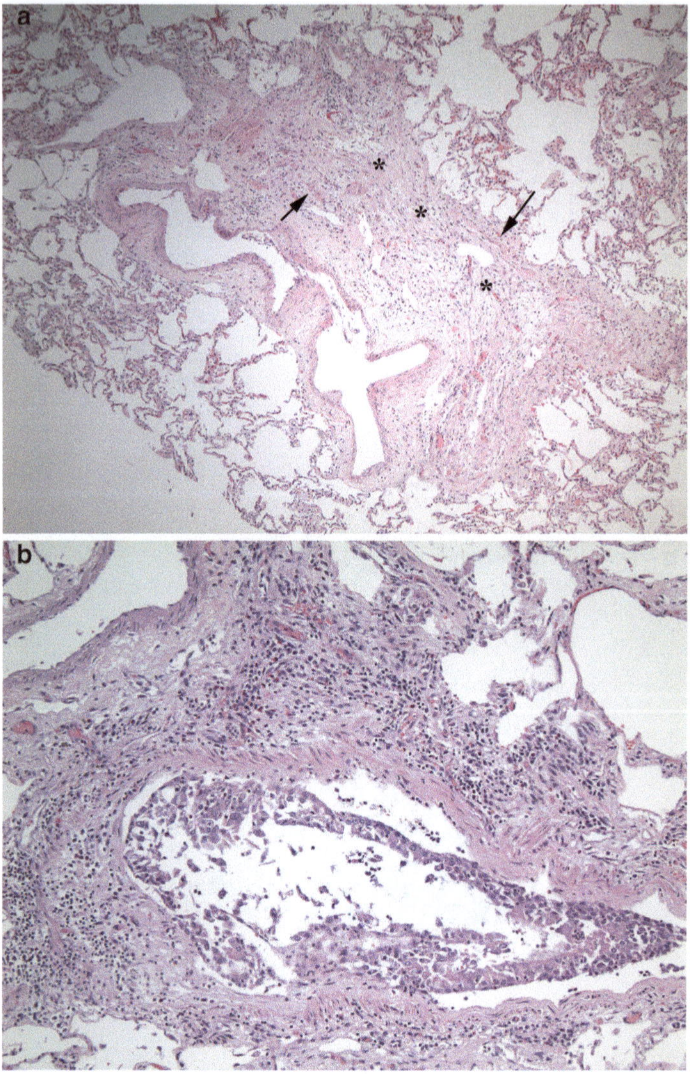

Fig. 2.5 Obliterative bronchiolitis, autopsy material. The patient was a 30-year-old female who had received a double lung transplant approximately 8 years earlier for cystic fibrosis. BOS was the cause of death. There was no evidence of acute cellular rejection (ACR). (**a**) Bronchovascular bundle showing complete occlusive fibrosis of the bronchiole (*asterisks*) (hematoxylin and eosin, original magnification ×40). Notice the residual fascicles of smooth muscle in the bronchiolar wall (*arrows*). (**b**) There is evidence of concomitant lymphocytic bronchiolitis (hematoxylin and eosin, original magnification ×100). This bronchiole shows circumferential submucosal inflammation, which is focally of moderate density. The epithelial sloughing is an artifact of autolysis

Recently, there has been increasing attention on the existence and possible role for antibody-mediated rejection (AMR) as a risk factor for OB/BOS [32]. This stems from the occurrence of OB in patients with no evidence of antecedent ACR [33], evidence of septal capillary injury in cases of otherwise unexplained graft dysfunction [34], complement deposition in capillary endothelium [35], and the uncommon but well-documented occurrence of graft dysfunction in patients who developed donor-specific anti-human leukocyte antigen (anti-HLA) antibodies and capillaritis on biopsy [36]. Despite tantalizing evidence of a possible link between AMR and lung allograft dysfunction there are persistent unresolved questions regarding its diagnosis and significance. Capillaritis has been proposed as a histologic marker of AMR in TBBx but distinguishing capillaritis from simple neutrophil margination (diapedesis) in small specimens is challenging at best. Bronchopneumonia must be rigorously excluded in this setting since neutrophil margination is common in acute infection. In the non-transplant setting necrotizing capillaritis is virtually always associated with clinical and histologic evidence of diffuse alveolar hemorrhage. Immunohistochemical stains for C4d are of limited value given that interpretation is plagued by nonspecific background staining of endothelial cells and elastic tissue. Furthermore, there is a poor correlation between linear C4d staining, the presence of necrotizing capillaritis, and the development of donor-specific HLA alloantibodies [37]. Thus, substantial difficulties remain before AMR can be embraced as a distinct clinicopathologic form of lung rejection.

Collagen fibrosis involving and expanding the bronchiolar submucosa is the histologic hallmark of OB. The fibrosis may be eccentric or concentric and in more advanced lesions results in complete obliteration of the airspace lumen. OB may be more difficult to recognize in the late fibrotic stage as the airways are completely scarred and therefore difficult to recognize. Key to identifying these focal scars as former airways includes the presence of an associated similar-caliber artery or the presence of residual fascicles of smooth muscle within the fibrosis. In most cases, the fibrosis is not accompanied by inflammation but persistence of mononuclear cell inflammation of the sort and character of LB may be noted in some cases. Indeed, LB and OB may coexist. Mucostasis and/or accumulation of foamy, lipid-laden histiocytes within peribronchiolar air spaces may be present as nonspecific markers of small airways dysfunction of any cause. Occasionally these finding are present in the absence of diagnostic small airways changes and are suggestive—but not diagnostic of—bronchiolar pathology.

Large Airway Inflammation/Lymphocytic Bronchitis (Fig. 2.6)

Lymphocytic bronchiolitis, as the name implies, affects the small airways—that is, the distal-most portions of the conducting bronchioles and the respiratory bronchioles of the allografted lung. The significance of LB with respect to lung rejection is now well established. Occasionally, similar appearing inflammation of the large conducting cartilaginous airways may also occur, with or without associated LB [38]. Unlike LB, much less is known about the significance of isolated large airway inflammation vis-à-vis rejection. Early studies found increased numbers of specialized Leu-7 (CD57)-positive T lymphocytes in the mucosa of donor bronchi with morphologic evidence of

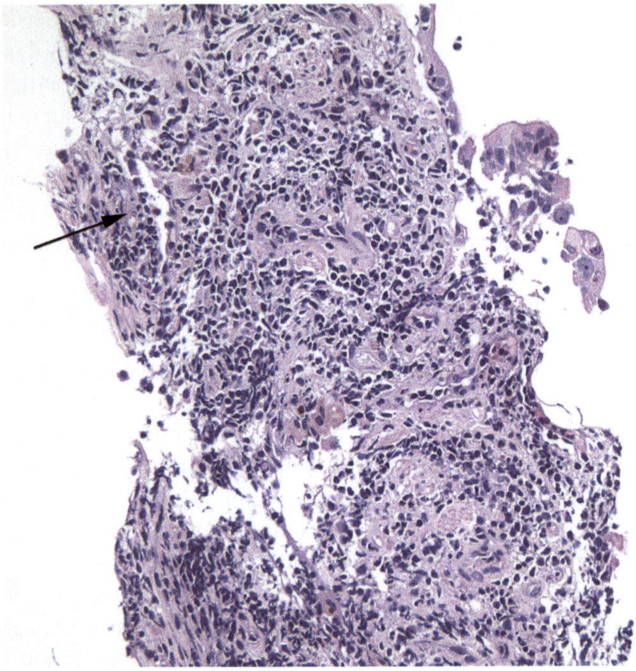

Fig. 2.6 Lymphocytic bronchitis, TBBx (hematoxylin and eosin, original magnification ×200). Dense mononuclear cell inflammation involving a bronchus. Both the wall and epithelium is involved; the latter shows evidence of injury in the form of sloughing and regenerative atypia. There is evidence of small airway involvement as well (lymphocytic bronchiolitis); a tangential portion of an affected bronchiole is seen in the section (*arrow*). Other fragments (not shown) also showed lymphocytic bronchiolitis. Cultures for microorganisms and other microbiological assays were negative for infection

airway injury and observed an association between lymphocytic bronchitis and subsequent OB [39–41]. In another study, Yousem and colleagues also found that "chronic inflammation of the bronchi" was associated with subsequent development of OB, with a sensitivity and specificity of 83 % and 100 %, respectively, although the number of cases was very small [42]. Large airway bronchial fibrosis has also been observed in some lung allografts with coexisting OB [43]. These studies suggested that bronchial mucosa may be a target for rejection prompting the use of the combined term "lymphocytic bronchitis/bronchiolitis" (LBB) to refer to the mononuclear cell infiltrates jointly affecting the bronchi and the bronchioles. As is true in small airways, inflammation in large airways is not specific for rejection and is commonly present with clinical (or subclinical) infection, aspiration, chronic obstructive pulmonary disease, and other inhalational injuries. Indeed, the ISHLT working formulation recognizes that large airway inflammation is most commonly associated with infection and aspiration and does not currently identify or grade "lymphocytic bronchitis" as such [21]. Bronchiectasis has also been described in lung transplant patients with BOS, although it is not known if this is a consequence of infection, rejection, ischemic injury, or some combination of these factors [44].

The significance of lymphocytic bronchitis in a TBBx depends upon not only the morphologic features but also the clinical context. To help distinguish lymphocytic bronchitis from nonspecific forms of chronic bronchitis the term should be limited to cases in which dense collections of lymphocytes are confined to the bronchial submucosa and submucosal glands, often infiltrating into the bronchial epithelium. With more intense degrees of inflammation, greater numbers of transformed lymphocytes, immunoblasts, and even eosinophils are present, and there may be evidence of epithelial injury including apoptosis, squamous metaplasia, or ulceration. Neutrophils should not be abundant and there should not be evidence of viral cytopathic change or aspiration, features which would point to another etiology. When narrowly defined in this way lymphocytic bronchitis is not a common finding and, when present, is often seen in combination with other findings typical of acute rejection, usually LB. Such cases should be graded conventionally as per ISHLT guidelines, with or without mention of the presence of lymphocytic bronchitis, since in any event clinical decision making will be based on the formal "A-B-C" rejection grade. Lymphocytic bronchitis is uncommon as a truly isolated finding, and when present without other corroborative histologic support for a diagnosis of rejection its significance is uncertain.

Non-rejection Findings

Normal (Bronchus-Associated Lymphoid Tissue) (Fig. 2.7)

The airways, as in other non-sterile mucosal sites with a more-or-less constant exposure to the external environment, possess a mucosa-associated lymphoid tissue (MALT tissue) specifically referred to as bronchus-associated lymphoid tissue (BALT). In the large airways, these comprise circumscribed submucosal aggregates (primary follicles) of lymphocytes. They are usually not very prominent, unless there has been antigenic stimulation, in which case there may be BALT hyperplasia which may be associated with germinal center formation (secondary follicles). The circumscription and submucosal localization of BALT follicular aggregates is not likely to be confused with lymphocytic bronchitis and bronchiolitis. However, in the intermediate and small airways, the lymphocytes may extend into the overlying epithelium ("lymphoepithelium"), which is focally attenuated as it is in other MALT sites. It is important not to confuse this normal finding with LB (or with any other pathology). The key features distinguishing BALT and lymphoepithelium from LB are that the lymphoid infiltrates of the latter are denser, are not circumscribed, and do not form primary or secondary follicles; establishing this may require assessment of multiple consecutive tissue levels. Furthermore, LB may be associated with epithelial damage including epithelial cell necrosis, mucosal ulceration, and squamous metaplasia, particularly when high grade (B2R). Lastly, LB is often associated with the perivascular lymphoid infiltrates of ACR.

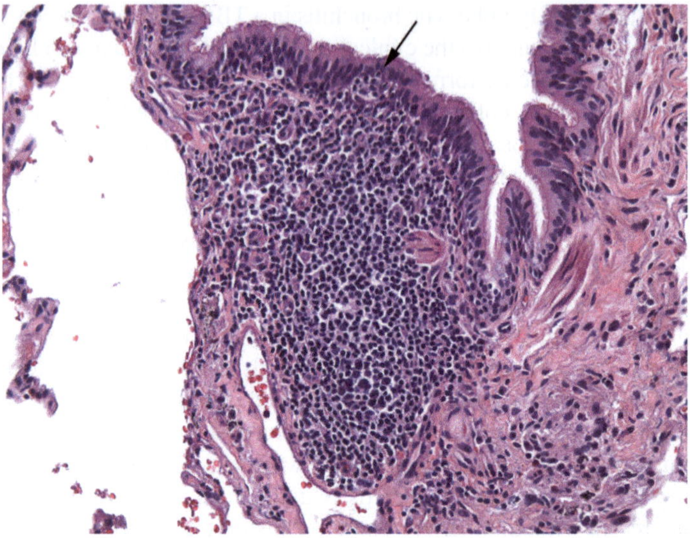

Fig. 2.7 Bronchus-associated lymphoid tissue, wedge biopsy (hematoxylin and eosin, original magnification ×200). BALT, a normal finding, comprises mucosal lymphoid aggregates associated with large and/or small airways. The aggregates are comprised of well-circumscribed subepithelial primary or secondary lymphoid follicles. In the small airways, as seen here, the lymphocytes may focally percolate among the epithelial cells ("lymphoepithelium," *arrow*). It may sometimes be difficult to distinguish BALT from bronchiolitis (of any cause) on TBBx, particularly when the sample is very small, fragmented, or crushed

Nonspecific Chronic Bronchiolitis

Chronic bronchiolitis is a histopathologic term referring to chronic inflammation involving bronchiolar and peribronchiolar interstitium with or without fibrosis [45]. Chronic bronchiolitis is a nonspecific finding; its significance is defined by the histopathologic and clinical context [46]. For example, chronic bronchiolitis is a common finding in other primary pathologic processes, such as hypersensitivity pneumonia. In hypersensitivity pneumonia, chronic bronchiolitis is only one component of a unique combination of equally nonspecific findings that is characteristic only when present collectively. Chronic bronchiolitis is uncommon as an isolated primary pathologic process and occurs in surprisingly heterogeneous clinical contexts. In smokers with evidence of obstructive airways disease, chronic bronchiolitis corresponds to the small airways disease thought to account for airflow limitation in patients with emphysema and chronic bronchitis [47]. Occasional unexplained chronic bronchiolitis occurs in nonsmokers with airflow limitation who lack other features of emphysema, chronic bronchitis, or asthma (i.e., idiopathic small airways disease). Chronic bronchiolitis does not by itself predict for physiologically significant obstructive airways disease, however, and in some patients may actually be affiliated with evidence of restrictive lung disease.

Given the nonspecific nature of chronic bronchiolitis and the wide range of potential causes and associations, attributing bronchiolitis to rejection in transplant patients requires careful integration of not only histopathologic but also clinical, physiologic, and radiologic data.

Opportunistic Infection

Infectious complications are a major obstacle to both short-term and long-term survival in lung transplantation. Non-CMV infections are the leading cause of morbidity and mortality in the first year status post-transplantation, and remain the second leading cause of mortality thereafter, preceded only by BOS [17]. Pneumonia, particularly bacterial pneumonia, is the most common infection affecting lung transplant patients, especially in the early post-transplant period, although mycobacterial, viral, and fungal pneumonia all occur at an increased frequency in lung transplant patients [48]. For the pathologist, the diagnosis of acute bronchopneumonia due to pyogenic bacteria or granulomatous infection is generally straightforward and not likely to be confused with acute rejection; the former entities are characterized by suppurative or granulomatous inflammation involving the airspaces, while acute rejection is typified by mononuclear/lymphocytic inflammation in the perivascular and peribronchiolar interstitium.

Certain infectious agents produce a *cellular interstitial pneumonia* that is more likely to be confused with acute rejection. In particular, two important opportunistic pathogens, CMV and *Pneumocystis jirovecii*, cause an infectious pneumonia that may show prominent chronic interstitial inflammation (i.e., chronic interstitial pneumonia) that closely resembles acute rejection [49, 50]. In a study of CMV and pneumocystis pneumonia diagnosed by open lung biopsy and TBBx, Tazelaar [50] noted perivascular lymphocytic infiltrates similar to those seen in acute rejection in 42 % of CMV cases and 21 % of pneumocystis cases. Such results reiterate the need for the pathologist to at least consider the possibility of infection in every transplant TBBx and to rigorously exclude—or include—infection with ancillary special stains in selected cases. A TBBx diagnosis of infection that includes perivascular lymphoid infiltrates does not preclude the possibility of concomitant rejection, however, and should be regarded as indeterminate ("AXBX") in this regard. If clinically warranted, a subsequent TBBx following appropriate antimicrobial treatment may be more helpful in evaluating for rejection without the confounding effects of infection. This serves as a reminder that the ultimate diagnosis in any individual patient should be the result of integration with all available clinical data, including those from microbiologic and serologic studies.

Among non-alloimmune risk factors for the development of OB/BOS, pulmonary infection due to CMV has been the most extensively studied, with relatively fewer reports analyzing non-CMV viruses, bacteria, and fungi including pneumocystis [14, 16]. Bacterial and pneumocystis pneumonia have not been clearly shown to be significant risk factors for OB/BOS, while studies assessing the significance of CMV pneumonia on the development of OB/BOS have shown inconsistent results

[14, 16]. At this time, pulmonary infections, in general, and viral respiratory pathogens, in particular, are considered to be possible risk factors for OB/BOS, perhaps by potentiating the effects of acute rejection.

Cytomegalovirus Pneumonia (Fig. 2.8)

The key to the diagnosis of CMV pneumonia is the recognition of characteristic viral cytopathic changes caused by CMV infection, of which there are three—cytomegaly, nuclear inclusions, and cytoplasmic inclusions. Cellular and nuclear enlargement (cytomegaly) is perhaps the most easily recognizable alteration. The intranuclear inclusions consist of centrally placed amorphous basophilic inclusions, usually with a clear halo separating them from the nuclear membrane. The cytoplasmic inclusions, which are not seen in every infected cell, are also basophilic and coarsely granular. The latter often stain positively with the Gomori methenamine silver (GMS) method. These viral cytopathic changes can affect virtually any cell, including pneumocytes, interstitial cells, and endothelial cells. While some cases may show numerous CMV virocytes, other cases may show only a few or rare infected cells, particularly in the limited samples that TBBx provides. An immunohistochemical stain for CMV is widely available and can be very helpful in confirming the diagnosis, especially in subtle cases. In addition to the characteristic altered cells, CMV pneumonia typically elicits a predominantly chronic inflammatory cell reaction involving the interstitium and the airways that may be nearly indistinguishable from ACR and LB. In more severe cases, it may also cause diffuse alveolar damage (DAD) and/or fibrinous airspace exudate.

As stated above, unless the viral cytopathic changes are recognized, the case is likely to be misdiagnosed as acute rejection. The viral changes caused by CMV must be distinguished from those due to herpes simplex virus (HSV). HSV infection does not result in significant cytomegaly, nor does it cause intracytoplasmic inclusions. In addition, HSV infection produces ground glass intranuclear inclusions that are usually prominently eosinophilic and with a margin of peripherally condensed chromatin.

Pneumocystis jirovecii Pneumonia (Fig. 2.9)

There are a number of histologic changes that can be seen in pneumocystis pneumonia. The classic change is the presence of an eosinophilic "frothy" alveolar exudate on hematoxylin and eosin (H&E) staining. On higher power, this exudate possesses a honeycomb-like or microcystic appearance, representing numerous organism cysts and it is pathognomonic for the disease. This frothy exudate may be associated with features of DAD including hyaline membranes. Granulomatous inflammation—necrotizing, non-necrotizing, or both—is an uncommon manifestation of pneumocystis pneumonia that is often associated with lymphocytic inflammation and clusters of histiocytes. Other less common changes include areas of necrosis, calcification, and a pulmonary alveolar proteinosis-like reaction.

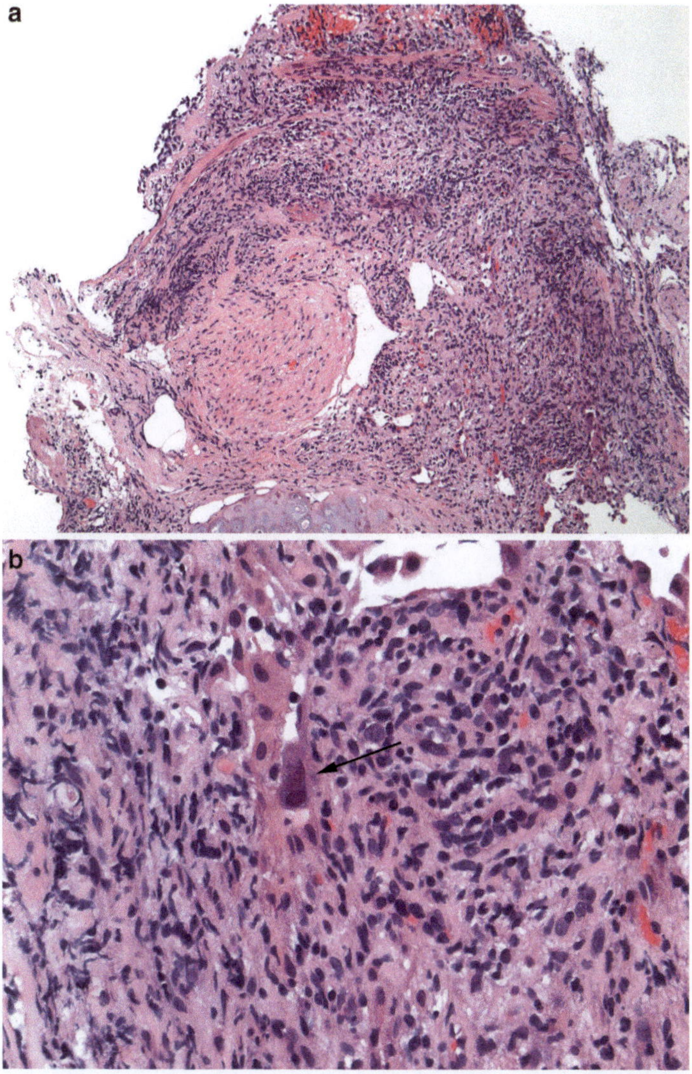

Fig. 2.8 Cytomegalovirus (CMV) pneumonia, TBBx. (**a**) On low power, there is a dense predominantly chronic inflammatory infiltrate involving the bronchus and subjacent alveolar tissue(hematoxylin and eosin, original magnification ×100). Such an appearance is reminiscent of high-grade ACR with lymphocytic bronchitis/bronchiolitis. (**b**) On higher magnification, an endothelial cell with CMV viral cytopathic change is seen (*arrow*) (hematoxylin and eosin, original magnification ×400). This comprises nucleomegaly and cytomegaly and basophilic ground glass nuclear inclusions. There may also be basophilic intracytoplasmic granules, although these are somewhat difficult to discern even at this magnification. An immunohistochemical stain for CMV was also positive (not shown). Note the marked lymphohistiocytic inflammation

TBBx is a sensitive technique for the detection of pneumocystis pneumonia. If the characteristic frothy eosinophilic alveolar exudates are present, then the diagnosis is straightforward and can be made even in the absence of special stains.

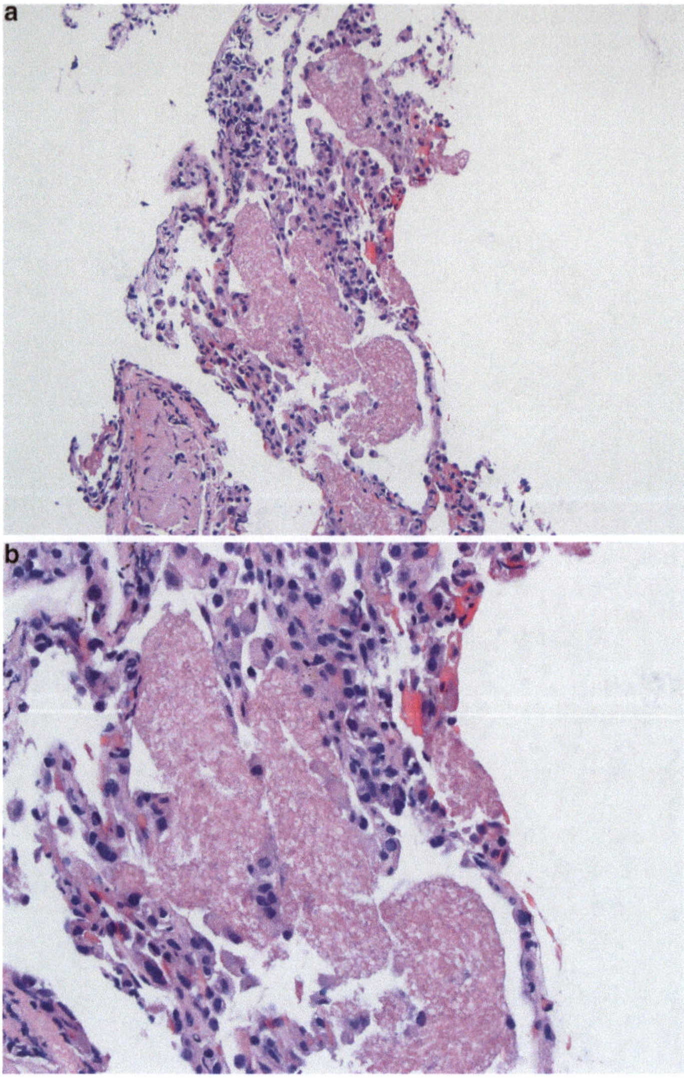

Fig. 2.9 *Pneumocystis jirovecii* pneumonia, TBBx. (**a**) This photomicrograph demonstrates frothy, eosinophilic alveolar exudates, the most helpful and characteristic feature of *Pneumocystis* pneumonia (hematoxylin and eosin, original magnification ×200). (**b**) These exudates have a distinctive microcystic appearance at high magnification (hematoxylin and eosin, original magnification ×400). (**c**) Silver stains, such as the Gomori methenamine silver (GMS) stain, demonstrate the yeast forms, which are 4–6 μm in diameter and helmet-shaped, crescentic, or spherical (GMS, original magnification ×600). Note the internal dot-like enhancement inside the cysts (*arrow*), a feature which helps distinguish *Pneumocystis* from *Histoplasma* spp. yeast forms

Occasionally, however, only hyaline membranes, a chronic interstitial pneumonia, or granulomas are present. For that reason, it is important to maintain a low threshold for performing special stains, especially stains such as a GMS stain that highlight pneumocystis organisms.

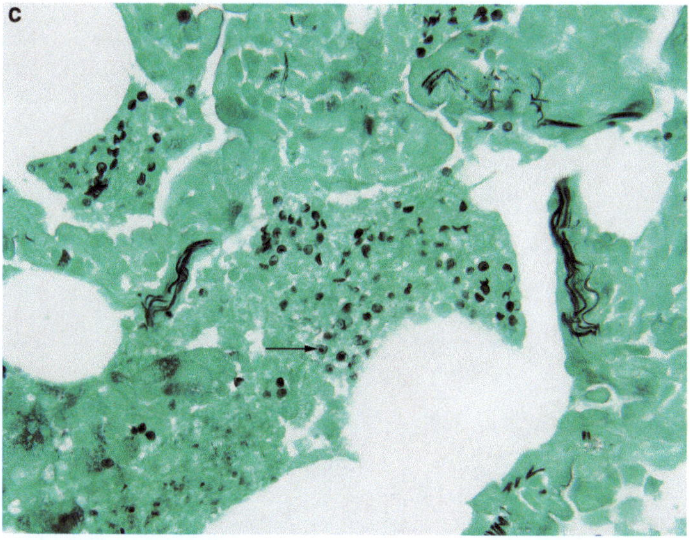

Fig. 2.9 (continued)

Bronchiolitis Obliterans-Organizing Pneumonia (Fig. 2.10)

Bronchiolitis obliterans-organizing pneumonia (BOOP), also termed organizing pneumonia (OP), is a nonspecific manifestation of acute lung injury. As such, it can be caused by or associated with a wide variety of insults and conditions, including infectious pneumonia, medications, aspiration of gastric contents, radiation, or connective tissue disease [51]. The etiology is usually not apparent on the basis of the histologic findings alone. BOOP may also be seen as a nonspecific secondary change in other primary processes. Idiopathic BOOP, also termed cryptogenic OP or COP, refers to a distinct syndrome of unknown cause with characteristic clinical and radiographic features and BOOP as an isolated finding on lung biopsy [52]. Spontaneous remission may occur, and in those patient requiring treatment it tends to be a steroid-responsive disease, although relapses are common. These features are in contrast to OB, which is typically insidious and progressive and not marked by relapses or remissions. BOOP is a fairly common finding in rejection biopsies [53], reemphasizing the importance of its distinction from OB by the reviewing pathologist. Indeed, in an earlier review of organizing pneumonia-like reactions in allograft biopsies, Yousem and colleagues described BOOP as most commonly occurring in the setting of acute rejection [53]. Several groups have also found BOOP to be a risk factor for OB/BOS [54, 55]. As such, BOOP has been proposed to be included in the histologic classification of lung rejection [56], although this has not been adopted.

BOOP is characterized by fusiform proliferations of spindled fibroblastic and myofibroblastic cells set within a pale-staining myxoid matrix containing abundant mucopolysaccharides (ground substance), a combination of findings sometimes

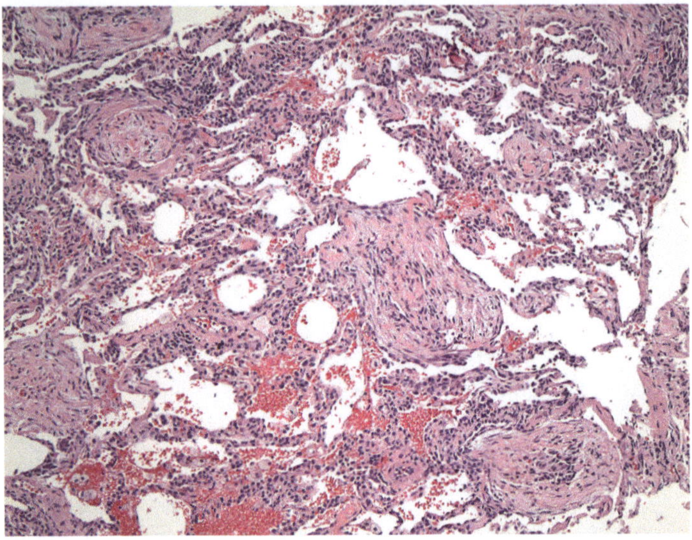

Fig. 2.10 Bronchiolitis obliterans-organizing pneumonia, TBBx (hematoxylin and eosin, original magnification ×100). Fibromyxoid plugs of spindled fibroblasts and myofibroblasts are present within the airspaces and lumens of distal airways. When encountering a TBBx with BOOP, the pathologist should search for more specific features that might suggest an underlying etiology, such as evidence of acute infection, viral changes, granulomas, or aspirated foreign material. Notice the presence of an associated cellular chronic interstitial pneumonia, a common associated finding in BOOP (of any cause), and one that should be distinguished from the perivascular mononuclear cell infiltrates of ACR

described as fibromyxoid plugs of "young" fibrosis. A key feature defining BOOP is the localization of these fibromyxoid plugs to the lumens of the distal bronchioles ("bronchiolitis obliterans") and alveolar airspaces and ducts ("organizing pneumonia"). This distribution accounts for its typical whorled and serpentine appearance. Involvement of the bronchiolar lumens causes small airway dysfunction, which in turn results in a variably prominent accumulation of foamy macrophages, sometimes referred to as endogenous lipoid pneumonia. BOOP may be accompanied by abundant airspace fibrin, lending an eosinophilic appearance to the process. Associated inflammation can be highly variable, from negligible to dense infiltrates, and is usually comprised of chronic inflammatory cells, mostly lymphocytes and plasma cells. The inflammatory cells can be found within the fibromyxoid tissue or alveolar septal walls or both. However, if alveolar septal and perivascular mononuclear infiltrates are prominent, then high-grade ACR should be strongly considered as the underlying etiology. Neutrophils and histiocytes may also be found, but if prominent, an infectious etiology should be suspected and the use of special stains for microorganisms may be helpful in further evaluating for that possibility.

The organizing phase of DAD may be indistinguishable from BOOP in small biopsies. BOOP can usually be distinguished by the intraluminal localization of the fibroblastic plugs and the absence of hyaline membranes but these helpful clues are not always easily discerned in TBBx. DAD typically occurs in the setting of the adult respiratory distress syndrome (ARDS) and for that reason can usually be separated from BOOP by correlating with the patient's clinical status in histologically challenging cases. BOOP is usually easily distinguishable from OB, even in small biopsies, as both the location (airspaces in the former, submucosa in the latter) and constitutive elements (fibromyxoid tissue in the former, collagen fibrosis in the latter) are distinctly different.

Aspiration Pneumonia (Fig. 2.11)

Patients who have undergone lung transplantation are at a significantly increased risk for gastroesophageal reflux and aspiration [57–59], possibly due to impaired cough reflex and mucociliary clearance mechanisms. While massive acute aspiration is not a clinically occult condition, chronic, low-level episodes of repeated aspiration pose a more difficult diagnostic challenge; in fact, chronic aspiration is often clinically unsuspected [60, 61]. Chronic gastroesophageal reflux and aspiration have been implicated as non-alloimmune risk factors for the development of OB/BOS [62], and anti-reflux therapy utilizing medical (macrolide antibiotics) and surgical (gastric fundoplication) modalities has resulted in improved lung function in several studies [63–66]. Thus, aspiration is a treatable cause of pulmonary allograft dysfunction and it is a diagnosis the pathologist is often in a unique position to make.

The morphologic features of particulate aspiration are sufficiently unique that the diagnosis can often be made on TBBx. Aspiration pneumonia is characterized by airway-centered granulomatous inflammation that is often necrotizing. The granulomas typically elicit an associated BOOP response, which is often quite prominent and is sometimes the dominant finding. Acute and chronic bronchitis and bronchiolitis are a nearly constant finding and thus the pathologist must take care before ascribing bronchiolitis to rejection or to infection. The defining feature of aspiration pneumonia is the presence of exogenous aspirated foreign material, either in an extracellular location or within giant cells or both. The aspirated material is of two major kinds—foodstuffs and inorganic crystalline "fillers" derived from oral medications; the presence of either substance in the appropriate histologic context is diagnostic. The foodstuffs have a varying appearance depending on the age of the process. They include recognizable skeletal muscle and plant cell walls derived from consumed meats and vegetables, respectively; the latter may be refractile and either weakly or strongly birefringent on polarized microscopy. Older organic material tends to have a pale, amorphous eosinophilic appearance, and is more difficult to recognize. The most common inorganic fillers include microcrystalline cellulose, which is strongly birefringent, and crospovidone, which has an amorphous densely basophilic appearance. These exogenous compounds must not be confused with various endogenous materials that can be found within giant cells, including blue bodies, asteroid bodies, and birefringent calcium salts. As mentioned above, the granulomas in aspiration sometimes show central suppurative necrosis, wherein the giant cells surround pockets of neutrophils. The latter feature, while nonspecific (as it can be seen with certain infections, Wegener granulomatosis, and rheumatoid

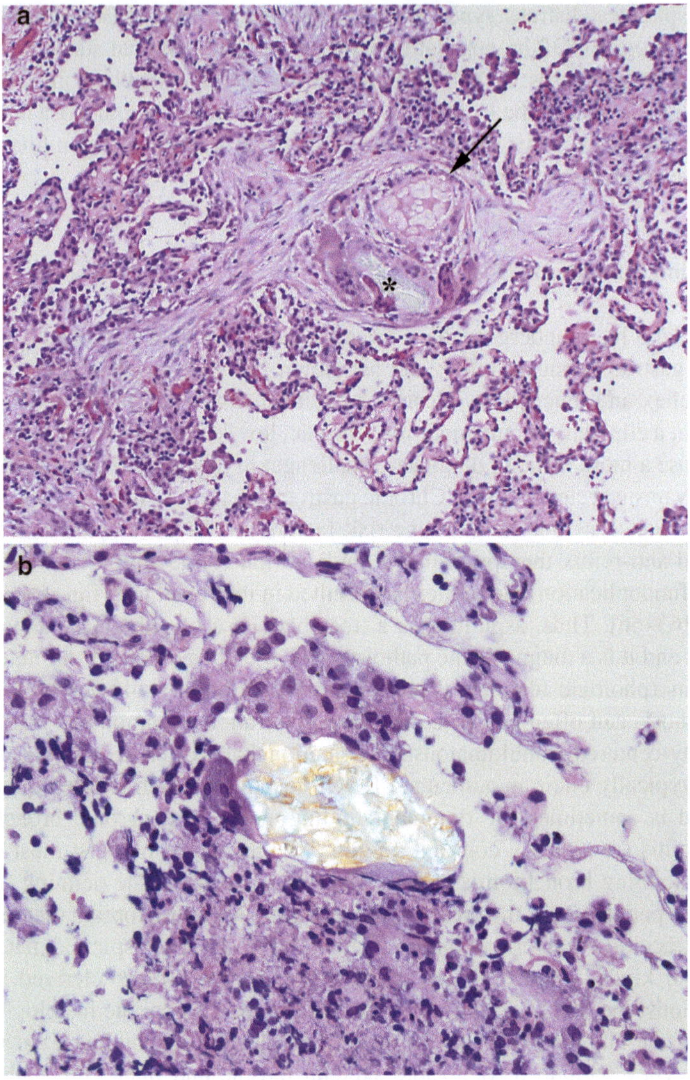

Fig. 2.11 Aspiration pneumonia, TBBx. (**a**) Intermediate magnification photomicrograph showing BOOP with granulomatous inflammation (hematoxylin and eosin, original magnification ×200). Multinucleated giant cells are engulfing aspirated exogenous substances. The amorphous pale-staining material within the upper giant cell (*arrow*) is partially digested foodstuff while the birefringent, cracked, crystalline material in the lower giant cell (*asterisk*) is microcrystalline cellulose, a common inorganic filler utilized in oral medications. (**b**) Polarized light microscopy can be helpful in identifying and/or confirming polarizable substances in suspected cases of aspiration (hematoxylin and eosin, original magnification ×600). Certain crystalline fillers, such as microcrystalline cellulose (as seen here) are strongly polarizable. Plant cell walls from aspirated foods vary greatly in their strength of polarization

nodules) is not common and is therefore a potential clue to the diagnosis. If suppurative granulomas are present in a TBBx, this should prompt the pathologist to search carefully for any associated exogenous aspirated substances. Occasionally, no aspirated material can be found, a problem more common in small biopsies, and a confident diagnosis of aspiration pneumonia may not be possible. In immunocompromised patients the differential diagnosis for otherwise unexplained granulomatous inflammation includes mainly opportunistic infections and should prompt appropriate special stains and microbiological assays. Organisms that may cause suppurative granulomatous inflammation resembling that seen in aspiration include, most commonly, *Nocardia*, *Actinomyces*, and *Blastomyces* species.

References

1. Estenne M, Maurer JR, Boehler A, Egan JJ, Frost A, Hertz M, et al. Bronchiolitis obliterans syndrome 2001: an update of the diagnostic criteria. J Heart Lung Transplant. 2002;21(3):297–310.
2. Gauhar UA, Gaffo AL, Alarcon GS. Pulmonary manifestations of rheumatoid arthritis. Semin Respir Crit Care Med. 2007;28(4):430–40.
3. Sung RYT, Chan RCK, Tam JS, Cheng AFB, Murray HGS. Epidemiology and etiology of acute bronchiolitis in Hong-Kong infants. Epidemiol Infect. 1992;108(1):147–54.
4. Aguerre V, Castanos C, Pena HG, Grenoville M, Murtagh P. Postinfectious bronchiolitis obliterans in children: clinical and pulmonary function findings. Pediatr Pulmonol. 2010;45(12):1180–5.
5. Takayama S, Ogawa T, Tominaga S, Yasui M, Ohno S, Ohkochi M, et al. [Penicillamine-induced bronchiolitis obliterans diagnosed by transbronchial lung biopsy]. Nihon Kokyuki Gakkai Zasshi. 2006;44(2):128–33.
6. Price SK, Hughes JE, Morrison SC, Potgieter PD. Fatal ammonia inhalation. A case report with autopsy findings. S Afr Med J. 1983;64(24):952–5.
7. Tasaka S, Kanazawa M, Mori M, Fujishima S, Ishizaka A, Yamasawa F, et al. Long-term course of bronchiectasis and bronchiolitis obliterans as late complication of smoke inhalation. Respiration. 1995;62(1):40–2.
8. Ettinger NA, Albin RJ. A review of the respiratory effects of smoking cocaine. Am J Med. 1989;87(6):664–8.
9. Kreiss K, Gomaa A, Kullman G, Fedan K, Simoes EJ, Enright PL. Clinical bronchiolitis obliterans in workers at a microwave-popcorn plant. N Engl J Med. 2002;347(5):330–8.
10. Harber P, Saechao K, Boomus C. Diacetyl-induced lung disease. Toxicol Rev. 2006;25(4):261–72.
11. Yousem SA. The histological spectrum of pulmonary graft-versus-host disease in bone-marrow transplant recipients. Hum Pathol. 1995;26(6):668–75.
12. Workman DL, Clancy Jr J. Interstitial pneumonitis and lymphocytic bronchiolitis/bronchitis as a direct result of acute lethal graft-versus-host disease duplicate the histopathology of lung allograft rejection. Transplantation. 1994;58(2):207–13.
13. Boehler A, Chamberlain D, Kesten S, Slutsky AS, Liu MY, Keshavjee S. Lymphocytic airway infiltration as a precursor to fibrous obliteration in a rat model of bronchiolitis obliterans. Transplantation. 1997;64(2):311–7.
14. Sharples LD, McNeil K, Stewart S, Wallwork J. Risk factors for bronchiolitis obliterans: a systematic review of recent publications. J Heart Lung Transplant. 2002;21(2):271–81.
15. Neuringer IP, Chalermskulrat W, Aris R. Obliterative bronchiolitis or chronic lung allograft rejection: a basic science review. J Heart Lung Transplant. 2005;24(1):3–19.

16. Scott AIR, Sharples LD, Stewart S. Bronchiolitis obliterans syndrome—risk factors and therapeutic strategies. Drugs. 2005;65(6):761–71.
17. Christie JD, Edwards LB, Kucheryavaya AY, Benden C, Dobbels F, Kirk R, et al. The registry of the International Society for Heart and Lung Transplantation: twenty-eighth adult lung and heart-lung transplant report-2011. J Heart Lung Transplant. 2011;30(10):1104–22.
18. Van Muylem A, Knoop C, Estenne M. Early detection of chronic pulmonary allograft dysfunction by exhaled biomarkers. Am J Respir Crit Care Med. 2007;175(7):731–6.
19. Yousem SA, Berry GJ, Brunt EM, Chamberlain D, Hruban RH, Sibley RK, et al. A working formulation for the standardization of nomenclature in the diagnosis of heart and lung rejection—Lung Rejection Study-Group. J Heart Transplant. 1990;9(6):593–601.
20. Yousem SA, Berry GJ, Cagle PT, Chamberlain D, Husain AN, Hruban RH, et al. Revision of the 1990 working formulation for the classification of pulmonary allograft rejection: Lung Rejection Study Group. J Heart Lung Transplant. 1996;15(1 Pt 1):1–15.
21. Stewart S, Fishbein MC, Snell GI, Berry GJ, Boehler A, Burke MM, et al. Revision of the 1996 working formulation for the standardization of nomenclature in the diagnosis of lung rejection. J Heart Lung Transplant. 2007;26(12):1229–42.
22. Radio S, Wood S, Wilson J, Lin H, Winters G, McManus B. Allograft vascular disease: comparison of heart and other grafted organs. Transplant Proc. 1996;28(1):496–9.
23. Yousem SA, Paradis IL, Dauber JH, Zeevi A, Duquesnoy RJ, Dalcol R, et al. Pulmonary arteriosclerosis in long-term human heart-lung transplant recipients. Transplantation. 1989;47(3):564–9.
24. Glanville AR. Bronchoscopic monitoring after lung transplantation. Semin Respir Crit Care Med. 2010;31(2):208–21.
25. Sandrini A, Glanville AR. The controversial role of surveillance bronchoscopy after lung transplantation. Curr Opin Organ Transplant. 2009;14(5):494–8.
26. Hopkins PM, Aboyoun CL, Chhajed PN, Malouf MA, Plit ML, Rainer SP, et al. Association of minimal rejection in lung transplant recipients with obliterative bronchiolitis. Am J Respir Crit Care Med. 2004;170(9):1022–6.
27. Tazelaar HD, Nilsson FN, Rinaldi M, Murtaugh P, McDougall JC, McGregor CG. The sensitivity of transbronchial biopsy for the diagnosis of acute lung rejection. J Thorac Cardiovasc Surg. 1993;105(4):674–8.
28. Scott JP, Fradet G, Smyth RL, Mullins P, Pratt A, Clelland CA, et al. Prospective study of transbronchial biopsies in the management of heart-lung and single lung-transplant patients. J Heart Lung Transplant. 1991;10(5):626–37.
29. Kramer MR, Stoehr C, Whang JL, Berry GJ, Sibley R, Marshall SE, et al. The diagnosis of obliterative bronchiolitis after heart-lung and lung transplantation: low yield of transbronchial lung biopsy. J Heart Lung Transplant. 1993;12(4):675–81 [Research Support, U.S. Gov't, P.H.S.].
30. Cagle PT, Brown RW, Frost A, Kellar C, Yousem SA. Diagnosis of chronic lung transplant rejection by transbronchial biopsy. Mod Pathol. 1995;8(2):137–42 [Comparative Study].
31. Weill D, McGiffin DC, Zorn GL, Alexander CB, Early LJ, Kirklin JK, et al. The utility of open lung biopsy following lung transplantation. J Heart Lung Transplant. 2000;19(9):852–7.
32. Glanville AR. Antibody-mediated rejection in lung transplantation: myth or reality? J Heart Lung Transplant. 2010;29(4):395–400.
33. Magro CM, Abbas AE, Seilstad K, Pope-Harman AL, Nadasdy T, Ross P. C3d and the septal microvasculature as a predictor of chronic lung allograft dysfunction. Hum Immunol. 2006;67(4–5):274–83.
34. Badesch DB, Zamora M, Fullerton D, Weill D, Tuder R, Grover F, et al. Pulmonary capillaritis: a possible histologic form of acute pulmonary allograft rejection. J Heart Lung Transplant. 1998;17(4):415–22.
35. Magro CM, Harman AP, Klinger D, Orosz C, Adams P, Waldman J, et al. Use of C4d as a diagnostic adjunct in lung allograft biopsies. Am J Transplant. 2003;3(9):1143–54.
36. Morrell MR, Patterson GA, Trulock EP, Hachem RR. Acute antibody-mediated rejection after lung transplantation. J Heart Lung Transplant. 2009;28(1):96–100.

37. Chantranuwat C, Qiao JH, Kobashigawa J, Hong L, Shintaku P, Fishbein MC. Immunoperoxidase staining for C4d on paraffin-embedded tissue in cardiac allograft endomyocardial biopsies: comparison to frozen tissue immunofluorescence. Appl Immunohistochem Mol Morphol. 2004;12(2):166–71.
38. Yousem SA. Lymphocytic bronchitis bronchiolitis in lung allograft recipients. Am J Surg Pathol. 1993;17(5):491–6.
39. Beschorner WE, Saral R, Hutchins GM, Tutschka PJ, Santos GW. Lymphocytic bronchitis associated with graft-versus-host disease in recipients of bone-marrow transplants. N Engl J Med. 1978;299(19):1030–6.
40. Hruban RH, Beschorner WE, Gupta PK, Baumgartner WA, Achuff SC, Traill TA, et al. Diagnosis of rejection of lung allografts. N Engl J Med. 1988;318(17):1129.
41. Hruban RH, Beschorner WE, Baumgartner WA, Achuff SC, Traill TA, Marsh BR, et al. Diagnosis of lung allograft rejection by bronchial intraepithelial Leu-7 positive T lymphocytes. J Thorac Cardiovasc Surg. 1988;96(6):939–46.
42. Yousem SA, Paradis IL, Dauber JA, Zeevi A, Rabinowich H, Duquesnoy R, et al. Large airway inflammation in heart-lung transplant recipients—its significance and prognostic implications. Transplantation. 1990;49(3):654–6.
43. Akindipe O, Fernandez-Bussy S, Jantz M, Lu L, Deem A, Swafford W, et al. Obliterative bronchiolitis in lung allografts removed at retransplant for intractable airway problems. Respirology. 2009;14(4):601–5.
44. Boehler A, Kesten S, Weder W, Speich R. Bronchiolitis obliterans after lung transplantation—a review. Chest. 1998;114(5):1411–26.
45. Visscher DW, Myers JL. Bronchiolitis: the pathologist's perspective. Proc Am Thorac Soc. 2006;3(1):41–7.
46. Ryu JH, Myers JL, Swensen SJ. Bronchiolar disorders. Am J Respir Crit Care Med. 2003;168(11):1277–92.
47. Hogg JC, Chu F, Utokaparch S, Woods R, Elliott WM, Buzatu L, et al. The nature of small-airway obstruction in chronic obstructive pulmonary disease. N Engl J Med. 2004;350(26):2645–53.
48. Remund KF, Best M, Egan JJ. Infections relevant to lung transplantation. Proc Am Thorac Soc. 2009;6(1):94–100.
49. Nakhleh RE, Bolman RM, Henke CA, Hertz MI. Lung-transplant pathology—a comparative-study of pulmonary acute rejection and cytomegaloviral infection. Am J Surg Pathol. 1991;15(12):1197–201.
50. Tazelaar HD. Perivascular inflammation in pulmonary infections: implications for the diagnosis of lung rejection. J Heart Lung Transplant. 1991;10(3):437–41.
51. Katzenstein A-LA, Askin FB. Katzenstein and Askin's surgical pathology of non-neoplastic lung disease. 4th ed. Philadelphia, PA: Elsevier Saunders; 2006.
52. Lohr RH, Boland BJ, Douglas WW, Dockrell DH, Colby TV, Swensen SJ, et al. Organizing pneumonia. Features and prognosis of cryptogenic, secondary, and focal variants. Arch Intern Med. 1997;157(12):1323–9.
53. Yousem SA, Duncan SR, Griffith BP. Interstitial and airspace granulation-tissue reactions in lung-transplant recipients. Am J Surg Pathol. 1992;16(9):877–84.
54. Milne DS, Gascoigne AD, Ashcroft T, Sviland L, Malcolm AJ, Corris PA. Organizing pneumonia following pulmonary transplantation and the development of obliterative Bronchiolitis. Transplantation. 1994;57(12):1757–62.
55. Girgis RE, Tu IP, Berry GJ, Reichenspurner H, Valentine VG, Conte JV, et al. Risk factors for the development of obliterative bronchiolitis after lung transplantation. J Heart Lung Transplant. 1996;15(12):1200–8.
56. Gabbay E, Dark JH, Ashcroft T, Corris PA. Cryptogenic organizing pneumonia is an important cause of graft dysfunction and should be included in the classification of pulmonary allograft rejection. J Heart Lung Transplant. 1998;17(2):230–1.

57. Young LR, Hadjiliadis D, Davis RD, Palmer SM. Lung transplantation exacerbates gastroesophageal reflux disease. Chest. 2003;124(5):1689–93.
58. Blondeau K, Merters V, Vanaudenaerde BA, Verleder GM, Van Raemdonck DE, Sifrim D, et al. Gastro-oesophageal reflux and gastric aspiration in lung transplant patients with or without chronic rejection. Eur Respir J. 2008;31(4):707–13.
59. D'Ovidio F, Keshavjee S. Gastroesophageal reflux and lung transplantation. Dis Esophagus. 2006;19(5):315–20.
60. Mukhopadhyay S, Katzenstein A-LA. Pulmonary disease due to aspiration of food and other particulate matter: a clinicopathologic study of 59 cases diagnosed on biopsy or resection specimens. Am J Surg Pathol. 2007;31(5):752–9.
61. Barnes TW, Vassallo R, Tazelaar HD, Hartman TE, Ryu JH. Diffuse bronchiolar disease due to chronic occult aspiration. Mayo Clin Proc. 2006;81(2):172–6.
62. Rinaldi M, Martinelli L, Volpato G, Pederzolli C, Silvestri M, Pederzolli N, et al. Gastroesophageal reflux as cause of obliterative bronchiolitis—a case-report. Transplant Proc. 1995;27(3):2006–7.
63. Cantu E, Appel JZ, Hartwig MG, Woreta H, Green C, Messier R, et al. Early fundoplication prevents chronic allograft dysfunction in patients with gastroesophageal reflux disease. Ann Thorac Surg. 2004;78(4):1142–51.
64. Davis RD, Lau CL, Eubanks S, Messier RH, Hadjiliadis D, Steele MP, et al. Improved lung allograft function after fundoplication in patients with gastroesophageal reflux disease undergoing lung transplantation. J Thorac Cardiovasc Surg. 2003;125(3):533–42.
65. Verleden GM, Dupont LJ. Azithromycin therapy for patients with bronchiolitis obliterans syndrome after lung transplantation. Transplantation. 2004;77(9):1465–7.
66. Yates B, Murphy DM, Forrest IA, Ward C, Rutherford RM, Fisher AJ, et al. Azithromycin reverses airflow obstruction in established bronchiolitis obliterans syndrome. Am J Respir Crit Care Med. 2005;172(6):772–5.

Chapter 3
Non-Bronchiolitis Obliterans Syndrome Forms of Chronic Lung Allograft Dysfunction

Gregory I. Snell, Bronwyn J. Levvey, and Glen P. Westall

Abstract The bronchiolitis obliterans syndrome (BOS) has been described as the clinical correlate of chronic lung allograft rejection and defined as irreversible airflow obstruction in the absence of other causes. However, it has become apparent that BOS does not explain all chronic lung allograft dysfunction (CLAD) and that a variety of other etiologies with a mixed obstructive and restrictive pattern on spirometry, or even a pure restrictive picture (restrictive allograft syndrome, or RAS), are also identifiable. Surgical, mechanical, vascular obstructive, infectious, and infiltrative processes, as well as a whole range of chronic lung allograft rejection entities need to be considered in making a diagnosis of CLAD. The performance of any lung allograft is really the sum-of-the-parts of all of these processes, and considering non-BOS CLAD in all its forms may potentially provide more therapeutic options than just considering BOS alone as the explanation for declining lung function.

Keywords Lung transplantation • Bronchiolitis obliterans syndrome • Chronic lung allograft dysfunction • Obliterative bronchiolitis • Restrictive lung allograft syndrome • Allograft rejection • Chronic rejection

G.I. Snell, M.B.B.S., F.R.A.C.P., M.D (✉) • G.P. Westall, M.D., Ph.D.
Department of Allergy, Immunology and Respiratory Medicine,
The Alfred Hospital, Melbourne, VIC 3004, Australia
e-mail: G.Snell@alfred.orf.au

B.J. Levvey, R.N., B.Ed. Stu, Grad. Dip. Clin. Epi.
Department of Allergy, Immunology and Respiratory Medicine,
The Alfred Hospital, Melbourne, VIC 3004, Australia

Faculty of Medicine, Nursing and Health Sciences, Monash University,
Melbourne, VIC, Australia

K.C. Meyer and A.R. Glanville (eds.), *Bronchiolitis Obliterans Syndrome in Lung Transplantation*, Respiratory Medicine 8, DOI 10.1007/978-1-4614-7636-8_3,

Introduction

The bronchiolitis obliterans syndrome (BOS) is credited with being the major cause of morbidity and mortality following lung transplantation (LTx) [1, 2]. Defined semantically as "irreversible airflow obstruction in the absence of other causes" and histologically as obliterative bronchiolitis (OB), BOS has been characterized as the likely clinical correlate of chronic LTx rejection [1]. BOS has been extensively dissected by LTx clinicians and scientists alike, and, indeed, this book aims to summarize this important work. Notwithstanding these endeavours, it has become apparent that BOS does not explain all chronic lung allograft dysfunction (CLAD) [3–5]. Indeed, the performance of any lung allograft is really the sum-of-the-parts of all surgical, physiological, and pathological processes. This is a very important concept for patients (who complain simply of poor exercise tolerance, not BOS) and clinicians (whose job is to investigate, treat, and hopefully reverse CLAD, whatever its cause).

There is no universally accepted consensus definition of CLAD, but its definition must include lung dysfunction as defined by decreased lung function testing, impaired gas exchange, or impaired exercise ability [2]. It is not even uniformly agreed if CLAD is a deviation from "normal" function (as referenced against a healthy non-transplant population) or the "best function" seen post-LTx in any given individual. Additionally, even following the "perfect transplant," healthy LTx recipients will (by the nature of the surgery) still have denervated airways and vessels, divided lymphatics and bronchial arteries, and changes in muscle composition [6, 7]. These features result in impaired ventilation/perfusion matching, issues of muscle fatigability, and even bronchial hyper-responsiveness [6].

This chapter will therefore focus on the non-BOS forms of CLAD, an area poorly characterized and under-investigated, yet with significant therapeutic potential if accurately identified.

The Causes, Associations, and Subtypes of CLAD

There is a long list of potential and proven causes of CLAD, with the commonest outlined in Fig. 3.1. These causes are additive, with an individual patient potentially having more than one cause or even different causes at different time points post-LTx. Some are reversible (i.e., mechanical issues), while some are irreversible (i.e., interstitial fibrosis). Although BOS is not in this list, its pathognemonic histopathological chronic allo-rejection correlate, OB, is. Additionally, as can be seen in following chapters, BOS is associated with a number of other non-alloimmune mechanisms, including infection (Chap. 11) and aspiration (Chap. 12), separately considered as contributors to CLAD.

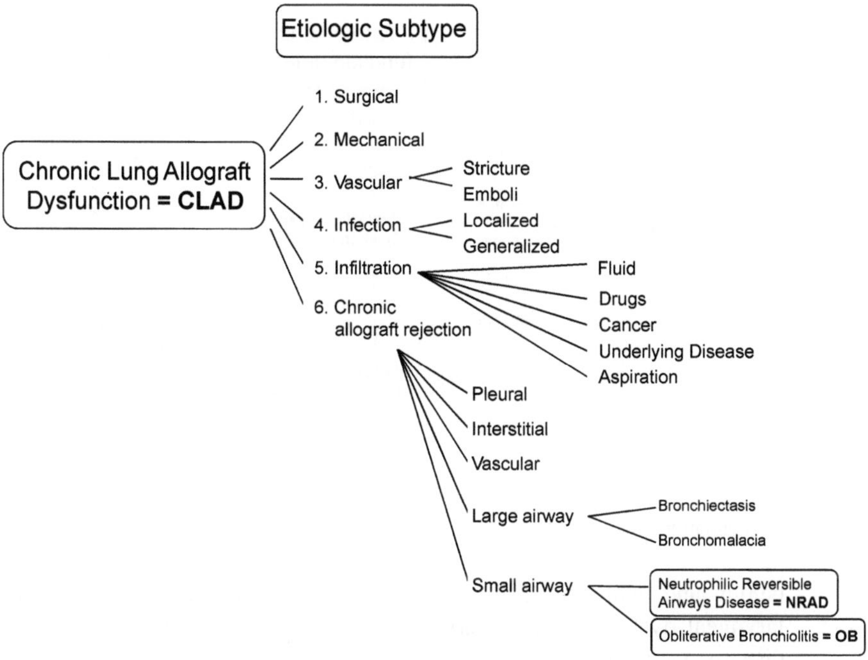

Fig. 3.1 Common etiologic subtypes of CLAD

CLAD Subtypes Based on Potential Etiology

The features of these subtypes are further outlined in Fig. 3.2, although, as noted, mixed subtypes may occur.

1. *Surgical subtype.* No actual allograft pathology is present; rather, the actual removal of lung tissue, either from the allograft or from the remaining native lung (in single-lung transplantation), will reduce overall measured lung volumes (i.e., bullectomy, lung volume reduction surgery, lobectomy for cancer, plication of diaphragm, diagnostic open lung biopsy, and so forth) [7]. These processes are considered as nonimmune and unlikely to progress.
2. *Mechanical subtype.* No actual allograft disease is present; rather, the measured lung function is reduced as a result of factors extrinsic to the allograft. Here the process is usually nonimmune and unlikely to progress:
   (a) Compression/decompression (i.e., obesity, abdominal distension with ascites/air, over/under inflation of native lung in single-lung transplantation [8], pneumothorax, bronchopleural fistula, pleural effusion [9], and so on).
   (b) Decreased graft inflation (i.e., pain due to fractured ribs/sternum, vertebral crush fracture, chest wall myopathy, diaphragmatic dysfunction or paralysis, thoracic radiotherapy, proximal (non-transplanted) bronchomalacia,

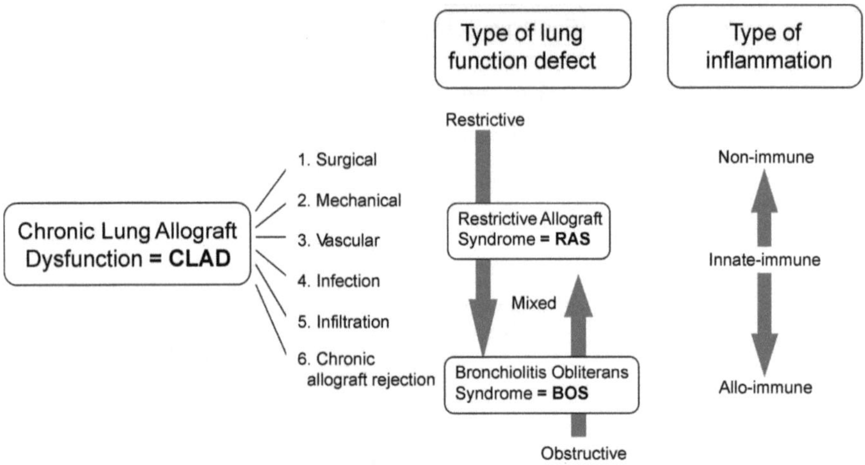

Fig. 3.2 Common patterns of lung function testing abnormalities and patterns of immune dysfunction/dysregulation seen in CLAD

benign and malignant airway stenosis [10], anastomotic strictures [11], laryngeal dysfunction or paralysis, cerebrovascular accident, Parkinson's disease, and so on).

3. *Graft vascular obstructive subtype*. No actual allo-inflammatory process is present, and, unless cancer is present, the process is usually not progressive.
   (a) Pulmonary arterial and venous anastomotic strictures.
   (b) Pulmonary thromboembolism [12], cancer emboli [13], and so on.
4. *Graft infection subtype*. Innate immune responses predominate. It usually resolves but can also lead to progressive airway damage or parenchymal fibrosis. Infections may be:
   (a) Localized (i.e., abscess or aspergilloma, anastomotic infection, empyema).
   (b) Generalized (i.e., post-bacterial, fungal, or viral pneumonia).
5. *Graft infiltration subtype*. Nonspecific, innate immune responses may be present with no actual alloimmune-mediated inflammatory processes and, if left untreated or if untreatable, progressive airway damage or parenchymal fibrosis is likely.
   (a) Pulmonary edema, from cardiac failure or renal failure.
   (b) Drugs, causing an interstitial drug reaction (e.g., sirolimus, everolimus, amiodarone [14]).
   (c) Neoplasia (lung primary or metastatic disease) [13].
   (d) Recurrence of native disease [15] (e.g., sarcoidosis, histiocytosis X, lymphangioleiomyomatosis, α (alpha)-1 anti-trypsin deficiency, non-transplant-related obliterative bronchiolitis, veno-occlusive disease, and collagen vascular diseases).
   (e) Chronic aspiration of gastric contents (see Chap. 12).

6. *Chronic allograft rejection subtype*. These are entities proven to be a consequence of, or at least strongly linked to, alloimmune-mediated inflammatory processes, and these are usually irreversible and progressive. The role of chronic ischemia, either as a primary feature of the LTx process due to absence of a reanastomosed bronchial blood supply [16], or as a secondary feature of chronic airway wall or parenchymal alloimmune-mediated vasculopathy, remains speculative [17].
   (a) Chronic pleural inflammation and thickening [9, 18, 19].
   (b) Chronic interstitial fibrosis. Chronic interstitial fibrosis has been seen in various forms after LTx [19–23]. An upper lobe progressive fibrotic disease was first reported by the Toronto Group in 2003 [21], and other centers have since also added case series [24, 25]. Both focal and diffuse interstitial patterns have been described [25]. The etiology of this particular CLAD subtype is unknown, but alloimmune factors are suspected [22, 24, 26]. In other instances, a nonspecific chronic interstitial fibrosis pattern such as fibrinoid organizing pneumonia (FOP) or bronchiolitis obliterans organizing pneumonia (BOOP) may arise as an outcome of an earlier documented acute lung injury [22, 23, 27, 28]. These entities have been recently considered for [22], but not formally incorporated into, the current official International Society for Heart and Lung Transplantation (ISHLT) Rejection Grading System [23].
   (c) Chronic vascular rejection (CVR). CVR is defined histologically by the presence of fibrointimal thickening of arteries and veins in the allograft [23]. Transbronchial biopsies are typically too small to assess the histologic changes of CVR, and the morphologic vascular changes are more likely to be visualized from open lung biopsy or postmortem samples [20]. It is currently unknown if CVR leads to OB or BOS or, alternatively, if the immunologic injury that occurs to the airway epithelium that leads to OB is actually responsible for the blood vessel changes of CVR. One hypothesis is that vascular injury from acute cellular rejection (an inflammatory lesion of small blood vessels) leads to ischemic injury of the airway [29], thereby explaining why acute cellular rejection is the leading risk factor for OB and BOS. While CVR is well described and has been incorporated into the recent revision to the classification and nomenclature for the diagnosis of lung rejection, there are only very few published case reports, including those that have assessed explanted lung tissue from re-transplantation cases performed for BOS [20, 23].
   (d) Chronic large airways inflammation (e.g., bronchiectasis, bronchomalacia, bronchial webs, etc. [11, 19, 30, 31]).
   (e) Chronic small airways inflammation, including follicular bronchiolitis [32], exudative bronchiolitis [33], neutrophilic reversible allograft dysfunction (NRAD) [34] (see Chap. 16), and OB (see Chap. 6).

CLAD Subtypes Based on Simple Lung Function

Inherent to the diagnosis of BOS is a pathological process resulting in irreversible airflow obstruction and a readily recognizable obstructive pattern on pulmonary function testing. Given that there is more to CLAD than BOS, not unsurprisingly, we are starting to describe other abnormal spirometric patterns that are associated with CLAD, such as restrictive lung function patterns. Figure 3.2 describes the general spirometric patterns that might be seen with CLAD. It is also notable that the proportion of obstruction versus restriction versus a mixed pattern in a particular post-LTx cohort will depend on the definitions and cutoff values used as well as the exact proportions of specific post-LTx complications seen an individual lung transplant center.

Notwithstanding these comments, recent publications from several groups indicate broadly consistent results. Based on a forced expiratory volume in one second (FEV_1), less than 80 % of a reference value baseline post-LTx, Sato and colleagues reported a 30 % incidence of CLAD [35], and 30 % of these recipients had a restrictive spirometric pattern, which has been lately something they defined as the restrictive allograft syndrome (RAS). Importantly they described a significantly inferior survival in this restrictive CLAD subtype. Verleden and coauthors [4] diagnosed 24 % of a large LTx cohort as having CLAD, with 28 % having the restrictive form, and this was again associated with statistically worse survival compared to the obstructive CLAD group. Additionally, Woodrow and colleagues have reported that 40 % of their LTx recipients had CLAD [5].

CLAD Subtypes Based on Chest Computerized Tomography Scans

Although each of these CLAD subtype studies has a slightly different population, proportion of single versus double LTx as well as variable CLAD and CT definitions, the CT findings are also of note. Sato et al. [3] reported 74 % and Verleden et al. [4] 85 % of the restrictive CLAD group as having lung infiltrates on CT scan. CLAD with the presence of CT infiltrates was associated with the worst outcomes in both series. Woodrow's series [5] defined "CLAD-BOS" and "CLAD-non-specific" groups according to CT changes, and they further subdivided the cohort into two CLAD BOS groups, one with obstruction (65 %) and one with restriction (35 %). In contrast to the other two series, survival outcomes were equivalent for each of these CLAD subgroups.

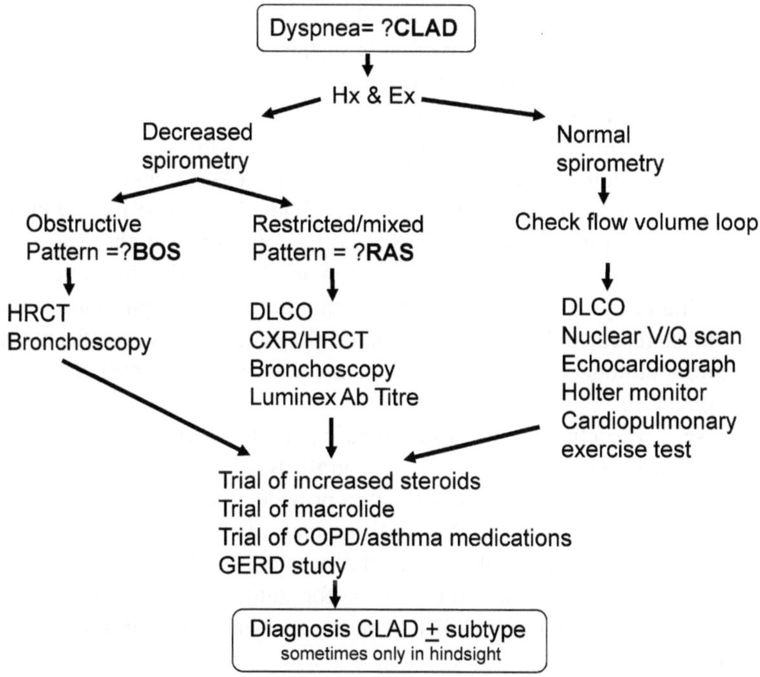

Fig. 3.3 A potential clinical decision pathway for investigating CLAD subtypes, RAS, and BOS. *HRCT* high-resolution computed tomography of chest, *Ab* antibody, *V/Q* scan, nuclear ventilation/perfusion scan, *DLCO* gas transfer test, *GERD* gastroesophageal reflux disease, *COPD* chronic obstructive pulmonary disease

CLAD Subtypes: Other Relevant Investigations and a Diagnostic Pathway

As pointed out above, CLAD has multiple potential causes or associations, many of which may have clinical relevance. Therefore, carefully targeted investigation of an individual patient with CLAD is therefore indicated to detect treatable conditions. Figure 3.3 outlines a potential clinical decision pathway when considering CLAD, RAS, and BOS. Although the exact extent and sequence of investigations will also need to take into account any recent relevant history and prior investigations, clinical decision making is triggered by the first recognition of an abnormal spirometric pattern (augmented easily with DLCO [gas transfer measurement], flow volume loop, and oxyhemoglobin saturation level).

Pure obstruction on pulmonary function testing warrants exclusion of unrecognized allograft infection and recurrent aspiration, but the detection of such may well lead to a diagnostic and even potentially therapeutic trial of steroids and a macrolide (with or without a change of baseline immunosuppression). Bronchoscopy with transbronchial biopsy and CT scan is mandated to exclude other processes, although these may well show no pathology until the more advanced stages of BOS have been reached [36]. If airflow obstruction is sustained, then BOS can be confirmed retrospectively as the CLAD subtype diagnosis.

The absence of a longitudinal change in spirometry in the setting of new symptoms of exercise limitation or dyspnea nonetheless warrants exclusion of airway complications, pulmonary emboli, pulmonary hypertension, and graft infiltrative diseases as the cause of CLAD in such an individual, and non-CLAD etiologies (anemia, cardiac dysfunction, etc.) must also be considered. A thoracic CT scan, nuclear perfusion scan, and an echocardiogram are the investigations that are likely to hold the highest yield in this situation. If symptoms progress, pulmonary function tests should be repeated despite results that did not initially show significant decline, and a cardiopulmonary exercise test [6] should be added to provide additional strategic direction.

Likewise, a restrictive or mixed spirometric pattern requires appropriate investigation to identify any treatable causes for graft dysfunction. Bronchoscopy with transbronchial biopsy and CT scan can often provide an initial direction for subsequent investigations, although the findings may also be nonspecific [20, 36]. This pattern of presentation also raises the possibility of CVR and warrants an immunological anti-donor antibody screen for antibody-mediated vasculopathy [37, 38]. Additionally, the possibility of recurrent aspiration warrants a pH study (see Chap. 12).

The Role of Alloimmunity in Non-BOS CLAD

It was first postulated that OB represented the histopathological process underlying chronic alloreactivity following LTx in 1984 [39]. Given that alloimmune responses may lead to histological patterns other than OB, one should consider the possibility that alternate alloimmune pathways may contribute to pathologies that are not specific to the airways.

Antibody-mediated rejection may lead to BOS through the elaboration of donor-specific antibodies directed against both HLA- and non-HLA peptides residing on airway epithelial cells. These same antibodies may also target HLA epitopes expressed elsewhere in the lung allograft, especially on cells that reside within the vasculature [22, 23] and interstitium, potentially causing CVR and interstitial fibrosis, respectively.

Autoimmune T- and B-cell responses, acting via an auto-reactive Th17 pathway that is directed against self-antigens (collagen V, K-α (alpha)1-tubulin) exposed in the injured lung, have been associated with OB. Of interest, the same Th17 pathway has been implicated in a non-transplant setting with the development of chronic autoimmune lung inflammation [40]. Encouragingly, targeting Th17 cells using humanized monoclonal antibodies to interleukin-17A have been shown to be efficacious in a number of autoimmune diseases [41], and such an intervention may provide a future treatment strategy in patients with CLAD.

Inherent to lung transplant surgery is loss of the bronchial circulation leading potentially to ischemia of the lung microvasculature. Hypoxia resulting from an impaired microcirculation may contribute to epithelial-to-mesenchymal transition (EMT), a recognized precursor of fibrosis. EMT has been associated with OB following LTx [42, 43] as well as with pulmonary fibrosis in a non-transplant setting [44]. Of note, the pro-angiogenic mediator, hypoxia inducible factor (HIF-1α (alpha)), which may have a role in the pathogenesis of pulmonary fibrosis, has also been implicated in the pathogenesis of OB [45].

Finally, the development of CLAD may be associated with pulmonary hypertension. While chronic hypoxia may contribute to pulmonary hypertension in some patients, the absence of neomuscularization in one autopsy study led the authors to speculate that alloimmune responses may be driving the development of pulmonary hypertension in patients with CLAD [46].

In summary, as we have come to recognize different CLAD phenotypes as defined by etiology, changes in lung function, and radiological patterns, we also need to consider CLAD in terms of the underlying pathogenic processes, many of which may be alloimmune in origin. As described above, many of the alloimmune processes implicated in the development of OB may also have a role in the development of non-airway pathologies associated with CLAD.

Future Directions

There is much to define, describe, and explore regarding the interrelationships of CLAD, RAS, and BOS. Indeed the clinical BOS 0–3 grading tool introduced by Estenne and coworkers [1] may now need to be extended to include a restrictive component to describe non-BOS CLAD. One could envisage a clinical RAS 0–3 grading tool that could be used in parallel to the BOS tool. Mechanisms of non-BOS CLAD also need to be explored with a new and specific focus on whole lung ischemia [17] and large-scale, longitudinal studies of antibody-mediated rejection [38].

Conclusion

The lung transplant community has had great insights over the last 15 years by focusing on BOS as a mode of allograft failure. However, it is now quite apparent that non-BOS CLAD is likely to be every bit as important to overall lung allograft function, noting that the level of allograft function directly translates to recipient quality of life and, ultimately, survival. The challenge is to go forward into the next 15 years and apply the lessons learned from the study of BOS to non-BOS CLAD.

Acknowledgement Support for this work comes from the Margaret Pratt Foundation.

References

1. Estenne M, Maurer JR, Boehler A, Egan JJ, Frost A, Hertz M, et al. Bronchiolitis obliterans syndrome 2001: an update of the diagnostic criteria. J Heart Lung Transplant. 2002;21(3):297–310.
2. Verleden SE, Verleden GM, Vanaudenaerde BM. Phenotyping BOS could improve understanding of mechanisms involved. J Heart Lung Transplant. 2010;30(1):112.
3. Todd JL, Palmer SM. Bronchiolitis obliterans syndrome: the final frontier for lung transplantation. Chest. 2011;140(2):502–8.
4. Verleden GM, Vos R, Verleden SE, De Wever W, De Vleeschauwer SI, Willems-Widyastuti A, et al. Survival determinants in lung transplant patients with chronic allograft dysfunction. Transplantation. 2011;92(6):703–8.
5. Woodrow JP, Shlobin OA, Barnett SD, Burton N, Nathan SD. Comparison of bronchiolitis obliterans syndrome to other forms of chronic lung allograft dysfunction after lung transplantation. J Heart Lung Transplant. 2010;29(10):1159–64.
6. Williams TJ, Snell GI. Early and long-term functional outcomes in unilateral, bilateral, and living-related transplant recipients. Clin Chest Med. 1997;18(2):245–57.
7. Fitton TP, Bethea BT, Borja MC, Yuh DD, Yang SC, Orens JB, et al. Pulmonary resection following lung transplantation. Ann Thorac Surg. 2003;76(5):1680–5.
8. Hadjiliadis D, Hutcheon MA. Detection of bronchiolitis obliterans syndrome (BOS) in single lung transplant recipients. J Heart Lung Transplant. 2003;22(7):829–30.
9. Ferrer J, Roldan J, Roman A, Bravo C, Monforte V, Pallissa E, et al. Acute and chronic pleural complications in lung transplantation. J Heart Lung Transplant. 2003;22(11):1217–25.
10. Kono C, Yamaguchi T, Yamada Y, Hoshi S, Amano H, Minami M, et al. [A case of bronchostenosis in the allograft after lung transplantation in pulmonary lymphangioleiomyomatosis]. Nihon Kokyuki Gakkai Zasshi. 2004;42(2):170–5.
11. Santacruz JF, Mehta AC. Airway complications and management after lung transplantation: ischemia, dehiscence, and stenosis. Proc Am Thorac Soc. 2009;6(1):79–93.
12. Kahan ES, Petersen G, Gaughan JP, Criner GJ. High incidence of venous thromboembolic events in lung transplant recipients. J Heart Lung Transplant. 2007;26(4):339–44.
13. Regueiro F, Roche P, Regueiro MV, Lozano R. The importance of histology in the evaluation of pulmonary transplantation: carcinomatous lymphangitis. Thorac Cardiovasc Surg. 2005;53(2):122–3.
14. Rossi SE, Erasmus JJ, McAdams HP, Sporn TA, Goodman PC. Pulmonary drug toxicity: radiologic and pathologic manifestations. Radiographics. 2000;20(5):1245–59.
15. Orens JB, Estenne M, Arcasoy S, Conte JV, Corris P, Egan JJ, et al. International guidelines for the selection of lung transplant candidates: 2006 update–a consensus report from the Pulmonary Scientific Council of the International Society for Heart and Lung Transplantation. J Heart Lung Transplant. 2006;25(7):745–55.
16. Esmore DS, Brown R, Buckland M, Briganti EM, Fetherston GJ, Rabinov M, et al. Techniques and results in bilateral sequential single lung transplantation. The National Heart & Lung Replacement Service. J Card Surg. 1994;9(1):1–14.
17. Snell GI, Westall GP. The contribution of airway ischemia and vascular remodelling to the pathophysiology of bronchiolitis obliterans syndrome and chronic lung allograft dysfunction. Curr Opin Organ Transplant. 2010;15(5):558–62.
18. Boffa DJ, Mason DP, Su JW, Murthy SC, Feng J, McNeill AM, et al. Decortication after lung transplantation. Ann Thorac Surg. 2008;85(3):1039–43.
19. Ng YL, Paul N, Patsios D, Walsham A, Chung TB, Keshavjee S, et al. Imaging of lung transplantation: review. AJR Am J Roentgenol. 2009;192(3 Suppl):S1–13.
20. Martinu T, Howell DN, Davis RD, Steele MP, Palmer SM. Pathologic correlates of bronchiolitis obliterans syndrome in pulmonary retransplant recipients. Chest. 2006;129(4):1016–23.

21. Konen E, Weisbrod GL, Pakhale S, Chung T, Paul NS, Hutcheon MA. Fibrosis of the upper lobes: a newly identified late-onset complication after lung transplantation? AJR Am J Roentgenol. 2003;181(6):1539–43.
22. Snell GI, Boehler A, Glanville AR, McNeil K, Scott JP, Studer SM, et al. Eleven years on: a clinical update of key areas of the 1996 lung allograft rejection working formulation. J Heart Lung Transplant. 2007;26(5):423–30.
23. Stewart S, Fishbein MC, Snell GI, Berry GJ, Boehler A, Burke MM, et al. Revision of the 1996 working formulation for the standardization of nomenclature in the diagnosis of lung rejection. J Heart Lung Transplant. 2007;26(12):1229–42.
24. Kroegel C, Reissig A, Foerster M. Pulmonary fibrosis of the upper lobes after lung transplantation is associated with selective CD8+ T lymphocyte expansion. AJR Am J Roentgenol. 2005;184(3):1024–5.
25. Pakhale SS, Hadjiliadis D, Howell DN, Palmer SM, Gutierrez C, Waddell TK, et al. Upper lobe fibrosis: a novel manifestation of chronic allograft dysfunction in lung transplantation. J Heart Lung Transplant. 2005;24(9):1260–8.
26. Sato M, Hirayama S, Matsuda Y, Wagnetz D, Hwang DM, Guan Z, et al. Stromal activation and formation of lymphoid-like stroma in chronic lung allograft dysfunction. Transplantation. 2011;91(12):1398–405.
27. Siddiqui MT, Garrity ER, Husain AN. Bronchiolitis obliterans organizing pneumonia-like reactions: a nonspecific response or an atypical form of rejection or infection in lung allograft recipients? Hum Pathol. 1996;27(7):714–9.
28. Gabbay E, Dark JH, Ashcroft T, Corris PA. Cryptogenic organizing pneumonia is an important cause of graft dysfunction and should be included in the classification of pulmonary allograft rejection. J Heart Lung Transplant. 1998;17(2):230–1.
29. Luckraz H, Goddard M, McNeil K, Atkinson C, Sharples LD, Wallwork J. Is obliterative bronchiolitis in lung transplantation associated with microvascular damage to small airways? Ann Thorac Surg. 2006;82(4):1212–8.
30. Herrera JM, McNeil KD, Higgins RS, Coulden RA, Flower CD, Nashef SA, et al. Airway complications after lung transplantation: treatment and long-term outcome. Ann Thorac Surg. 2001;71(3):989–93. discussion 93–4.
31. Keating DT, Westall GP, Pham A, Whitford HM, Williams TJ, Snell GI. Proliferating bronchial webs after lung transplantation. Ann Thorac Surg. 2011;92(5):1893–6.
32. Vos R, Vanaudenaerde BM, De Vleeschauwer SI, Van Raemdonck DE, Dupont LJ, Verbeken EK, et al. Follicular bronchiolitis: a rare cause of bronchiolitis obliterans syndrome after lung transplantation: a case report. Am J Transplant. 2009;9(3):644–50.
33. McManus TE, Milne DG, Whyte KF, Wilsher ML. Exudative bronchiolitis after lung transplantation. J Heart Lung Transplant. 2008;27(3):276–81.
34. Verleden GM, Vos R, De Vleeschauwer S, Verleden S, Dupont L, Nevens F, et al. Neutrophilic reversible airways dysfunction after lung transplantation: a case report. Transplant Proc. 2011;43(5):2078–81.
35. Sato M, Waddell TK, Wagnetz U, Roberts HC, Hwang DM, Haroon A, et al. Restrictive allograft syndrome (RAS): a novel form of chronic lung allograft dysfunction. J Heart Lung Transplant. 2010;30(7):735–42.
36. Glanville AR. Bronchoscopic monitoring after lung transplantation. Semin Respir Crit Care Med. 2009;31(2):208–21.
37. Girnita AL, McCurry KR, Zeevi A. Increased lung allograft failure in patients with HLA-specific antibody. Clin Transpl. 2007:231–9.
38. Glanville AR. Antibody-mediated rejection in lung transplantation: myth or reality? J Heart Lung Transplant. 2009;29(4):395–400.
39. Burke CM, Theodore J, Dawkins KD, Yousem SA, Blank N, Billingham ME, et al. Post-transplant obliterative bronchiolitis and other late lung sequelae in human heart-lung transplantation. Chest. 1984;86(6):824–9.

40. Baraut J, Michel L, Verrecchia F, Farge D. Relationship between cytokine profiles and clinical outcomes in patients with systemic sclerosis. Autoimmun Rev. 2010;10(2):65–73.
41. Hueber W, Patel DD, Dryja T, Wright AM, Koroleva I, Bruin G, et al. Effects of AIN457, a fully human antibody to interleukin-17A, on psoriasis, rheumatoid arthritis, and uveitis. Sci Transl Med. 2010;2(52):52;72.
42. Willis BC, Borok Z. Epithelial-mesenchymal transition: potential role in obliterative bronchiolitis? Thorax. 2009;64(9):742–3.
43. Ward C, Forrest IA, Murphy DM, Johnson GE, Robertson H, Cawston TE, et al. Phenotype of airway epithelial cells suggests epithelial to mesenchymal cell transition in clinically stable lung transplant recipients. Thorax. 2005;60(10):865–71.
44. Coward WR, Saini G, Jenkins G. The pathogenesis of idiopathic pulmonary fibrosis. Ther Adv Respir Dis. 2010;4(6):367–88.
45. Jiang X, Khan MA, Tian W, Beilke J, Natarajan R, Kosek J, et al. Adenovirus-mediated HIF-1alpha gene transfer promotes repair of mouse airway allograft microvasculature and attenuates chronic rejection. J Clin Invest. 2011;121(6):2336–49.
46. Saggar R, Ross DJ, Saggar R, Zisman DA, Gregson A, Lynch 3rd JP, et al. Pulmonary hypertension associated with lung transplantation obliterative bronchiolitis and vascular remodeling of the allograft. Am J Transplant. 2008;8(9):1921–30.

Chapter 4
The Role of Thoracic Imaging in the Diagnosis of BOS and Related Disorders

Jeffrey P. Kanne

Abstract Imaging plays a critical role in evaluating patients before and after lung transplantation. Chest radiography is usually the initial imaging test performed to evaluate transplant recipients with signs and symptoms of respiratory tract infection or acute graft dysfunction. However, the utility of chest radiography in patients with bronchiolitis obliterans syndrome (BOS) is very limited. Computerized tomography (CT) is more sensitive than radiography for lung abnormalities and may show findings of air trapping, consistent with the presence of constrictive bronchiolitis. This chapter reviews the current state of imaging of patients with documented or suspected BOS and illustrates the radiographic and CT findings.

Keywords Bronchiolitis obliterans syndrome • Constrictive bronchiolitis • Computerized tomography • Chest radiography • Hyperpolarized helium • Magnetic resonance imaging

Introduction

Bronchiolitis obliterans syndrome (BOS) is a major cause of morbidity and mortality following lung transplantation and is the leading cause of death among transplant recipients surviving longer than 1 year [1–3]. The incidence of BOS ranges from 25 to 50 % [4–6]. BOS is the clinical manifestation of constrictive bronchiolitis and is characterized by progressive airflow obstruction. Because of the inherent limitations of specimens obtained from transbronchial biopsy and the

J.P. Kanne, M.D. (✉)
Department of Radiology, University of Wisconsin School of Medicine and Public Health, 600 Highland Avenue, MC 3252, Madison, WI 53792-3252, USA
e-mail: kanne@wisc.edu

K.C. Meyer and A.R. Glanville (eds.), *Bronchiolitis Obliterans Syndrome in Lung Transplantation*, Respiratory Medicine 8, DOI 10.1007/978-1-4614-7636-8_4,

heterogeneous distribution of constrictive bronchiolitis in the lungs, histologic confirmation of constrictive bronchiolitis can be difficult to achieve [4, 7].

Prompt diagnosis of BOS is essential, because early treatment with increased immunosuppression may preserve allograft function [8]. Unfortunately, early detection of BOS is difficult, because pulmonary function testing may lack sensitivity for detecting small but potentially important decline in pulmonary function. In particular, for single-lung transplant recipients, alteration in ventilation in the native lung can mask abnormalities in the allograft. Furthermore, because the distribution of constrictive bronchiolitis is usually patchy within the lung allograft, surveillance transbronchial biopsy lacks sufficient sensitivity for detecting acute rejection and constrictive bronchiolitis [8–10].

Imaging remains central in evaluating patients both before and after lung transplantation. In the immediate postoperative period, chest radiography can help assess placement of life support devices, track evolution of postoperative pneumothoraces and pleural effusions, and detect complications such as implantation response, atelectasis, aspiration, pneumonia, and acute rejection. Computerized tomography (CT) is usually reserved for further characterizing complications such as anastomotic dehiscence or stricture, pulmonary thromboembolism, or suspected empyema.

Later in the post-transplant period, imaging, particularly chest radiography, is often employed when patients present with signs and symptoms of respiratory tract infection or graft dysfunction. CT may be performed when radiographic findings are inconclusive or nonspecific or to assess delayed anastomotic complications such as stricture. In this chapter, the role of imaging in evaluating patients with BOS will be discussed.

Radiography

Chest radiography is frequently the first imaging test used to assess lung transplant recipients with suspected infection, acute rejection, or other causes of acute respiratory illness or graft dysfunction. Chest radiography often suffices for patients presenting with pneumonia, pleural effusion, or congestive heart failure. However, chest radiography is usually unrevealing in patients with mild or developing BOS because the sensitivity and specificity of chest radiography for small airways diseases are low, especially with mild to moderate degrees of airflow limitation. Many patients with BOS will have a normal radiograph. With more advanced airflow obstruction, pulmonary hyperinflation may become evident, and regions of attenuated pulmonary vascularity may be apparent [11–14]. Sometimes bronchial wall thickening or a nodular or reticulonodular pattern may be seen [15].

In a study of eleven patients with pathologically proven constrictive bronchiolitis following heart–lung transplant, Skeens et al. [14] described abnormalities in all patients and findings of central airway dilation in nine of the eleven patients. Four distinct radiographic patterns were described: diffuse linear-nodular pattern (five patients), discrete nodular opacities (two patients), confluent nodular opacities (one patient), and diffuse alveolar opacities (three patients). In all patterns, a basal predominance of findings occurred. CT scans were available for two patients and confirmed the presence of bronchiectasis. Nine of the study patients had pulmonary function testing before chest radiography showing varying degrees of airflow obstruction. Two of the patients initially had normal chest radiographs at the time during which pulmonary function began to decline. Conclusions from this study include that chest radiographic findings occurring in patients with BOS are highly nonspecific, and patients with early decline in graft function may have normal radiographs.

Computerized Tomography

CT, particularly high-resolution CT (HRCT), is superior to chest radiography for detecting signs of BOS. Furthermore, CT can further elucidate other abnormalities detected on chest radiography. The hallmark of constrictive bronchiolitis on HRCT is a mosaic pattern of lung attenuation characterized by regions of reduced lung attenuation accompanied by a decrease in the caliber of pulmonary vessels supplying these regions (Fig. 4.1). Expiratory image shows evidence of air trapping manifesting characterized by increased attenuation of normal lung and persistent low attenuation of entire lobules with air trapping (Fig. 4.2) [16–26]. Other reported findings associated with BOS include bronchial dilation and bronchial wall thickening (Figs. 4.3, 4.4, 4.5, and 4.6). While nonspecific, these larger airway findings are more often associated with more advanced disease [23].

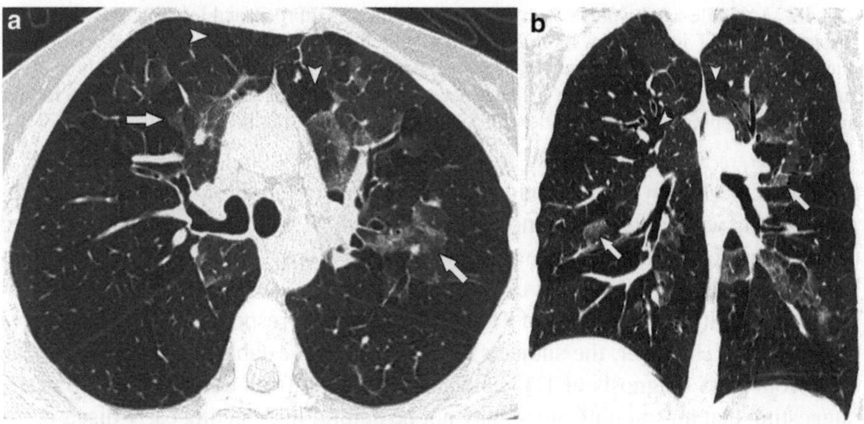

Fig. 4.1 A 36-year-old woman with double-lung transplant and BOS. Transverse (**a**) and coronal reformatted (**b**) HRCT images show hyperinflated lungs with a mosaic pattern of attenuation, characterized by areas of ground-glass attenuation (*arrows*) and hyperlucency (*arrowheads*). Note the patchy distribution of the abnormalities

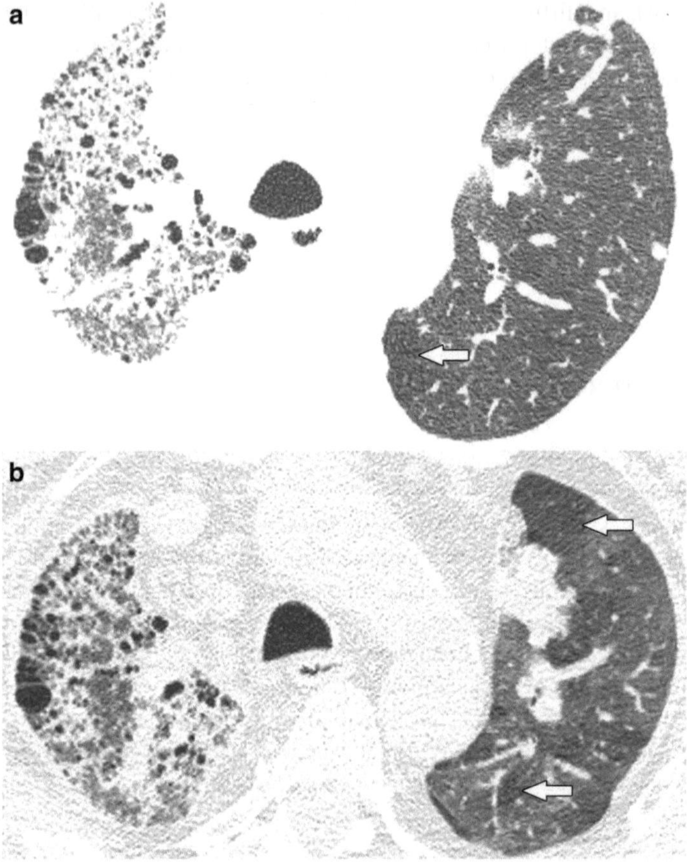

Fig. 4.2 A middle-aged woman with idiopathic pulmonary fibrosis and left lung transplant. (**a**) Inspiratory HRCT image shows a relatively normal left lung allograft with a subtle area of low attenuation (*arrow*) on this image with narrow window width settings. The native right lung is diffusely fibrotic. (**b**) Expiratory HRCT image accentuates the heterogeneity of the lung with lobular areas of air trapping (*arrows*). Courtesy of Sudhakar Pipavath, MD, Seattle, WA

Mosaic perfusion or attenuation related to constrictive bronchiolitis and alterations of lung ventilation is common in patients with BOS. Leung et al. [22] reviewed HRCT scans of 11 lung transplant recipients with biopsy-proven constrictive bronchiolitis and reported that the presence of air trapping on expiratory CT has a sensitivity, specificity, and accuracy of 91 %, 80 %, and 86 %, respectively, for constrictive bronchiolitis. However, the subjects in this study had established BOS with mean time from BOS diagnosis of 1.3 years and mean time from transplant of 4.8 years, suggesting that air trapping alone may not be helpful in detecting early disease.

Two additional studies showed that air trapping is the most sensitive predictor of BOS in lung transplant recipients [16, 25]. Bankier et al. [16] concluded that a threshold of 32 % air trapping on expiratory CT was 83 % sensitive, 89 % specific,

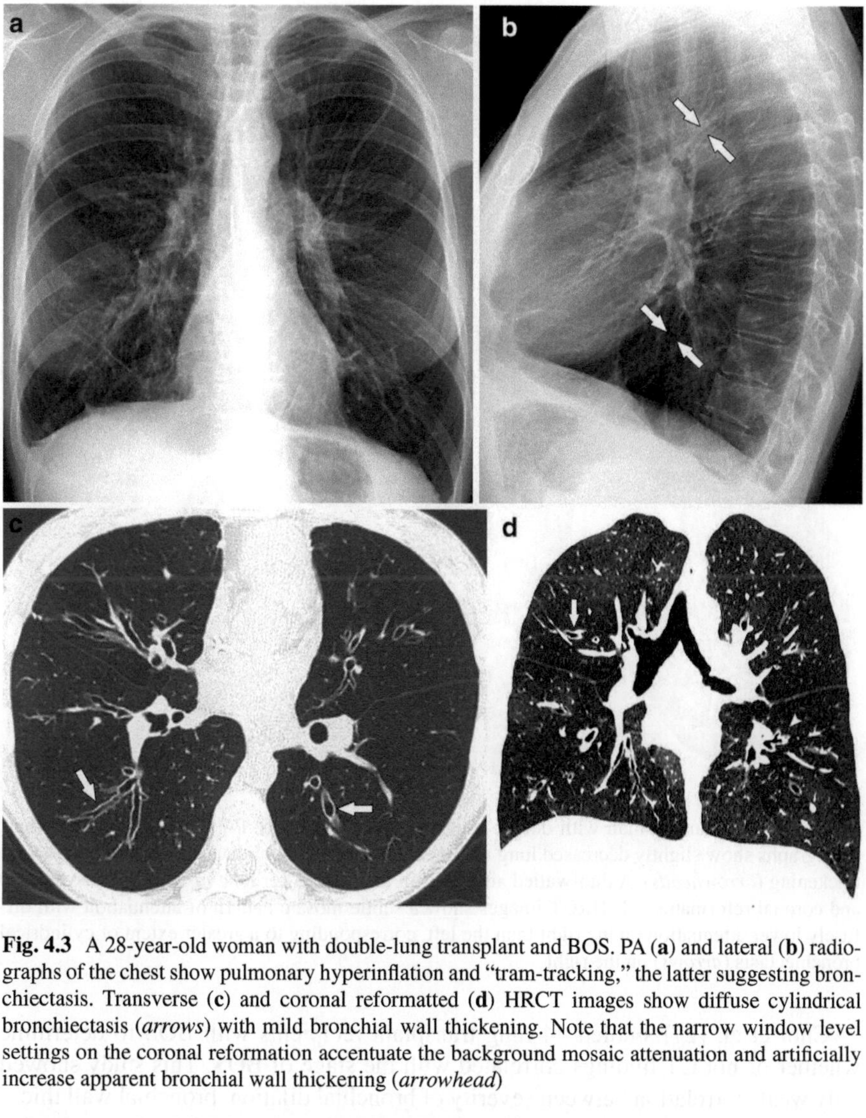

Fig. 4.3 A 28-year-old woman with double-lung transplant and BOS. PA (**a**) and lateral (**b**) radiographs of the chest show pulmonary hyperinflation and "tram-tracking," the latter suggesting bronchiectasis. Transverse (**c**) and coronal reformatted (**d**) HRCT images show diffuse cylindrical bronchiectasis (*arrows*) with mild bronchial wall thickening. Note that the narrow window level settings on the coronal reformation accentuate the background mosaic attenuation and artificially increase apparent bronchial wall thickening (*arrowhead*)

and 88 % accurate for distinguishing patients with BOS from those without BOS. Furthermore, the presence of air trapping on expiratory CT may predict the development of BOS following lung transplantation. In a retrospective study, Siegel et al. [25] compared 21 pediatric lung transplant recipients with BOS to 41 pediatric lung transplant recipients without BOS and considered to have normal airways and reported sensitivity, specificity, and positive predictive value for expiratory CT of 100 %, 71 %, and 64 %, respectively, for BOS. Mean FEV_1 in the BOS cohort was 58 % of predicted value (range, 29–77 %). The degree of expiratory air trapping was measured subjectively, in keeping with clinical practice patterns at the time.

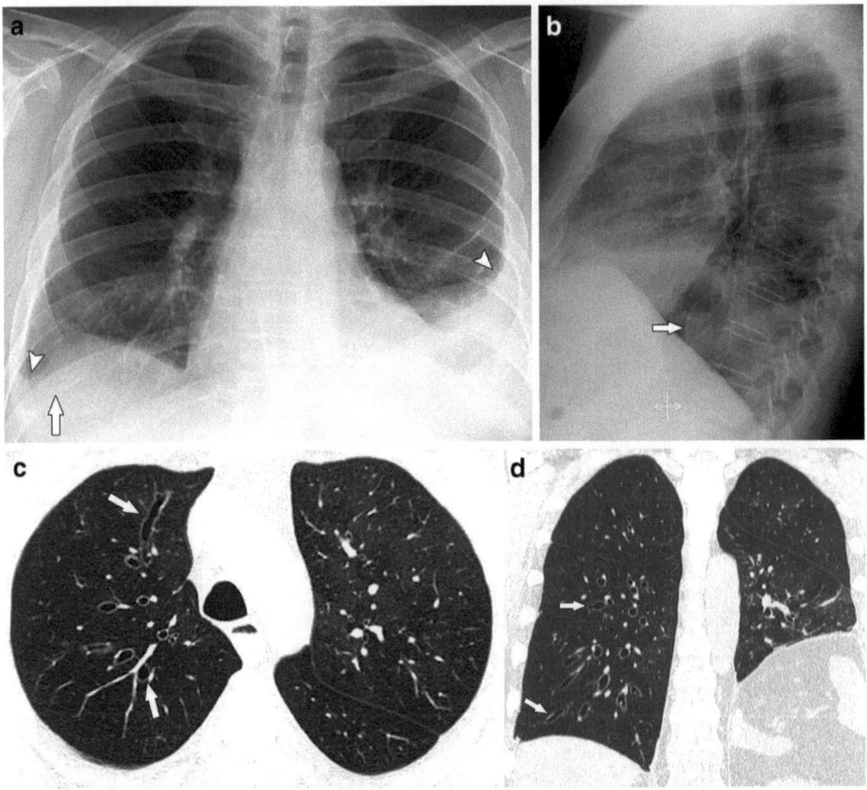

Fig. 4.4 A 57-year-old man with double-lung transplant and BOS. PA (**a**) and lateral (**b**) chest radiographs show slightly decreased lung volumes, elevated left hemidiaphragm, and mild pleural thickening (*arrowheads*). A thin-walled air cyst is in the right lower lobe (*arrows*). Transverse (**c**) and coronal reformatted (**d**) HRCT images show a subtle mosaic pattern of attenuation with diffusely lower attenuation on the right than the left, corresponding to a greater extent of cylindrical bronchiectasis (*arrows*) on the right

Choi et al. [27] studied 44 lung transplant recipients with BOS to determine whether or not CT findings correlated with the stage of BOS. This study showed only weak correlation between severity of bronchial dilation, bronchial wall thickening, and mosaic attenuation on CT with clinical stage of BOS. The study also showed no correlation between air trapping and severity of BOS in both single- and double-lung transplant recipients, a finding supported by earlier studies [20, 22]. This contrasts to the 32 % threshold reported by Bankier et al. [16]. Differing results among these studies may be accounted for by different acquisition techniques during expiratory CT and variations in coaching of patients in executing a full expiration.

Worthy et al. [24] studied 15 consecutive lung transplant recipients with pathologically proven constrictive bronchiolitis and 18 control subjects (5 post-transplant and 13 healthy subjects) with HRCT. Of the patients with constrictive bronchiolitis,

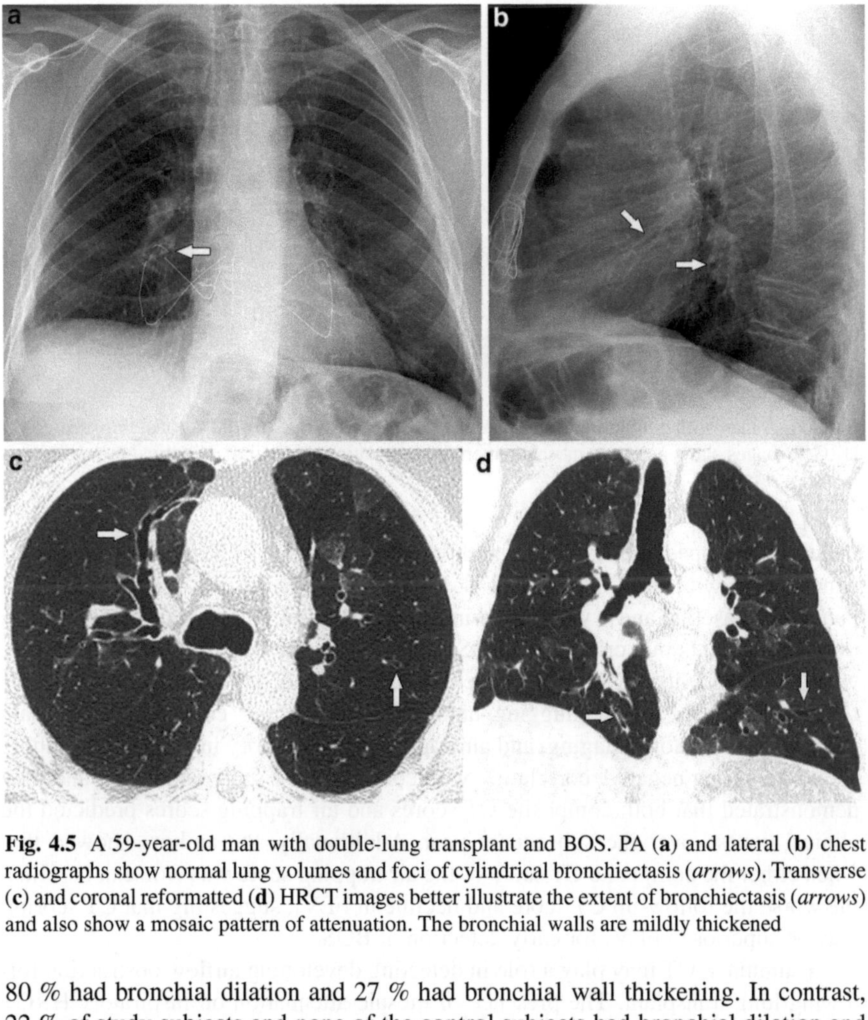

Fig. 4.5 A 59-year-old man with double-lung transplant and BOS. PA (**a**) and lateral (**b**) chest radiographs show normal lung volumes and foci of cylindrical bronchiectasis (*arrows*). Transverse (**c**) and coronal reformatted (**d**) HRCT images better illustrate the extent of bronchiectasis (*arrows*) and also show a mosaic pattern of attenuation. The bronchial walls are mildly thickened

80 % had bronchial dilation and 27 % had bronchial wall thickening. In contrast, 22 % of study subjects and none of the control subjects had bronchial dilation and bronchial wall thickening, respectively. Furthermore, Lentz et al. [21] studied HRCT scans of 16 heart–lung transplant recipients and showed the degree of lower lobe bronchial dilation correlated with the severity of BOS as measured by pulmonary function testing and increases with worsening pulmonary function.

With end-stage constrictive bronchiolitis, air trapping may be so severe that the mosaic pattern of attenuation is no longer present and little change in lung attenuation and volume is apparent between inspiratory and expiratory CT. Moreover, diffuse panlobular emphysema can mimic extensive air trapping on CT [28, 29]. However, the clinical context often suffices to distinguish the two.

Two studies of serial HRCT scans following lung transplantation have been published. In a study of 13 lung transplant recipients by Ikonen et al. [18], 126 HRCT scans were obtained over a mean follow-up period of 23 months. Eight of the study

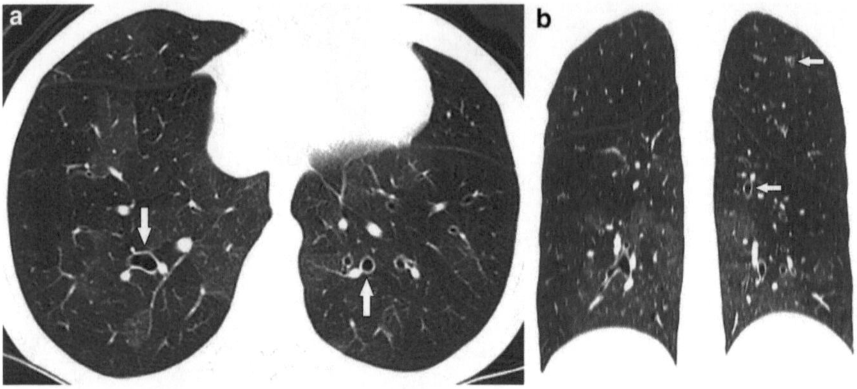

Fig. 4.6 A man with double-lung transplant and BOS. Transverse (**a**) and coronal reformatted (**b**) HRC T images show a diffuse mosaic pattern of attenuation with mild cylindrical bronchiectasis (*arrows*)

patients developed BOS, and the authors showed that HRCT findings developed concurrently with BOS. De Jong et al. [30] reported the results of CT scans of 38 patients at baseline and 1 year following single- or double-lung transplant. Sixteen of the 38 patients met criteria for BOS stages 1–3 at the time of baseline CT scan, with only 6 patients having BOS stage 2 or 3. Two blinded CT readers scored scans for bronchiectasis, mucus plugging, airway wall thickening, consolidation, mosaic pattern on inspiratory imaging, and air trapping on expiratory imaging. The authors showed a strong negative correlation with composite CT score and FEV_1, and they demonstrated that both composite CT scores and air trapping scores predicted the clinical course over the subsequent year. Additionally, the authors showed that when either the composite CT score or the air trapping score was worse at baseline, the worse the follow-up CT score and decline in FEV_1, suggesting that CT scoring may be superior to FEV_1 for early detection of BOS.

In summary, CT may play a role in detecting developing airflow obstruction following lung transplant. The presence of mosaic attenuation on inspiratory HRCT and air trapping on expiratory CT are suggestive of airflow obstruction. However, published data are limited to relatively small cohorts with varying severity of BOS. Emerging techniques in quantitative CT with more standardized image acquisition protocols and automated or semi-automated analyses of lung attenuation may provide more insight into the precise role of HRCT in screening lung transplant recipients for signs of developing airflow obstruction.

Magnetic Resonance Imaging

Magnetic resonance imaging (MRI) of the lungs using hyperpolarized helium (^3He) has been shown to be sensitive for detecting disturbances of ventilation in patients with a variety of lung diseases [31–34]. One study of nine lung transplant recipients,

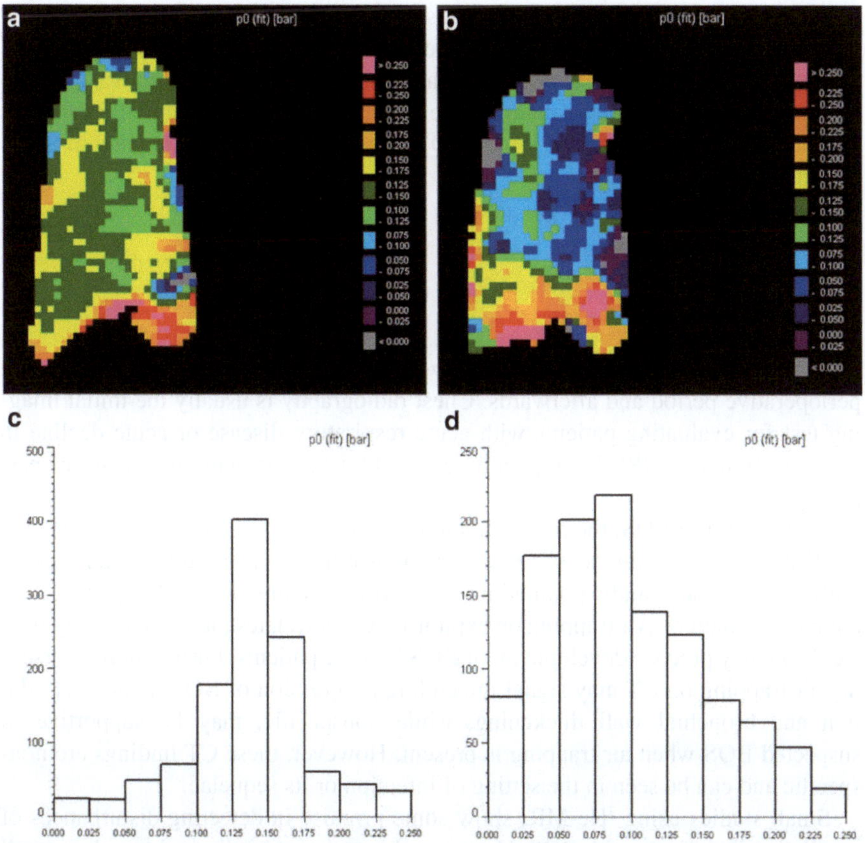

Fig. 4.7 A 42-year-old woman with right lung allograft and BOS. (**a**) Intrapulmonary pO_2 map obtained during normal graft function. (**b**) pO_2 map following the development of BOS with post-transplant FEV_1 decline of 30 % shows diminished pO_2 and increased heterogeneity. (**c, d**) pO_2 histogram during normal graft function and after development of BOS, respectively. With kind permission from Dr. Klaus Kurt Gast and Springer Science+Business Media: European Radiology, Oxygen-sensitive ^{3}He-MRI in bronchiolitis obliterans after lung transplantation, 18 (3), 2008, 530–537, Gast KK, Biedermann A, Herweling A, Schreiber WG, Schmiedeskamp J, Mayer E, et al., Figure 4

five of whom had BOS, showed a greater incidence of ventilation defects in grafts of patients with BOS [35]. Of the five subjects with BOS, MRI showed abnormalities before airflow obstruction was detected by pulmonary function testing. Another study of twelve lung transplant recipients, six with BOS and eight without BOS, using oxygen-sensitive ^{3}He-MRI (Fig. 4.7) showed overall decreased intrapulmonary pO_2 and increased heterogeneity of pO_2 in patients with BOS compared to those without BOS [36]. Unfortunately, the utility of these techniques is limited because of their relatively high expense and limited number of centers with gas polarizers.

Further advances in pulmonary MRI using other inhaled gases such as xenon and oxygen may prove to be useful alternatives to ^{3}He in evaluating patients with BOS. Although at this time MRI of the lungs may not suffice as the sole noninvasive diagnostic tool for assessing transplant recipients for BOS, it could potentially guide the bronchoscopist to the areas of lowest pO_2 in order to maximize the yield of transbronchial biopsy.

Conclusion

Imaging plays an important role in follow-up of lung transplant patients, both in the perioperative period and afterwards. Chest radiography is usually the initial imaging test for evaluating patients with acute respiratory disease or acute decline in graft function, and HRCT is typically reserved for patients with inconclusive chest radiographs.

With regard to BOS, the role of imaging in the setting of BOS remains unclear. Published data are limited to relatively small retrospective studies, and lack of uniformity among study populations and HRCT acquisition techniques further complicate matters. Air trapping on expiratory CT correlates the most strongly with BOS and may precede development of BOS in some patients. Furthermore, worsening air trapping on CT may signal impending progression of BOS. Bronchial dilation and bronchial wall thickening, while nonspecific, may be supportive of suspected BOS when air trapping is present. However, these CT findings are nonspecific and can be seen in the setting of infection or its sequelae.

Small studies using ^{3}He-MRI show some promise in detecting disturbances of ventilation in patients with BOS. However, this technique is limited to only a small number of centers possessing the proper equipment and necessary expertise. Newer MRI techniques using more readily available gases such as xenon and oxygen have the potential to increase the role that MRI plays in evaluating lung transplant recipients. Further investigations into these techniques are needed.

References

1. Reichenspurner H, Girgis RE, Robbins RC, Yun KL, Nitschke M, Berry GJ, et al. Stanford experience with obliterative bronchiolitis after lung and heart-lung transplantation. Ann Thorac Surg. 1996;62(5):1467–72. discussion 72–3.
2. Burke CM, Theodore J, Dawkins KD, Yousem SA, Blank N, Billingham ME, et al. Post-transplant obliterative bronchiolitis and other late lung sequelae in human heart-lung transplantation. Chest. 1984;86(6):824–9.
3. Glanville AR, Baldwin JC, Burke CM, Theodore J, Robin ED. Obliterative bronchiolitis after heart-lung transplantation: apparent arrest by augmented immunosuppression. Ann Intern Med. 1987;107(3):300–4.

4. Kramer MR, Stoehr C, Whang JL, Berry GJ, Sibley R, Marshall SE, et al. The diagnosis of obliterative bronchiolitis after heart-lung and lung transplantation: low yield of transbronchial lung biopsy. J Heart Lung Transplant. 1993;12(4):675–81.
5. Nathan SD, Ross DJ, Belman MJ, Shain S, Elashoff JD, Kass RM, et al. Bronchiolitis obliterans in single-lung transplant recipients. Chest. 1995;107(4):967–72.
6. Reichenspurner H, Girgis RE, Robbins RC, Conte JV, Nair RV, Valentine V, et al. Obliterative bronchiolitis after lung and heart-lung transplantation. Ann Thorac Surg. 1995;60(6): 1845–53.
7. Cooper JD, Billingham M, Egan T, Hertz MI, Higenbottam T, Lynch J, et al. A working formulation for the standardization of nomenclature and for clinical staging of chronic dysfunction in lung allografts. International Society for Heart and Lung Transplantation. J Heart Lung Transplant. 1993;12(5):713–6.
8. Chamberlain D, Maurer J, Chaparro C, Idolor L. Evaluation of transbronchial lung biopsy specimens in the diagnosis of bronchiolitis obliterans after lung transplantation. J Heart Lung Transplant. 1994;13(6):963–71.
9. Estenne M, Maurer JR, Boehler A, Egan JJ, Frost A, Hertz M, et al. Bronchiolitis obliterans syndrome 2001: an update of the diagnostic criteria. J Heart Lung Transplant. 2002;21(3):297–310.
10. Pomerance A, Madden B, Burke MM, Yacoub MH. Transbronchial biopsy in heart and lung transplantation: clinicopathologic correlations. J Heart Lung Transplant. 1995;14(4):761–73.
11. Garg K, Lynch DA, Newell JD, King Jr TE. Proliferative and constrictive bronchiolitis: classification and radiologic features. AJR Am J Roentgenol. 1994;162(4):803–8.
12. Morrish WF, Herman SJ, Weisbrod GL, Chamberlain DW. Bronchiolitis obliterans after lung transplantation: findings at chest radiography and high-resolution CT. The Toronto Lung Transplant Group. Radiology. 1991;179(2):487–90.
13. Sweatman MC, Millar AB, Strickland B, Turner-Warwick M. Computed tomography in adult obliterative bronchiolitis. Clin Radiol. 1990;41(2):116–9.
14. Skeens JL, Fuhrman CR, Yousem SA. Bronchiolitis obliterans in heart-lung transplantation patients: radiologic findings in 11 patients. AJR Am J Roentgenol. 1989;153(2):253–6.
15. Breatnach E, Kerr I. The radiology of cryptogenic obliterative bronchiolitis. Clin Radiol. 1982;33(6):657–61.
16. Bankier AA, Van Muylem A, Knoop C, Estenne M, Gevenois PA. Bronchiolitis obliterans syndrome in heart-lung transplant recipients: diagnosis with expiratory CT. Radiology. 2001;218(2):533–9.
17. Hansell DM, Rubens MB, Padley SP, Wells AU. Obliterative bronchiolitis: individual CT signs of small airways disease and functional correlation. Radiology. 1997;203(3):721–6.
18. Ikonen T, Kivisaari L, Harjula AL, Lehtola A, Heikkila L, Kinnula VL, et al. Value of high-resolution computed tomography in routine evaluation of lung transplantation recipients during development of bronchiolitis obliterans syndrome. J Heart Lung Transplant. 1996;15(6):587–95.
19. Ikonen T, Kivisaari L, Taskinen E, Piilonen A, Harjula AL. High-resolution CT in long-term follow-up after lung transplantation. Chest. 1997;111(2):370–6.
20. Lee ES, Gotway MB, Reddy GP, Golden JA, Keith FM, Webb WR. Early bronchiolitis obliterans following lung transplantation: accuracy of expiratory thin-section CT for diagnosis. Radiology. 2000;216(2):472–7.
21. Lentz D, Bergin CJ, Berry GJ, Stoehr C, Theodore J. Diagnosis of bronchiolitis obliterans in heart-lung transplantation patients: importance of bronchial dilatation on CT. AJR Am J Roentgenol. 1992;159(3):463–7.
22. Leung AN, Fisher K, Valentine V, Girgis RE, Berry GJ, Robbins RC, et al. Bronchiolitis obliterans after lung transplantation: detection using expiratory HRCT. Chest. 1998;113(2): 365–70.
23. Loubeyre P, Revel D, Delignette A, Wiesendanger T, Philit F, Bertocchi M, et al. Bronchiectasis detected with thin-section CT as a predictor of chronic lung allograft rejection. Radiology. 1995;194(1):213–6.

24. Worthy SA, Park CS, Kim JS, Muller NL. Bronchiolitis obliterans after lung transplantation: high-resolution CT findings in 15 patients. AJR Am J Roentgenol. 1997;169(3):673–7.
25. Siegel MJ, Bhalla S, Gutierrez FR, Hildebolt C, Sweet S. Post-lung transplantation bronchiolitis obliterans syndrome: usefulness of expiratory thin-section CT for diagnosis. Radiology. 2001;220(2):455–62.
26. Padley SP, Adler BD, Hansell DM, Muller NL. Bronchiolitis obliterans: high resolution CT findings and correlation with pulmonary function tests. Clin Radiol. 1993;47(4):236–40.
27. Choi YW, Rossi SE, Palmer SM, DeLong D, Erasmus JJ, McAdams HP. Bronchiolitis obliterans syndrome in lung transplant recipients: correlation of computed tomography findings with bronchiolitis obliterans syndrome stage. J Thorac Imag. 2003;18(2):72–9.
28. Guest PJ, Hansell DM. High resolution computed tomography (HRCT) in emphysema associated with alpha-1-antitrypsin deficiency. Clin Radiol. 1992;45(4):260–6.
29. Foster Jr WL, Gimenez EI, Roubidoux MA, Sherrier RH, Shannon RH, Roggli VL, et al. The emphysemas: radiologic-pathologic correlations. Radiographics. 1993;13(2):311–28.
30. de Jong PA, Dodd JD, Coxson HO, Storness-Bliss C, Pare PD, Mayo JR, et al. Bronchiolitis obliterans following lung transplantation: early detection using computed tomographic scanning. Thorax. 2006;61(9):799–804.
31. Altes TA, Powers PL, Knight-Scott J, Rakes G, Platts-Mills TA, de Lange EE, et al. Hyperpolarized 3He MR lung ventilation imaging in asthmatics: preliminary findings. J Magn Reson Imaging. 2001;13(3):378–84.
32. van Beek EJ, Hill C, Woodhouse N, Fichele S, Fleming S, Howe B, et al. Assessment of lung disease in children with cystic fibrosis using hyperpolarized 3-Helium MRI: comparison with Shwachman score, Chrispin-Norman score and spirometry. Eur Radiol. 2007;17(4):1018–24.
33. Salerno M, de Lange EE, Altes TA, Truwit JD, Brookeman JR, Mugler 3rd JP. Emphysema: hyperpolarized helium 3 diffusion MR imaging of the lungs compared with spirometric indexes–initial experience. Radiology. 2002;222(1):252–60.
34. van Beek EJ, Wild JM, Kauczor HU, Schreiber W, Mugler 3rd JP, de Lange EE. Functional MRI of the lung using hyperpolarized 3-helium gas. J Magn Reson Imaging. 2004;20(4):540–54.
35. Gast KK, Zaporozhan J, Ley S, Biedermann A, Knitz F, Eberle B, et al. (3)He-MRI in follow-up of lung transplant recipients. Eur Radiol. 2004;14(1):78–85.
36. Gast KK, Biedermann A, Herweling A, Schreiber WG, Schmiedeskamp J, Mayer E, et al. Oxygen-sensitive 3He-MRI in bronchiolitis obliterans after lung transplantation. Eur Radiol. 2008;18(3):530–7.

Chapter 5
Making a Confident Diagnosis of Obliterative Bronchiolitis

A. Whitney Brown and Steven D. Nathan

Abstract Bronchiolitis obliterans syndrome (BOS) is a dreaded complication of lung transplantation. Despite the fact that over 50 % of lung transplant recipients will eventually be diagnosed with BOS, it remains a challenging diagnosis to make with complete certainty. This diagnostic dilemma is a product of the inherent limitations of spirometry, the parameter upon which the diagnosis relies, as well as the many confounding diagnoses that must be considered and excluded before the diagnosis of BOS can be made. This chapter seeks to explore the diagnostic challenges surrounding BOS with the aim of establishing a diagnostic framework to assist the clinician with making a more confident diagnosis of BOS.

Keywords Bronchiolitis obliterans syndrome • Chronic lung allograft dysfunction • Forced expiratory volume in one second • Obliterative bronchiolitis • Spirometry

Introduction

Obliterative bronchiolitis (OB) was first described in heart–lung transplant recipients in 1984 and is well recognized as a major cause of morbidity and mortality after lung transplantation [1]. It is largely felt to be the pathologic correlate of chronic allograft rejection, although there is increasing recognition of non-alloimmune causes, such as chronic gastroesophageal reflux disease. Bronchiolitis obliterans syndrome (BOS) was proposed as a clinical entity in 1993 to describe progressive airflow limitation resulting from small airway obstruction (OB) after lung

A.W. Brown, M.D. • S.D. Nathan, M.D. (✉)
Advanced Lung Disease and Lung Transplant Program,
Inova Fairfax Hospital, Falls Church, VA, USA
e-mail: steven.nathan@inova.org

K.C. Meyer and A.R. Glanville (eds.), *Bronchiolitis Obliterans Syndrome in Lung Transplantation*, Respiratory Medicine 8, DOI 10.1007/978-1-4614-7636-8_5,

Table 5.1 Original and revised classifications of BOS[a]

Original classification		Revised classification	
BOS 0	$FEV_1 \geq 80$ % of baseline	BOS 0	$FEV_1 > 90$ % of baseline and $FEF_{25-75} > 75$ % of baseline
		BOS 0-p	FEV_1 81–90 % of baseline and/or $FEF_{25-75} \leq 75$ % of baseline
BOS 1	FEV_1 66–80 % of baseline	BOS 1	FEV_1 66–80 % of baseline
BOS 2	FEV_1 51–65 % of baseline	BOS 2	FEV_1 51–65 % of baseline
BOS 3	$FEV_1 \leq 50$ % of baseline	BOS 3	FEV_1 =or<50 % of baseline

BOS bronchiolitis obliterans syndrome, *FEF_{25-75}* mid-expiratory flow rate, *FEV_1* forced expiratory volume in 1 s

[a]Adapted from The Journal of Heart and Lung Transplantation, 21/3, Estenne M, Maurer JR, Boehler A, Egan JJ, Frost A, Hertz M, et al., Bronchiolitis obliterans syndrome 2001: an update of the diagnostic criteria, 297–310, Copyright 2002, with permission from Elsevier

transplantation [2]. The definition of BOS relies upon pulmonary function rather than histology owing to the unacceptably low sensitivity of histology for the detection of OB. BOS as a clinical syndrome is defined as a decrement of 20 % or more in forced expiratory volume in 1 s (FEV_1) compared to post-transplant baseline FEV_1 individualized for each patient. By definition, 3 or more months must have elapsed from the time of transplantation before the diagnosis of BOS can be made. Progressive stages of BOS are defined according to the magnitude of the decrease in FEV_1 [2]. The classification system for BOS was refined in 2002 to include a "potential BOS stage" to identify patients with a 10–20 % drop in FEV_1 and/or a >25 % drop in mid-expiratory flow rate (FEF_{25-75}) who are at risk for progression to BOS in order to facilitate earlier detection and potential intervention (Table 5.1) [3]. For the most part, however, BOS is characterized by irreversible loss of lung function for which there is no effective treatment.

Clinical Presentation and Evaluation

Many factors can influence lung function; therefore, BOS is a diagnosis of exclusion made only after other entities have been ruled out. There are natural fluctuations in spirometry due to factors including, but not limited to, patient effort, the time of day, and coaching. Therefore, the post-transplant baseline FEV_1 as well as the "BOS qualifying" FEV_1 must be repeated and confirmed on two occasions separated by 3 weeks or more [3].

BOS can present with an asymptomatic decline in FEV_1 detected at a routine clinic visit, or with the onset of a symptom such as progressive dyspnea on exertion.

In the symptomatic patient, the onset of symptoms is often insidious and gradual. For patients who present with dyspnea, the initial evaluation should include a routine physical examination with pulse oximetry, spirometry, a 6-min walk test (or other assessment of exertional oxygen requirement), and radiographic imaging of the chest (either chest radiograph or computed tomography [CT] as clinically appropriate). If spirometry is reduced from baseline, then a diagnostic bronchoscopy with airway inspection, bronchoalveolar lavage (BAL), and transbronchial biopsies is warranted in most cases.

In the absence of an alternative diagnosis such as pneumonia, acute rejection, airway stenosis, or bronchomalacia, further testing, such as a surgical lung biopsy for unexplained pulmonary infiltrates or an assessment for antibody-mediated rejection, may be considered depending on the clinical circumstances. When other etiologies have been appropriately evaluated and excluded, a diagnosis of BOS may be inferred if repeat spirometry (at least 3 weeks from initial reduced spirometry) demonstrates a persistent loss of 20 % or more from the baseline post-transplant FEV_1.

Another scenario that is not uncommon is the onset of BOS following an identifiable insult to the allograft such as pneumonia or acute rejection. Despite appropriate treatment of the infection or acute rejection, a subset of patients fail to recover to within 20 % of their previous baseline FEV_1 after several weeks, and their spirometry values evolve to meet diagnostic criteria for BOS. In this pathway to BOS, the initial insult may act as an immunogenic trigger that disrupts immune homeostasis and leads to progressive small airway obstruction and loss of lung function. Although there is a small subset of patients who appear to rebound from a decrement of >20 % in FEV_1 after several weeks or months (the concept of "de-BOS"), the majority of those patients will again meet criteria for BOS within several months ("re-BOS"). It is unclear whether the "de-BOS" patients have better long-term outcomes compared to patients with sustained BOS [4].

Screening

In the asymptomatic patient, a drop in lung function may be the only clue to the onset of BOS. For this reason, spirometry is an essential part of routine testing at post-transplant clinic visits. As these visits may get less frequent over time, the potential role for home spirometry monitoring becomes more significant [5]. A persistent drop in home spirometry, although not sufficient to make a diagnosis of BOS, may alert the patient and clinician to a problem that requires further evaluation in clinic. Ultimately, the use of equipment and techniques that meet American Thoracic Society standards for lung function testing [6] is necessary to make a confident diagnosis of BOS [3].

In addition to the FEV_1 and FEF_{25-75}, attention should be paid to the forced vital capacity (FVC) and FEV_1/FVC ratio on spirometric assessment as well. A preserved

FEV_1/FVC ratio (≥70 %) on spirometry can suggest the presence of a restrictive process that may provide an alternative explanation for a decrease in FEV_1. The diagnosis of restriction, by convention, should then be confirmed with lung volume testing, and ideally with body plethysmography, to assess for confounding gas trapping and hyperinflation. Common conditions that can reduce FEV_1 in the setting of restrictive physiology include, but are not limited to, obesity, muscle weakness, and pleural effusion.

Six-minute walk testing performed at regular intervals after transplant (such as quarterly or semiannually) may be helpful to assess for subtle changes in exercise tolerance that patients may not detect or report. Specifically, an increase in dyspnea on exertion (reflected in Borg scores), a decrease in exercise tolerance (reflected in overall walk distance), or a new or increased oxygen requirement with exertion are perceptible and quantifiable with serial 6-min walk testing over time. Although insufficient to make a diagnosis of BOS, these findings may alert the clinician to a changing clinical picture and prompt further diagnostic testing and increased clinical vigilance. In addition, 6-min walk test results, particularly walk distance, may hold prognostic value for long-term outcomes in post-transplant patients with BOS [7].

Imaging

Chest imaging, particularly CT, is an essential part of the diagnostic evaluation for BOS, with its primary utility resting in the detection of findings suggestive of alternative, potentially reversible diagnoses. Routine posteroanterior and lateral chest X-ray is neither sensitive nor specific for the diagnosis of BOS. The chest radiograph is typically unrevealing in the early stages of OB. As the disease progresses, decreased peripheral vascular markings, slight volume loss, and subsegmental atelectasis may become manifest [8]. Later findings are nonspecific and may include alveolar opacities related to infection and pleural-based opacities in the mid- to upper lung zones representing fibrosis [9].

CT findings include bronchial wall thickening, bronchiectasis, small nodular and linear branching opacities in a bronchiolar distribution, a mosaic pattern of lung attenuation, and air trapping (Fig. 5.1). Air trapping has historically been regarded as the most sensitive and accurate radiologic indicator of OB [10]. Because air trapping may only be seen on expiratory images, it is particularly important to obtain scans during expiration, especially when the inspiratory images are normal [9]. The use of high-resolution computed tomography (HRCT) has gained interest as the presence of certain structural changes may facilitate the earlier detection of BOS than functional measurements such as FEV_1 in some cases.

Although air trapping on expiratory HRCT appears to be the most sensitive and specific radiologic indicator of OB in the lung transplant population, it is far from perfect. In an early study of 21 patients after lung transplantation, air trapping was found in 10 of 11 (91 %) patients with biopsy-proven OB compared to 2 of 10

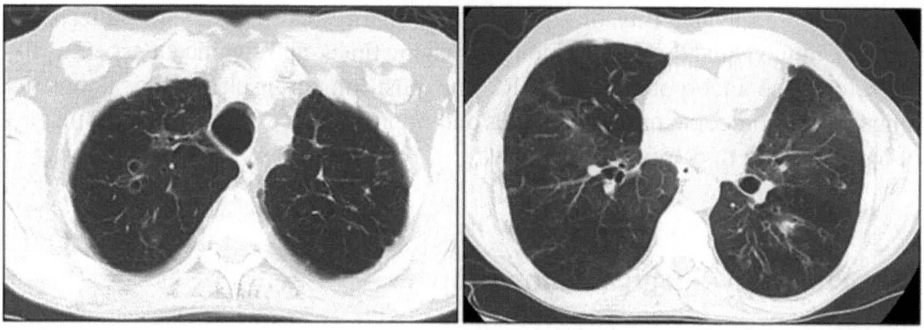

Fig. 5.1 Chest CT demonstrating bilateral bronchiectasis: a radiographic finding seen in the context of BOS after lung transplantation

(20 %) patients without OB ($p<0.002$). Air trapping was found to have a sensitivity of 91 %, a specificity of 80 %, and an accuracy of 86 % for OB. In contrast, the sensitivity, specificity, and accuracy of bronchiectasis and mosaic pattern for OB in that same study were 36 %, 80 %, and 57 %, and 64 %, 90 %, and 70 %, respectively [10]. Subsequent studies have investigated air trapping on expiratory HRCT and have shown similar results, with sensitivities ranging from 74 to 83 % and specificities of 67–89 % [11–13]. In yet another study, air trapping was found to have a fairly low sensitivity of only 44 %, but this was accompanied by a specificity of 100 % [14].

Composite CT scoring systems that include a combination of factors such as mosaic pattern of attenuation, airway wall thickening, mucus plugging, consolidation, and bronchiectasis have been developed. Both air trapping and composite CT scoring systems appear to have a significant association with FEV_1 at the time of the scan, as well as with decline in FEV_1 in the year following the CT scan [15]. Although there is good interobserver and intra-observer agreement for the air-trapping CT score, there is a relatively low interobserver agreement for the composite CT scoring system [15]. For this reason, the adoption of a universal CT scoring system that can be utilized as an adjunct to spirometry in the diagnosis of BOS remains problematic. Although there are certainly CT findings that can be consistent with or supportive of BOS, a paucity of findings can also be found in the context of patients with BOS. Thus, because HRCT findings cannot be solely relied upon to detect BOS, they are not part of the current diagnostic criteria.

The role of magnetic resonance imaging (MRI) in the detection of OB has been investigated. Hyperpolarized helium-3 (HP ^{3}He) MRI holds promise as a more sensitive alternative to HRCT with high spatial and temporal resolution [16–18]. ^{3}He MRI is attractive because of its ability to provide information on respiratory disease morphology as well as function (including the detection of ventilation defects) [19]. Additionally, MRI does not involve radiation exposure, an important consideration in lung transplant recipients owing to their considerable exposure to serial chest imaging over time. The logistic challenges of HP ^{3}He MRI are not insignificant and include limited availability of equipment (primarily restricted to specialized MR centers), limited quantities of ^{3}He, longer imaging times, and significant expense [19]. Therefore, the incorporation of MRI into post-lung transplant clinical practice hinges on the outcome of larger studies and improved accessibility, and routine use of MRI is likely to be several years away.

Bronchoscopy/Surgical Lung Biopsy

Suboptimal sensitivity limits the role of transbronchial lung biopsy (TBBx) in the diagnosis of OB, and this was one of the primary reasons that the physiologic measure of FEV_1 was adopted as the surrogate marker of BOS and used to define the entity of BOS and its clinical staging. Pathologic findings on TBBx to support OB in the setting of BOS are helpful, but if OB lesions are absent, this is likely due to inadequate sampling and/or the patchy nature of the disease. The primary role for TBBx in the evaluation of BOS is to exclude other histologic findings that might suggest an alternative pathologic process.

In an early study of TBBx, the sensitivity for the detection of OB was poor (27.7 %), although specificity was 75 %. Almost a third of TBBx specimens from patients with OB were unsatisfactory [20]. Likewise, another study concluded that although TBBx could suggest or diagnose OB in some cases, inadequate sampling was the major reason for a negative biopsy [21]. The Toronto experience revealed that the sensitivity and specificity of TBBx (average of 7.6 tissue fragments) for OB was 17.1 % and 94.5 %, respectively. The positive predictive value was 65.5 %, while the negative predictive value was 65.2 % [22].

Surgical lung biopsy is a more reliable method for diagnosing OB, but repeated sampling is unrealistic. However, surgical lung biopsy remains an important diagnostic tool in the evaluation of unexplained pulmonary infiltrates after lung transplantation when BAL and TBBx have failed to yield a clear diagnosis, or if the patient has failed to respond to seemingly appropriate therapy. The procurement of larger pieces of lung tissue enables the pathologist to differentiate between the various forms of rejection, infection, and other more unusual processes. In a study of open lung biopsy after lung transplantation, a novel, clinically unsuspected diagnosis was made in 14/48 biopsies (29 %), and all of these resulted in therapy changes. Thirty-two biopsies (67 %) confirmed clinical diagnoses, and new therapy was initiated in 30 of these patients. Two patients (4 %) had non-diagnostic biopsies, while four biopsies (8 % including the two non-diagnostic biopsies) did not result in any therapeutic changes. Complications occurred in three patients, all of whom had an air leak for greater than 7 days [23]. The incidence of persistent bronchopleural fistula would likely be lower with the increased and widespread use of video-assisted thoracoscopic surgery over the last several years. Therefore, in the setting of unexplained pulmonary infiltrates after lung transplantation, surgical lung biopsy renders a new, unsuspected diagnosis in nearly one-third of patients and often leads to targeted therapy [23].

Similar findings were noted by the Toronto group who published their 10-year experience [24]. Specifically, they reported the discovery of a new diagnosis that resulted in a change of therapy in 1 of 11 "early" (within 45 days of transplant) open lung biopsies performed for pulmonary infiltrates and clinical compromise. In contrast, a new diagnosis was established in 8 of 27 biopsies obtained "late" (>45 days) post-transplant. Indications for late biopsies were acute or progressive pulmonary disease with associated clinical findings, progressive loss of pulmonary function, radiologic compromise without clinical findings, persistent poor graft function, and persistent lymphocytosis in BAL. Pathologic diagnoses included OB, BOS organizing pneumonia (now known as cryptogenic organizing pneumonia (COP)), malignant lymphoma, chronic vascular rejection, and *Burkholderia cepacia* infection. Overall, surgical lung biopsy is of little value in the perioperative period, but it appears to yield useful information in approximately 30 % of patients when performed more than 45 days after transplant [24].

Biomarkers

Despite the need for markers to predict decline in lung function after lung transplant, there are no validated biomarkers that can aid in the diagnosis of BOS. The two potential biomarkers that have been studied most in this setting are BAL fluid neutrophil count and fraction of nitric oxide in exhaled breath (FeNO). However, neither has been adapted into routine clinical practice.

In lung transplant recipients with BOS, BAL neutrophilia is present and correlates highly with the presence of interleukin-8 (IL-8). Additionally, there is a trend toward higher levels of neutrophils and IL-8 in BAL from patients who subsequently develop BOS as compared to those who do not [25]. These findings suggest that there may be a role for BAL neutrophilia and elevation in IL-8 to predict the development of future BOS among lung transplant recipients. To further support this notion, azithromycin reduces airway neutrophilia and IL-8 mRNA in patients with BOS, and azithromycin has been shown to improve the FEV_1 in patients with BOS, particularly those with higher BAL neutrophilia and IL-8 levels. There are also data to support the implementation of azithromycin soon after transplantation as a preemptive strategy before BOS criteria are fulfilled [26]. Thus although BAL neutrophilia and elevation of IL-8 are not part of the current diagnostic criteria for BOS, if identified, such BAL findings may provide support for the diagnosis of BOS and predict response to treatment with azithromycin. While measurement of IL-8 from BAL fluid is not universally available in the clinical setting, BAL cell count with differential is routinely available and may be used as an adjunct in the evaluation of possible BOS.

The FeNO is an established biomarker of airway inflammation that has been studied extensively in asthmatics [27]. It has gained interest as a tool for the early detection of BOS in lung transplantation with the hypothesis that elevated FeNO may predict the onset or worsening of BOS. NO is produced by residential and inflammatory cells in the airways in response to endogenous and exogenous stimuli. In a longitudinal study of FeNO in 50 lung transplant recipients, the mean FeNO in patients with unstable BOS (defined as ≥15 % decline in FEV_1 over 6 months) was significantly higher than in stable BOS-free patients and stable BOS patients (<5 % decline in FEV_1 over 6 months). Measurements of FeNO showed little day-to-day variability when subjects were clinically stable [28].

In a second study investigating the role of FeNO in the early diagnosis of BOS after lung transplantation, 611 FeNO measurements in 166 consecutive patients were classified depending on BOS stage at the time of assessment and follow-up. Before the onset of an unstable clinical course, FeNO was significantly increased in comparison to those with stable lung function. The positive and negative predictive value of FeNO > 20 ppb for BOS was 69.0 % and 96.9 %, respectively [29]. Serial measurements demonstrated significantly lower mean individual variation in stable recipients as compared to stable patients transitioning to an unstable course. The robust negative predictive value of persistently low FeNO readings for future BOS suggests clinical utility of this marker as part of continuous risk stratification after lung transplantation [29]. Portable NO analyzers are now available, making routine FeNO testing a possibility in some clinical settings, but it remains mostly a research tool at this time.

Confounding Diagnoses

There are numerous reasons for lung function decline after lung transplantation other than BOS. A myriad of potential confounding diagnoses must be considered before a confident diagnosis of BOS can be made. In some cases, these conditions may coexist with BOS, further complicating the clinical picture. Potential contributing factors to loss of lung function can be conceptualized in several broad categories that capture both allograft-related and non-allograft-related processes over time (Table 5.2).

Allograft Rejection

Among the most important causes of impaired allograft function after lung transplantation are other forms of rejection. Rejection can be categorized into three broad types: acute cellular rejection, antibody-mediated rejection, and OB/BOS. Additionally, lymphocytic bronchiolitis is gaining recognition as a distinct clinical entity that can manifest with reduced lung function after transplant. In fact, in one study, the severity of lymphocytic bronchiolitis was associated with an increased risk of BOS and death after lung transplantation independent of acute vascular rejection [30]. These other etiologies of rejection must be considered and treated, if present, before a diagnosis of BOS can be made.

Table 5.2 Confounding conditions in the diagnosis of BOS

Category of lung function loss	Conditions
Allograft rejection	Acute cellular
	Antibody-mediated
	Lymphocytic bronchiolitis
	Bronchiolitis obliterans syndrome (BOS)
Chronic lung allograft dysfunction (CLAD)	Restrictive allograft syndrome (RAS)
	Bronchiolitis obliterans syndrome (BOS)
Parenchymal disease of the allograft	Cryptogenic organizing pneumonia (COP)
	Acute fibrinous and organizing pneumonia (AFOP)
	Diffuse alveolar damage (DAD)
	Drug toxicity (i.e., amiodarone, sirolimus)
Underlying lung disease	Recurrence in allograft (i.e., sarcoidosis)
	Native lung complications (i.e., bronchiectasis, hyperinflation)
Infection/inflammation	Bronchitis
	Pneumonia
	Bronchiectasis with persistent airway infection (NTM, fungal, gram negatives)
	Aspiration
Airway disease	Bronchomalacia
	Anastomotic stenosis/stricture
	Vanishing airway syndrome
	Other airway stenosis
Ventilatory disorders	Pain (rib/sternal/vertebral fracture)
	Muscle weakness/deconditioning
	Neuromuscular disease
	Extrinsic restriction by contralateral lung
	Chest wall pathology (kyphoscoliosis)
	Pleural disease (effusion, fibrosis)
	Pneumothorax/bronchopleural fistula
	Diaphragmatic dysfunction (paresis/paralysis)
	Obesity
	Abdominal distension/ascites
Cardiac disease	Ischemic heart disease
	Non-ischemic cardiomyopathy
	Diastolic dysfunction
	Pulmonary hypertension
Malignancy	Post-transplant lymphoproliferative disorder (PTLD)
	Lung cancer of native lung
Aging	Normal age-related loss of lung function (expected loss of ~30 mL/year in FEV_1)

Chronic Lung Allograft Dysfunction

The concept of chronic lung allograft dysfunction (CLAD) has been introduced in the literature in recent years. Although this term has been used in a variety of ways, it is not synonymous with chronic rejection or BOS. Rather, it is more accurately

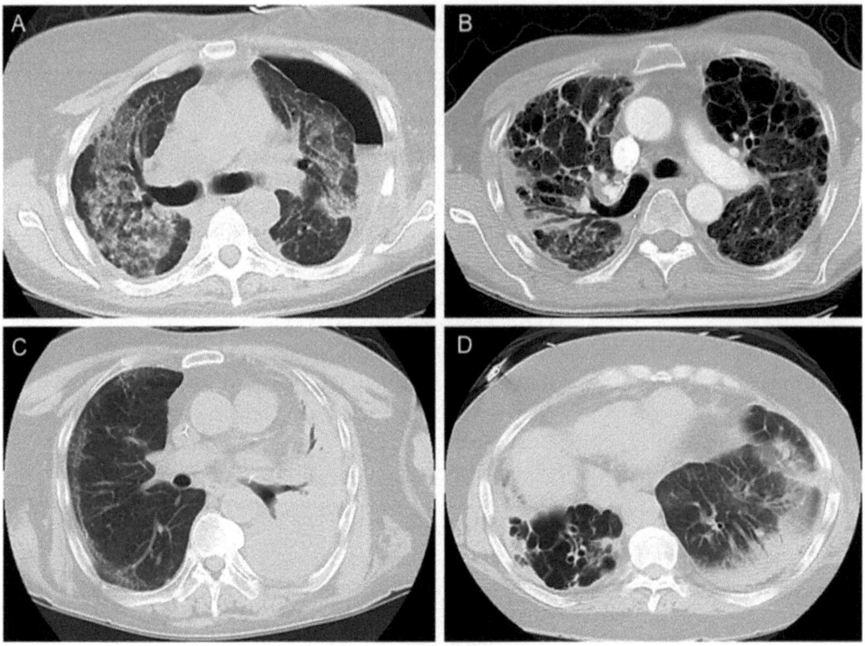

Fig. 5.2 Spectrum of parenchymal changes in patients with CLAD. (**a**) Bilateral alveolar/interstitial infiltrates in a COPD patient 18 months after bilateral lung transplantation. A small hydropneumothorax is also present on the left. (**b**) Pleuroparenchymal disease (*right*) with bullous disease (*left*) 5–6 years post-bilateral lung transplantation in an IPAH patient. (**c**) Diffuse allograft consolidation and opacification in an NSIP patient 2 years after left single-lung transplantation. (**d**) Peripheral consolidation in a sarcoid patient 18 months after left single-lung transplantation

defined as delayed loss of allograft function with a variety of potential etiologies, both reversible and irreversible in nature. An important subtype of CLAD is restrictive allograft syndrome (RAS). RAS has been characterized as a form of lung allograft dysfunction that can lead to irreversible decline of FEV_1 in the setting of restrictive physiology (preserved FEV_1/FVC ratio) and peripheral lung allograft fibrosis [31]. Additionally, loss of lung function (either in a restrictive or obstructive pattern on spirometry) in the setting of persistent pulmonary infiltrates without a clear pathologic explanation, is likely another subtype of CLAD (Fig. 5.2) and may be considered a distinct clinical phenotype from classical BOS [32].

Diffuse Parenchymal Lung Disease of the Allograft

Classic diffuse parenchymal lung diseases can affect the lung allograft as well, although less frequently. COP, acute fibrinous and organizing pneumonia (AFOP), diffuse alveolar damage (DAD), and drug toxicity are among these diagnostic possibilities. These entities usually manifest as cough and dyspnea in the setting of

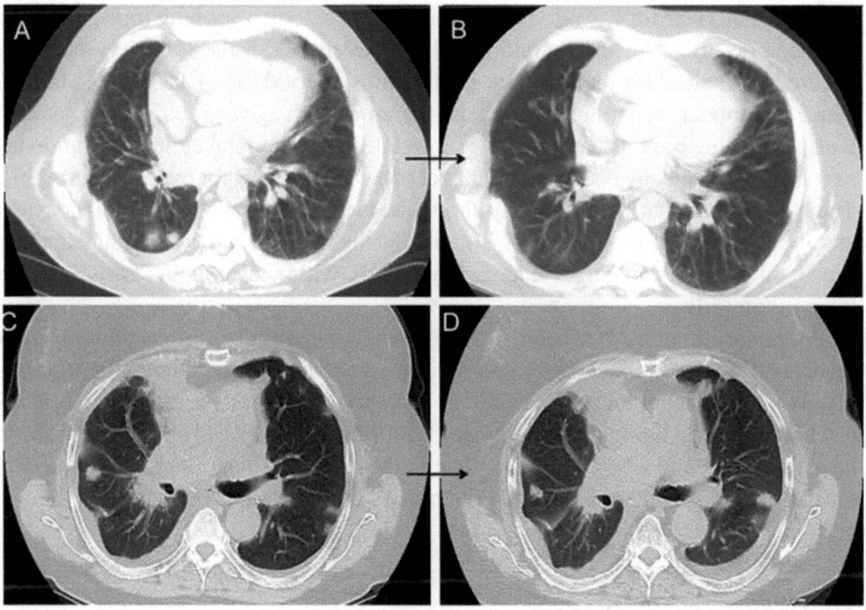

Fig. 5.3 Chest CT demonstrating cryptogenic organizing pneumonia (COP) after transplantation. (**a**) Right single-lung transplant for IPF with COP 1-year post-transplant. (**b**) Response seen after 6 weeks of augmented glucocorticoid therapy. (**c**) COP 2 years after bilateral lung transplantation for COPD. (**d**) Unresponsive to augmentation of glucocorticoid therapy after 6 months

diffuse pulmonary infiltrates and may require surgical lung biopsy for a conclusive diagnosis. COP (previously known as BOOP) is marked histologically by the presence of myxomatous connective tissue plugs in the lumen of bronchioles with extension into the alveoli, and COP may be found in association with acute rejection or ongoing infection [33]. Radiographically, COP is characterized by multiple patchy alveolar opacities (Fig. 5.3). AFOP is a rare variant of lung injury with a dominant histological finding of intra-alveolar fibrin (fibrin "balls") and patchy organizing pneumonia without hyaline membranes [34]. Both COP and AFOP are usually treated with augmentation of immunosuppression, in particular glucocorticosteroids, but may not respond completely in the setting of preexisting heavy immunosuppression [35, 36].

DAD is a fairly common finding after lung transplantation. In a recent review of transbronchial lung biopsies after lung transplantation, DAD was observed in 320 of 720 (44.4 %) patients at least once. Early onset DAD (within 3 months of transplant) was associated with significantly higher 90-day mortality and earlier onset of BOS. New-onset DAD after 3 months appeared to increase the risk for RAS [37].

The diagnosis of drug-induced pneumonitis after lung transplant is particularly challenging owing to the numerous diagnoses that must be considered first in the immunosuppressed patient. The clinical course and prognosis rely upon prompt identification and removal of the insulting agent with corresponding clinical improvement over time. Amiodarone pulmonary toxicity after lung transplantation has been described in the literature and is relevant given the relatively common occurrence of atrial fibrillation in the postoperative period [38]. Classically, the incidence of amiodarone pulmonary toxicity increases with age and is higher in patients with underlying lung disease. Toxicity correlates with the total cumulative amiodarone dose and typically occurs at doses exceeding 400 mg/day for over 2 months [39]. The BAL in patients with this may show elevated neutrophils, CD8 lymphocytes, and the presence of foamy cells with lamellar inclusions. Biopsy findings include septal thickening, interstitial edema, and lipids within endothelial cells and the interstitium [40].

Pulmonary toxicity has been recognized as a potentially serious complication associated with sirolimus therapy in solid organ transplant recipients. In approximately 95 % of reported cases, sirolimus discontinuation or dose reduction resulted in clinical and radiologic improvement within a few weeks [41]. Although there have only been a few case reports to date in the lung transplant literature, clinicians must remain vigilant to its potential pulmonary complications.

Underlying Lung Disease

In some cases, the underlying lung disease leading to lung transplantation can reemerge after transplant. There is a small but tangible possibility of primary disease recurrence in the allograft, particularly in systemic diseases such as sarcoidosis and lymphangioleiomyomatosis (LAM), although recurrence has also been seen with pulmonary alveolar proteinosis, Langerhans cell histiocytosis, diffuse panbronchiolitis, and talc granulomatosis. Confirmation of suspected primary disease recurrence requires a pathologic diagnosis, usually with TBBx or surgical lung biopsy.

Sarcoidosis is the most common disease to recur after lung transplantation [42]. Recurrent sarcoidosis most commonly manifests radiographically as either a solitary pulmonary nodule or numerous miliary nodules [42] (Fig. 5.4). Interestingly, the majority of sarcoid patients with disease recurrence in the allograft have no sarcoid-related pulmonary symptoms, and recurrence may not have any significant influence on lung function, at least in the short-term [43]. In sarcoidosis, it appears that sarcoid granulomas in the transplanted lung are derived from recipient's immune cells through colonization of the lung allograft [44].

In a multicenter study, patients with sarcoidosis were studied for biopsy-proven disease recurrence after single-lung, heart–lung, or bilateral lung transplantation. Disease recurrence was diagnosed in 16/45 patients (35.5 %) with a mean time post-transplant to diagnosis of 361.2 days (range 21–1,672) [45]. The frequency of acute rejection and infections was comparable to other disease groups. Nine patients (three with recurrence, six without) developed OB. One patient death was attributed

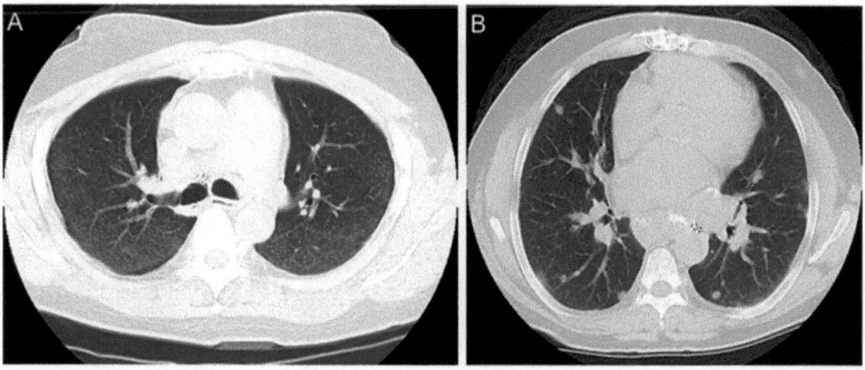

Fig. 5.4 Chest CT demonstrating biopsy-proven recurrence of sarcoidosis after bilateral lung transplantation. (**a**) Diffuse miliary pattern seen 4 years after transplant. (**b**) Bilateral pulmonary nodules seen 11 years after transplant. Reproduced with permission of the European Respiratory Society. Eur Respir J June 2012 39: 1520–1533; published ahead of print January 12, 2012, doi:10.1183/09031936.00175511

to sarcoidosis in the allograft and the native lung. Mean time to death after transplant for the disease recurrence group was 1,483 days (64–3,280) vs. 1,128 days (32–2,547) for those without recurrence. It is possible that recurrent sarcoidosis after lung transplantation may confer a slight survival advantage, but this remains speculative and warrants further study [45]. In LAM, disease recurrence has been reported in approximately 10 % of cases after lung transplantation and is usually discovered as an incidental finding 1–5 years post-transplant [42]. Data suggest that histologically benign LAM cells can migrate or metastasize in vivo to the transplanted lung [46]. Bilateral lung transplantation does not prevent recurrence due to nodal involvement.

In single-lung transplant recipients, acute or progressive hyperinflation of the native lung, particularly in chronic obstructive pulmonary disease (COPD), can cause extrinsic restriction of the allograft due to a herniation across the midline (Fig. 5.5). In most situations, it is unclear if it is the progressive dynamic hyperinflation of the native lung that compresses the allograft or if there is progressive restriction of the allograft with the native lung "filling the space." Lung volume reduction of the native lung has been performed in select cases with mixed results [47].

Yet another (although less likely) cause for decreased lung function due to underlying lung disease is progression of interstitial lung disease, even in the setting of immunosuppression, after single-lung transplantation. This is exemplified by a case report of an exacerbation of fibrotic nonspecific interstitial pneumonitis (NSIP) in the native lung causing respiratory failure after single-lung transplant [48]. Cases such as these support the possibility of acute exacerbations of interstitial lung disease leading to loss of lung function after single-lung transplant.

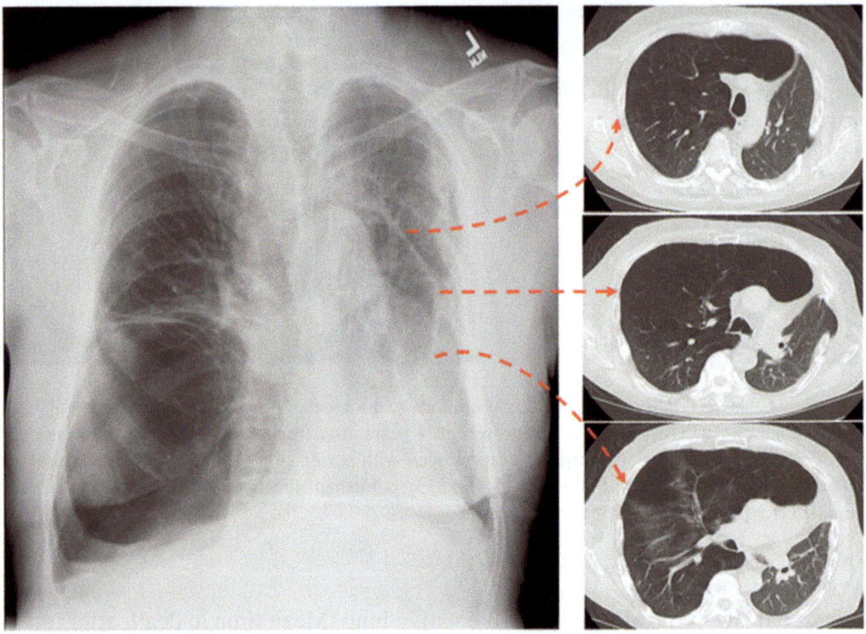

Fig. 5.5 Chest radiograph with corresponding CT images taken at three different levels demonstrating hyperinflation of native COPD lung and volume loss of allograft after left single-lung transplantation

Infection

The presence of infection can cause loss of lung function as well as progressive dyspnea in the lung transplant recipient. Infection can present as tracheobronchitis or pneumonia, with potential etiologies including a broad spectrum of viruses, bacteria, fungi, and non-tuberculous mycobacteria. Because these pathogens can be difficult to culture with routine sputum sampling, BAL is necessary in most cases. In the setting of active infection, a diagnosis of BOS is not possible and should be reassessed after appropriate antimicrobial treatment.

Aspiration, and the resulting infection or inflammatory response, can result in progressive allograft dysfunction. The reader is encouraged to refer to the chapter that addresses this important issue.

Airway Disease

Diseases of the airway are another cause for worsening dyspnea, with bronchomalacia, anastomotic stenosis, or stricture as possible complications in lung transplant recipients. Interestingly, although strictures invariably occur at the site of the

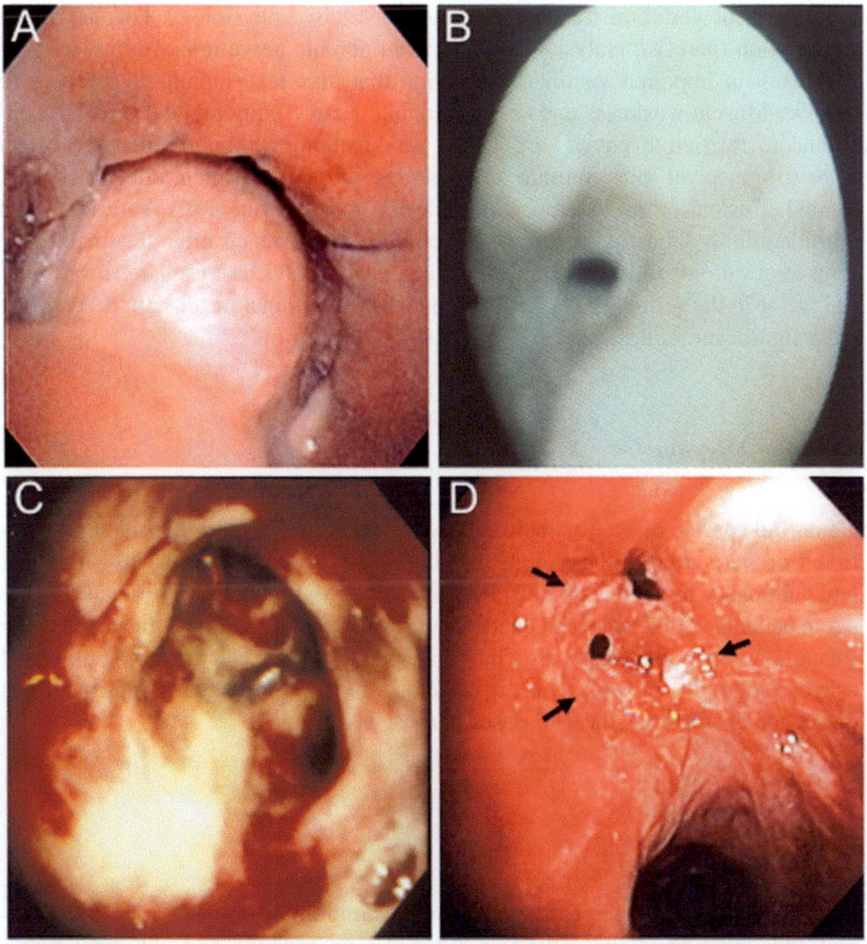

Fig. 5.6 Spectrum of airway pathology after lung transplantation. (**a**) Bronchomalacia post-transplant with invagination of posterior membranous portion of the right mainstem bronchus seen at the anastomosis. (**b**) Post-transplant stricture at the anastomosis. (**c**) Bronchocentric mycosis (aspergillus). (**d**) "Vanishing airway" syndrome with pinhole apertures seen at the origin of the left upper lobe. The *black arrows* outline the borders of the left upper lobe

anastomosis, they may occur more distally, either in isolated fashion or as part of the so-called "vanishing airway" syndrome (Fig. 5.6). While obstructive physiology on spirometry may raise the suspicion for airway disease, bronchoscopy is usually required to make these diagnoses.

Other Restrictive Disorders

Disorders of ventilation are numerous and vary in their degree of reversibility. Postoperative (post-thoracotomy or post-sternotomy) or later-onset chest pain from a rib or vertebral fracture can cause restrictive physiology. Diaphragmatic dysfunction (paresis/paralysis) resulting from phrenic nerve injury during surgery can result in impaired ventilatory function that may take months to improve or resolve. Muscle weakness and deconditioning occur commonly and can also contribute to restrictive physiology. Chest wall pathology (kyphoscoliosis) present prior to transplant may continue to cause restrictive impairment after transplant. Pleural effusions or the development of fibrosis (as is present in RAS) are additional considerations. Obesity, an extremely common occurrence after treatment with long-term steroids following transplantation, must always be considered as a potential factor in the setting of restriction. Likewise, abdominal distension, particularly from significant ascites, can cause a similar picture.

Cardiac Disease

Comorbid cardiac disease is increasingly common in the aging transplant population. Coronary artery disease, non-ischemic cardiomyopathy, diastolic dysfunction, and pulmonary hypertension must be considered as alternate or additional diagnoses in patients with dyspnea on exertion and reduced FVC and/or diffusing capacity for carbon monoxide (DL_{CO}) after lung transplant. Routine electrocardiography and echocardiography, as well as heart catheterization when clinically indicated, can detect and characterize these diseases in most cases.

Malignancy

Lung cancer, either of the native lung (most common) or the allograft, might warrant consideration in the setting of reduced lung function and abnormal radiographic findings after lung transplant. This is particularly salient because many recipients and an increasing number of donors are ex-smokers. New pulmonary nodules or suspicious infiltrates should be evaluated appropriately [49] to exclude the possibility of malignancy in this immunosuppressed population. Post-transplant lymph proliferative disorder with thoracic organ involvement is another significant concern in the setting of immunosuppression. Evaluation for the presence of Epstein-Barr viremia and histopathologic evaluation of pulmonary nodules or unexplained infiltrates may reveal this diagnosis, which should be of particular concern in the context of an EBV-negative recipient who received an organ from an EBV-positive donor.

Aging

Lung function declines slowly through adult life, even in healthy persons. Studies have shown an FEV_1 loss of 28–42 mL/year in never smokers, and up to 55 mL/year in current smokers [50–52]. This annual loss may accelerate after age 70 [53, 54]. It is conceivable that age-related decline in FEV_1 may impact both allograft and native lung function after lung transplantation, and at least partially explain a loss of FEV_1 over time after transplantation, particularly in long-term survivors.

These non-BOS conditions, although extremely important to identify and address, often do not exist in isolation and do not preclude the coexistence of BOS.

Limitations of the Current Diagnostic Criteria

The diagnosis of a disease or syndrome is only as good as its established criteria. Although revised in 2002 to improve the sensitivity for the detection of BOS with the addition of the potential BOS "0p" category [3], the specificity of the diagnosis remains undesirably low, making a confident diagnosis of BOS difficult to achieve.

There are many ways to conceptualize the many diagnostic tests and confounders that must be considered when diagnosing BOS. Figure 5.7 is an example of a potential diagnostic algorithm that may be helpful in this setting.

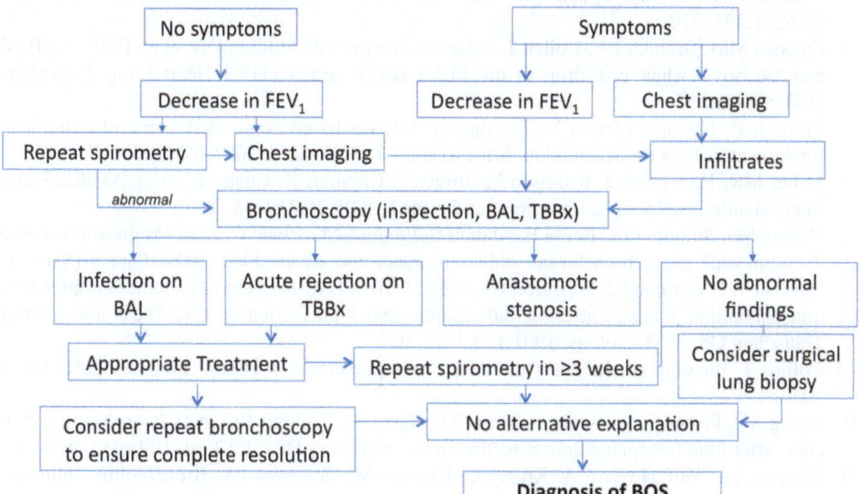

Fig. 5.7 BOS after lung transplantation: a diagnostic algorithm

Conclusion

OB remains an enigmatic diagnosis. Attempts to define a physiologic correlate in the form of BOS have enabled patients to be diagnosed without the need for a surgical lung biopsy. However, this has inadvertently resulted in multiple entities or phenotypes of chronic allograft dysfunction being labeled within the rubric of this physiologic entity. Recent attempts to provide further clarification should result in a new consensus statement endorsed by most of the major Respiratory and Transplant Societies. This will hopefully provide a standardized blueprint whereby all of these newly recognized and future entities can be more accurately categorized. Hopefully, this will further enable and facilitate an accurate diagnosis of OB without having to revert to reliance on surgical lung biopsies.

References

1. Burke CM, Theodore J, Dawkins KD, Yousem KD, Blank N, Billigham ME, et al. Post-transplant obliterative bronchiolitis and other late lung sequelae in human heart-lung transplant recipients. Chest. 1984;86:824–9.
2. Cooper JD, Billingham M, Egan T, Hertz MI, Higenbottam T, Lynch J, et al. A working formulation for the standardization of nomenclature and for clinical staging of chronic dysfunction in lung allografts. International Society for Heart and Lung Transplantation. J Heart Lung Transplant. 1993;12:713–6.
3. Estenne M, Maurer JR, Boehler A, Egan JJ, Frost A, Hertz MI, et al. Bronchiolitis obliterans syndrome 2001: an update of the diagnostic criteria. J Heart Lung Transplant. 2002;21:297–310.
4. Fregoso MM, Brenner RL, Collen J, Reffett T, Brown AW, Shlobin OA, et al. BOS, "DeBos" and "ReBos": when is a drop in the FEV1 really permanent? J Heart Lung Transplant. 2011;30(4S):S53.
5. Morlion B, Knoop C, Paiva M, Estenne M. Internet-based home monitoring of pulmonary function after lung transplantation. Am J Respir Crit Care Med. 2002;165(5):694–7.
6. Miller MR, Hankinson J, Brusasco V, Burgos F, Casaburi R, Coates A, et al. ATS/ERS task force: standardisation of spirometry. Eur Respir J. 2005;26:319–38.
7. Nathan SD, Shlobin OA, Reese E, Ahmad S, Fregoso M, Athale C, et al. Prognostic value of the 6min walk test in bronchiolitis obliterans syndrome. Respir Med. 2009;103(12):1816–21.
8. Morrish WF, Herman SJ, Weisbrod GL, Chamberlain DW. Bronchiolitis obliterans after lung transplantation: findings at chest radiography and high resolution CT. The Toronto Lung Transplant Group. Radiology. 1991;179:487–90.
9. Collins J. Imaging of the chest after lung transplantation. J Thorac Imaging. 2002;17(2):102–12.
10. Leung AN, Fisher K, Valentine V, Girgis RE, Berry GJ, Robbins RC, et al. Bronchiolitis obliterans after lung transplantation: detection using expiratory HRCT. Chest. 1998;113:365–70.
11. Bankier AA, Van Muylem A, Knoop C, Estenne M, Gevenois PA. Bronchiolitis obliterans syndrome in heart-lung transplant recipients: diagnosis with expiratory CT. Radiology. 2001;218(2):533–9.
12. Lee ES, Gotway MB, Reddy GP, Golden JA, Keith FM, Webb WR. Early bronchiolitis obliterans following lung transplantation: accuracy of expiratory thin-section CT for diagnosis. Radiology. 2000;216(2):472–7.

13. Berstad AE, Aalokken TM, Kolbenstvedt A, Bjortuft O. Performance of long-term CT monitoring in diagnosing bronchiolitis obliterans after lung transplantation. Eur J Radiol. 2006;58(1):124–31.
14. Konen E, Gutierrez C, Chaparro C, Murray CP, Chung T, Crossin J, et al. Bronchiolitis obliterans syndrome in lung transplant recipients: can thin-section CT findings predict disease before its clinical appearance? Radiology. 2004;231(2):467–73.
15. de Jong PA, Dodd JD, Coxson HO, Storness-Bliss C, Paré PD, Mayo JR, et al. Bronchiolitis obliterans following lung transplantation: early detection using computed tomographic scanning. Thorax. 2006;61:799–804.
16. Gast KK, Viallon M, Eberle B, Lill J, Puderbach M, Hanke A, et al. MR Imaging in lung transplant recipients using hyperpolarized ^{3}He: comparison with CT. J Magn Reson Imaging. 2002;15:268–74.
17. Gast KK, Zaporozhan J, Ley S, Biedermann A, Knitz F, Eberle B, et al. ^{3}He-MRI in follow-up of lung transplant recipients. Eur Radiol. 2004;14:78–85.
18. Gast KK, Biedermann A, Herweling A, Schreiber WG, Schmiedeskamp J, Mayer E, et al. Oxygen-sensitive ^{3}He-MRI in bronchiolitis obliterans after lung transplantation. Eur Radiol. 2008;18:530–7.
19. Fain S, Schiebler ML, McCormack DG, Parraga G. Imaging of lung function using hyperpolarized helium-3 magnetic resonance imaging: review of current and emerging translational methods and applications. J Magn Reson Imaging. 2010;32(6):1398–408.
20. Pomerance A, Madden B, Burke MM, Yacoub MH. Transbronchial biopsy in heart and lung transplantation: clinicopathologic correlations. J Heart Lung Transplant. 1995;14(4):761–73.
21. Cagle PT, Brown RW, Frost A, Kellar C, Yousem SA. Diagnosis of chronic lung transplant rejection by transbronchial biopsy. Mod Pathol. 1995;8(2):137–42.
22. Chamberlain D, Maurer J, Chaparro C, Idolor L. Evaluation of transbronchial lung biopsy specimens in the diagnosis of bronchiolitis obliterans after lung transplantation. J Heart Lung Transplant. 1994;13(6):963–71.
23. Weill D, McGiffin DC, Zorn GL, Alexander CB, Early LJ, Kirklin JK, et al. The utility of open lung biopsy following lung transplantation. J Heart Lung Transplant. 2000;19(9):852–7.
24. Chaparro C, Maurer JR, Chamberlain DW, Todd TR. Role of open lung biopsy for diagnosis in lung transplant recipients: ten-year experience. Ann Thorac Surg. 1995;59(4):928–32.
25. DiGiovine B, Lynch III JP, Martinez FJ, Flint A, Whyte RI, Iannettoni MD, et al. Bronchoalveolar lavage neutrophilia is associated with obliterative bronchiolitis after lung transplantation: role of IL-8. J Immunol. 1996;157:4194–202.
26. Verleden GM, Vanaudenaerde BM, Dupont LJ, Van Raemdonck DE. Azithromycin reduces airway neutrophilia and interleukin-8 in patient with bronchiolitis obliterans syndrome. Am J Respir Crit Care Med. 2006;174(5):566–70.
27. Taylor DR, Pinjenburg MW, Smith AD, De Jongste JC. Exhaled nitric oxide measurements: clinical application and interpretation. Thorax. 2006;61(9):817–27.
28. Brugiere O, Thabut G, Mal H, Marceau A, Dauriat G, Marrash-Chahla R, et al. Exhaled NO may predict the decline in lung function in bronchiolitis obliterans syndrome. Eur Respir J. 2005;25(5):813–9.
29. Neurohr C, Huppmann P, Leuschner S, von Wulffen W, Meis T, Leuchte H, Munich Lung Transplant Group, et al. Usefulness of exhaled nitric oxide to guide risk stratification for bronchiolitis obliterans syndrome after lung transplantation. Am J Transplant. 2011;11(1):129–37.
30. Glanville AR, Aboyoun CL, Havryk A, Plit M, Rainer S, Malouf MA. Severity of lymphocytic bronchiolitis predicts long-term outcome after lung transplantation. Am J Respir Crit Care Med. 2008;177(9):1033–40.
31. Sato M, Waddell TK, Wagnetz U, Roberts HC, Hwang DM, Haroon A, et al. Restrictive allograft syndrome (RAS): a novel form of chronic lung allograft dysfunction. J Heart Lung Transplant. 2011;30:735–42.
32. Woodrow JP, Shlobin OA, Barnett SD, Burton N, Nathan SD. Comparison of bronchiolitis obliterans syndrome to other forms of chronic lung allograft dysfunction after lung transplantation. J Heart Lung Transplant. 2010;10:1159–64.

33. Siddiqui MT, Garrity ER, Husain AN. Bronchiolitis obliterans organizing pneumonia-like reactions: a nonspecific response or an atypical form of rejection or infection in lung allograft recipients? Hum Pathol. 1996;27(7):714–9.
34. Beasley MB, Franks TJ, Galvin JR, Gochuico B, Travis WD. Acute fibrinous and organizing pneumonia: a histological pattern of lung injury and possible variant of diffuse alveolar damage. Arch Pathol Lab Med. 2002;126(9):1064–70.
35. Chaparro C, Chamberlain D, Maurer J, Winton T, Dehoyos A, Kesten S. Bronchiolitis obliterans organizing pneumonia (BOOP) in lung transplant recipients. Chest. 1996;110(5):1150–4.
36. Bierach JB, Meyer KC, Kanne J, Torrealba J. Acute fibrinous and organizing pneumonia following lung transplantation: a report of four cases. Chest. 2010;138:548A.
37. Sato M, Hwang DM, Ohmori-Matsuda K, Chaparro C, Waddell TK, Singer LG, et al. Revisiting the pathologic finding of diffuse alveolar damage after lung transplantation. J Heart Lung Transplant. 2012;31(4):354–63.
38. Diaz-Guzman E, Mireles-Cabodevila E, Arrossi A, Kanne JP, Budev M. Amiodarone pulmonary toxicity after lung transplantation. J Heart Lung Transplant. 2008;27(9):1059–63.
39. Jessurun GA, Boersma WG, Crijns HJ. Amiodarone-induced pulmonary toxicity. Predisposing factors, clinical symptoms and treatment. Drug Safety. 1998;18:339–44.
40. Myers JL, Kennedy JI, Plumb VJ. Amiodarone lung: pathologic findings in clinically toxic patients. Hum Pathol. 1987;18:349–54.
41. Garrean S, Massad MG, Tshibaka M, Hanhan Z, Caines AE, Benedetti E. Sirolimus-associated interstitial pneumonitis in solid organ transplant recipients. Clin Transplant. 2005;5:698–703.
42. Collins J, Hartman MJ, Warner TF, Muller NL, Kazerooni EA, McAdams HP, et al. Frequency and CT findings of recurrent disease after lung transplantation. Radiology. 2001;219:503–9.
43. Judson MA. Lung transplantation for pulmonary sarcoidosis. Eur Respir J. 1998;11:738–44.
44. Milman N, Andersen CB, Burton CM, Iversen M. Recurrent sarcoid granulomas in a transplanted lung derive from recipient immune cells. Eur Respir J. 2005;26:549–52.
45. Burke M, Stewart S, Ashcroft T, Corbishley C, Bishop P, Kjellstrom C. Biopsy diagnosis of disease recurrence after transplantation for pulmonary sarcoidosis: a multicenter study. J Heart Lung Transplant. 2001;20:154–5.
46. Karbowniczek M, Astrinidis A, Balsara BR, Testa JR, Lium JH, Colby TV, et al. Recurrent lymphangiomyomatosis after transplantation: genetic analyses reveal a metastatic mechanism. Am J Respir Crit Care Med. 2003;167(7):976–82.
47. Estenne M. Effect of lung transplant and volume reduction surgery on respiratory muscle function. J Appl Physiol. 2009;107(3):977–86.
48. Yang D, Wilson JM, Bai C, Yee J, Wilcox PG, Khalil N, et al. Acute exacerbation of pulmonary fibrosis following single lung transplantation. Can Respir J. 2012;19(1):e3–4.
49. MacMahon H, Austin JHM, Gamsu G, Herold CJ, Jett JR, Naidich DP, et al. Guidelines for management of small pulmonary nodules detected on CT scans: a statement from the Fleischner Society. Radiology. 2005;237(2):395–400.
50. Griffith KA, Sherrill DA, Siegel EM, Manolio TA, Bonekat HW, Enright PL. Predictors of loss of lung function in the elderly. Am J Respir Crit Care Med. 2001;163(1):61–8.
51. Sherman CB, Xu X, Speizer FE, Ferris BG, Weiss ST, Dockery DW. Longitudinal lung function decline in subjects with respiratory symptoms. Am Rev Respir Dis. 1992;146:855–9.
52. Lange P, Groth S, Nybee J, Mortensen J, Appleyard M, Jensen G, et al. Effects of smoking and changes in smoking habits on the decline of FEV1. Eur Respir J. 1989;2:811–6.
53. Knudson RJ, Lebowitz MD, Holberg CJ, Burrows B. Changes in the normal maximal expiratory flow–volume curve with growth and aging. Am Rev Respir Dis. 1983;127:725–34.
54. Knudson RJ. Aging of the respiratory system. Curr Pulmonol. 1989;10:1–24.

Chapter 6
The Role of Alloimmune T Cell Responses in Obliterative Bronchiolitis

Tereza Martinu

Abstract Obliterative bronchiolitis (OB) is the pathology thought to result from chronic lung allograft rejection. Anti-donor alloimmune T cells have been considered to be the main culprits in development of OB, although non-transplant and non-alloimmune etiologies of OB have also been identified. This chapter reviews basic concepts of transplant immunology, generation of alloimmune T cells, and T cell-mediated tissue injury. It further discusses the evidence supporting a role of alloimmune T cells in OB, based on human data and available animal models. Interactions between alloimmune T cells and other arms of the immune system immune system, such as the antibody response and innate immune cells, are described. New concepts in lung transplant immunology and recent landmark studies are reviewed, including data on regulatory T cells, Th17 responses, and local intrapulmonary immune events, which may have important implications for the future direction of basic lung transplant immunology research and development of therapeutics.

Keywords Alloimmune • Allorecognition • Alloantigen • T cell • Adaptive immunity • Lung transplant • Obliterative bronchiolitis • Chronic rejection • Cytokine • Major histocompatibility complex

Introduction

Post-lung transplant obliterative bronchiolitis syndrome (BOS) is equated with chronic lung allograft rejection. Consequently, the general dogma is that allograft long-term exposure to alloreactive T cells is key in the development of OB, the

T. Martinu, M.D. (✉)
Department of Medicine, Duke University Medical Center, 106 Research Drive, MSRB2, Suite 2073, DUMC Box 103000, Durham, NC 27710, USA
e-mail: tereza.martinu@duke.edu

K.C. Meyer and A.R. Glanville (eds.), *Bronchiolitis Obliterans Syndrome in Lung Transplantation*, Respiratory Medicine 8, DOI 10.1007/978-1-4614-7636-8_6,

pathologic manifestation of BOS. In fact, chronic rejection leads to occlusive fibrosis in other transplanted organs, such as chronic vasculopathy in heart transplant [1], arteriopathy along with bile duct vanishing disease in liver transplant [2], and arteriopathy with glomerulopathy in kidney transplant [3]. However, the lung's propensity to develop chronic rejection appears stronger than that of other organs, and the incidence of OB remains high in spite of improved immunosuppressive agents. One has to therefore wonder whether alloreactive T cell responses are in fact necessary and/or sufficient for development of OB. This very question will be analyzed and discussed in detail in this chapter. The lung is immunologically unique by its exposure to the environment, its extraordinary abundance of immune cells, and its susceptibility to recurrent injury and infections. Alloreactive T cells therefore function within a complex milieu of inflammatory and injurious stimuli that modulate or are modulated by rejection. While this chapter focuses on T cell-mediated alloreactivity, B cell-mediated responses and innate immune recognition of nonself molecular patterns are also important contributors to alloimmunity and are covered in other chapters.

The Alloimmune Response

Solid organ rejection is primarily based on host recognition of nonself donor antigens, which constitutes the alloimmune response. This alloimmune response is driven primarily by T cell recognition of foreign major histocompatibility complex (MHC) proteins, called human leukocyte antigens (HLA) in humans.

Major Histocompatibility Complex/Human Leukocyte Antigen

The MHC is the most polymorphic gene cluster in the vertebrate genome, and MHC molecules expressed on the surface of cells are highly variable between individuals of each species. The extraordinary diversity of MHC polymorphisms constitutes the main obstacle to transplantation, as the donor organ is quickly recognized as nonself on the basis of MHC differences with the recipient [4]. The MHC complex is divided into class I genes and class II genes, and more recently class III genes have been described [5]. MHC genes are expressed co-dominantly, meaning that an individual will express all MHC genes inherited from both parent. Each MHC molecule is composed of an extracellular peptide-binding cleft, a transmembrane domain, and a cytoplasmic domain (Fig. 6.1). It is the peptide-binding cleft that is polymorphic, allowing it to bind a large variety of antigenic peptides. MHC class I molecules are expressed on most nucleated cells. MHC class II molecules are expressed constitutively on antigen-presenting cells (APC), including dendritic cells (DC), macrophages, and B cells, but can be upregulated on these and other cells under inflammatory conditions [5].

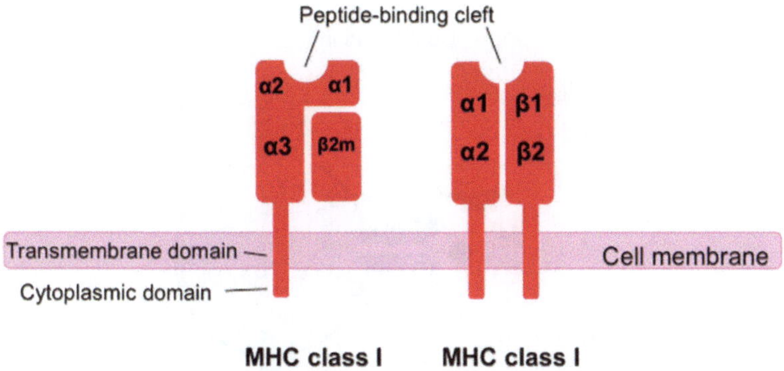

Fig. 6.1 Structure of major histocompatibility complex (MHC) molecules. The MHC class I molecule is composed of a polymorphic heavy α (alpha) chain and a non-polymorphic light β (beta) 2-microglobulin (β2m) chain. The α chain has a small cytoplasmic domain, a transmembrane-spanning domain, and an extracellular domain that is composed of three segments (α1, α2, and α3) and forms a peptide-binding cleft that presents antigen to CD8 T cells. The MHC class II molecule is a heterodimer with an α and a β chain. Both chains have an extracellular domain that includes two segments (α1, α2 and β1, β2), a transmembrane domain, and a cytoplasmic domain. The α1 and β1 domains together form the peptide-binding cleft that presents peptide to CD4 T cells

MHC molecules in mice are referred to as H-2 antigens, and these are recognized as the counterparts of HLA in humans. In humans, HLA genes are located on the short arm of chromosome 6 and are traditionally divided into two classes based on historic differentiation. The classical HLA class I genes include A, B, and C loci. The classical HLA class II genes include DR, DQ, and DP genes [5].

Alloantigen

An alloantigen is defined as a molecule on the allograft that is recognized as foreign by the recipient's alloreactive immune cells or antibodies. Most alloantigens are made up of polymorphic MHC peptides. Two individuals are allogeneic if they differ in their MHC molecules; twins or congenic mouse strains are identical in their MHC loci and are therefore syngeneic. In certain transplant settings, HLA matching can be performed to decrease allorecognition. In the case of lung transplantation, given the scarcity of organs and short time available for lung implantation, HLA matching is not usually performed, leading to a higher number of HLA mismatches compared to other organ transplantations [4].

T Cell Response to Antigen

T and B lymphocytes constitute the adaptive immune system in vertebrates, which is characterized by specificity, memory, and clonal expansion. In other words, T and

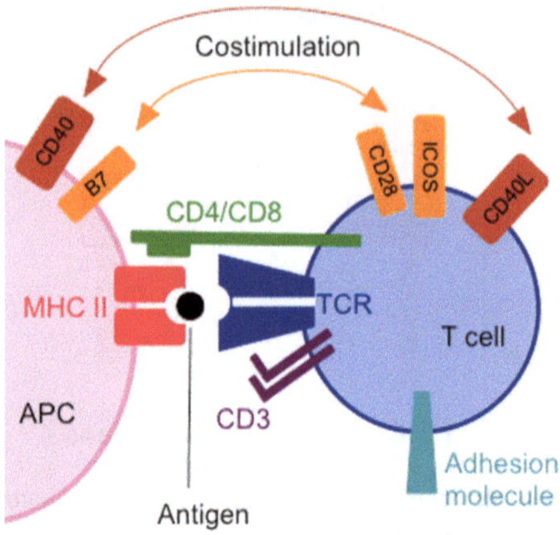

Fig. 6.2 T cell recognition of antigen. The antigen-presenting cell (APC) processes antigen and presents an antigenic peptide inside the peptide-binding cleft of its MHC molecule. The T cell receptor (TCR) binds this peptide with the help of the CD4 or CD8 coreceptor. The CD3 accessory protein helps with signal transduction. CD28, inducible T cell costimulator (ICOS), and CD40 ligand (CD40L) are costimulatory molecules expressed on the surface of T cells. They bind to costimulatory molecules B7 (of which there are many subtypes) and CD40 expressed by the APC. Adhesion molecules are also present on the surface of T cells and facilitate homing to tissue

B cells have the capacity to recognize specifically a large number of different peptides, generate memory cells with higher responsiveness to repeat stimuli, and rapidly produce clones of identical cells that can carry out the immune response. T cells recognize specific antigen through their T cell receptor (TCR), which is highly variable owing to somatic rearrangements. T cells also express several invariant signal transduction molecules that participate in antigen responses, such as CD3, coreceptors CD4 or CD8, costimulatory molecules CD28, ICOS, and CD40L, as well as adhesion molecules.

After emerging from the bone marrow, immature nonfunctional T cells first encounter MHC-bound peptides in the thymus, presented by thymic APC. Immature T cells that are able to bind self-MHC with adequate affinity receive a survival signal: this is called positive selection and leads to self-MHC restriction, meaning mature T cells should only bind to a foreign peptide when it is bound to a self-MHC. T cells that recognize self-peptides presented on self-MHC get deleted: this is called negative selection and protects against autoimmunity. The resulting mature T cells are, therefore, schooled to recognize foreign-peptide-self-MHC complexes.

After the selection process in the thymus, naïve T cells enter the circulation. T cells are recruited to sites of antigen presentation by responding to recruiting cytokines such as interleukin-2 (IL-2), which binds to the IL-2 receptor on T cells. There is also an abundance of cytokines that have been shown to cause chemotaxis or directional movement of T cells, and these are called chemokines. After binding to a foreign-antigen-self-MHC complex via their TCR (Fig. 6.2), naïve T cells are

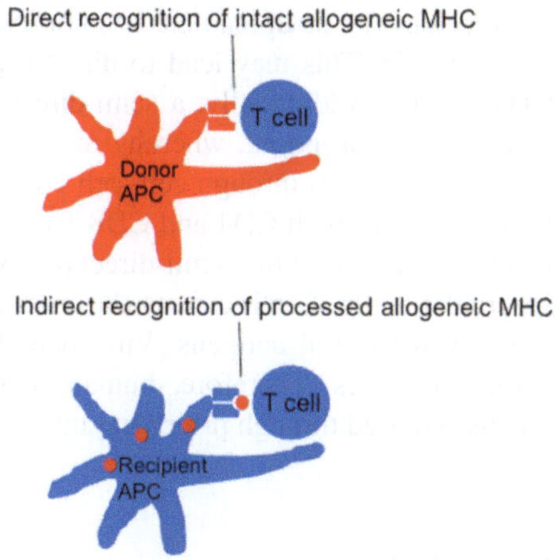

Fig. 6.3 Direct and indirect allorecognition. In the direct allorecognition pathway, T cells recognize intact allogeneic MHC molecules on donor cells. In the indirect allorecognition pathway, T cells recognize allogeneic MHC peptides processed and presented to them by recipient APC

activated, undergo clonal expansion, and become memory T cells. After encounters with known antigen, memory T cells proliferate and become effector T cells that produce pro-inflammatory signals and kill target cells [5].

T Cell Allosensitization

Even without prior exposure to alloantigen, naïve alloreactive T cells exist in the circulation, able to recognize an alloantigen-self-MHC complex. The frequency of naïve alloreactive T cells in humans is about 0.1 %, which is about a 1,000 times more frequent than any other T cell specificity. This high prevalence of alloreactive T cells has puzzled immunologists for decades and is now thought to be due to the inherent high affinity of the TCR for HLA molecules and the lack of thymic deletion of T cells that recognize allogeneic MHC [5, 6].

In general, T cells recognize antigens in the context of self-MHC (as opposed to B cells that can recognize soluble antigens as well) [5]. Nevertheless, in transplantation, unconventional recognition of antigen presented by nonself-MHC has been described through primary binding to the nonself-MHC molecule or primary binding to the antigen [6]. Consequently, there are two pathways for T cell allosensitization (Fig. 6.3). In the indirect pathway, recipient APC internalize and process donor antigens from dead cells and present alloantigen in the context of self-MHC to T cells. In the direct pathway, donor T cells directly recognize foreign MHC-peptide complexes on donor cells [4, 6–8]. The general thought is that the direct allosensitization pathway takes place early, potentiated by the greater presence of recipient MHC class II-expressing APC in the organ. Later, after transplant, as donor APC die out and there is increased donor cell injury, the indirect pathway takes over and remains active throughout the life of the allograft [9]. Furthermore, MHC expression is altered under inflammatory stimulation post-transplantation, and MHC class

II molecules can be upregulated on non-APC cells, such as epithelial or endothelial cells [10–12]. This may lead to direct recognition of structural allograft cells by CD4 T cells. Additionally, a semi-direct pathway of alloantigen recognition has recently been proposed, whereby recipient APC may acquire intact donor MHC-peptide complexes through cell–cell contact or exosomes, enabling recipient APC to interact with both CD4 and CD8 T cells simultaneously [13]. However, to date, no clear evidence of this semi-direct pathway occurring in lung transplant has been reported. Finally, T cells can also be cross-reactive to alloantigen through molecular mimicry with viral antigens. Viral peptides can resemble the variable region of MHC molecules. Therefore, humans may have clones of alloreactive memory T cells acquired through prior viral infections [14].

T Cell Subsets

CD4 vs. CD8 T Cells

T cells always express CD3 but differentially express the coreceptors CD4 or CD8. CD4 helper T cells (Th) recognize MHC class II molecules and require interaction with professional APC. As their name implies, the main function of CD4 Th cells is to help other cells by producing cytokines for CD8 T cell stimulation and activation of other inflammatory cells. CD8 T cells, called cytotoxic T cells (Tc), recognize MHC class I antigen. They can bind to any type of cell and have the ability to kill target cells by direct delivery of cytotoxic granules containing enzymes, such as granzyme B, that induce apoptosis [5]. In spite of this classical paradigm, CD4 and CD8 T cells have each been individually found to be sufficient for rejection of solid organs in animal models: CD4 T cells are capable of causing cytotoxic damage, and CD8 T cells can be activated by non-CD4-dependent mechanisms [15].

T Cell Polarization

The specific interaction of the APC with the T cell and the associated cytokine milieu determines subsequent T cell differentiation and polarization towards a certain phenotype characterized by a specific cytokine signature. This has been best described for CD4 helper T cells, but is now also known to take place in the case of CD8 cytotoxic T cells, which can assume similar phenotypes.

Th1 polarization is triggered usually by intracellular bacteria and viruses via APC production of IL-12 and interferon-γ (IFN-γ). IFN-γ activates the transcription factor T-box-expressed-in-T cells (T-bet), leading to Th1 differentiation and their own production of additional IFN-γ and IL-2. Th2 cells are known to produce IL-4, IL-5, and IL-13 and have been implicated in allergic responses. Th17 cells are potentiated by IL-23, produce IL-17, IL-21, and IL-22, and classically play a role in autoimmune diseases. Regulatory T cells (Treg) differentiate upon induction of the forkhead-box-protein-3 (FOXP3) transcription factor, make immunosuppressive IL-10, and are capable of suppressing other T cells [5]. Other Th polarization pathways have been described but are outside of the scope of this chapter.

Initial studies implicated mainly Th1 cells in the pathogenesis of organ rejection. However, more recent research has identified an important role for Th2, Th17, and Treg cells in organ transplantation and will be discussed further below. Alloreactive T cells are capable of polarization towards all four phenotypes [15].

Role of Allogeneic T Cell Responses in Human OB and BOS

There is no doubt that alloreactive T cells cause acute allograft rejection. However, while it is accepted that BOS represents chronic rejection of the lung allograft and that alloreactivity plays a role in its pathogenesis, the exact contribution of alloreactivity to OB is not entirely clear. T cells have been clearly identified in OB biopsies and are part of the active OB pathology grade (Fig. 6.4) [16]. The most important piece of evidence towards alloreactivity is, perhaps, the fact that OB, a relatively rare pathologic entity, is prevalent in lung as well as bone marrow transplant (BMT) recipients: alloreactivity is the common feature of those two patient populations. In BMT, T cell-depleted allogeneic stem cell transplant (SCT) is associated with a lower incidence of BOS than non-T cell-depleted allogeneic SCT [17]. Acute graft-versus-host disease, the hallmark of alloimmune recognition in BMT, increases the risk of subsequent BOS [17]; this is similar to the situation in lung transplantation whereby acute rejection increases the risk of BOS. What has puzzled the lung

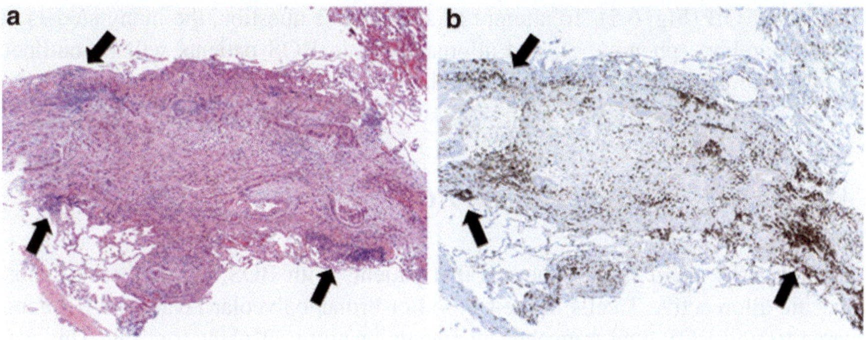

Fig. 6.4 Photomicrograph of an active OB lesion with infiltrating T cells. The tissue was obtained by bronchoscopic transbronchial biopsy from a lung transplant recipient. The pathology is described as active OB or a grade C1a lesion. (**a**) Shows a bronchiole obliterated with fibrous tissue and inflammatory cells, with a significant component of mononuclear cells (*arrows*) (hematoxylin and eosin stain). (**b**) Shows an adjacent section stained with anti-CD3 antibodies, showing clear T cell clusters within and on the periphery of the OB lesion (*arrows*) (peroxidase immunohistochemical stain). Courtesy of Dr. David Howell, Duke University Medical Center, Department of Pathology

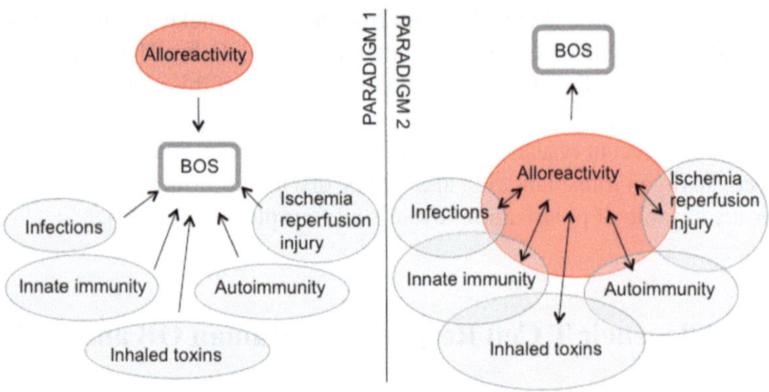

Fig. 6.5 Two paradigms of the role of alloreactivity in development of BOS. In paradigm 1, alloreactivity is just one of the many direct contributors to BOS and is capable of causing BOS by itself. In paradigm 2, other factors interact with each other and potentiate alloreactivity. Alloreactivity in turn augments the lung's response to other factors. The overall resulting injury causes BOS. Based on available data, paradigm 2 is closer to reality, with an ongoing crosstalk between various injurious pathways that all contribute to the disease

transplant community for decades has been the relative resistance of BOS to immunosuppression. Additionally, OB develops in non-transplant settings (e.g., toxin exposures, autoimmune diseases, respiratory syncytial virus infections), implying that alloreactivity is not absolutely necessary for development of this pathology. In reality, it is most probable that OB represents a common endpoint caused by a number of alloimmune and non-alloimmune injuries. The question then remains whether alloreactive T cell injury represents one of the insults that directly lead to OB or whether the allogeneic milieu increases susceptibility to other injuries that in turn cause OB (Fig. 6.5). To attempt to address this question, the many studies of T cell numbers, phenotypes, and alloreactivity in BOS patients will be outlined below. Animal studies will be discussed later.

Alloreactive T Cells in Human BOS

Several early, small studies showed that patients with BOS had increased donor-specific alloreactive T cells in their blood or bronchoalveolar lavage (BAL) compared to non-BOS lung transplant recipients or non-transplant controls. This was determined by measuring cell proliferation in cultures of BAL cells with donor splenocytes [18–20]. The largest of those studies included 28 patients and showed increased proliferation of peripheral blood and BAL lymphocytes upon exposure to donor spleen cells in BOS patients vs. non-BOS [20]. A more recent analysis found elevated anti-HLA antibodies and specific anti-donor-HLA T cell IFN-γ production in five BOS compared to five non-BOS patients [21]. However, at least one manuscript describes reduced T cell alloreactivity against donor cells in lung transplant patients compared to pre-transplant controls, unrelated to BOS or acute rejection [22]. The timing of the T cell alloreactivity measurement may be important. A study performed in kidney transplant recipients demonstrated that early post-transplant changes in donor-specific cytotoxic T cell activity were more predictive of graft survival than late changes [23]. It is possible that alloreactivity may wane with time and may be less active by the time BOS has fully developed.

Indirect Alloantigen Recognition and BOS

A number of studies suggest that indirect allorecognition is important for development of BOS. The assumption is that long-term presentation of donor alloantigens by recipient APC maintains persistent allorecognition over time and constitutes a mechanism for chronic rejection. Relevant manuscripts are listed and explained below.

Analysis of TCR variable gene repertoires in the peripheral blood showed oligoclonal expansion (i.e., cells with identical TCR genes) of circulating CD4 (but not CD8) T cells in a small cohort of lung transplant patients with BOS as compared to non-BOS. Therefore, it is possible that alloimmune responses in BOS are driven by indirect recognition of a small number of dominant alloantigens by recipient CD4 T cells [24, 25]. In a study of T cell alloproliferation in 8 OB patients compared to 11 stable patients, peripheral blood lymphocytes were hyperresponsive to alloantigen in the indirect route with concurrent direct hyporesponsiveness to donor cells. The investigators co-cultured recipient peripheral CD4 T cells with either a mixture of recipient APC and donor peptides (to test indirect allorecognition) or directly with donor APC (to test direct allorecognition). Proliferative responses were compared to responses to third-party (allogeneic but not donor) antigens [26].

Furthermore, a series of four smaller studies (5–7 patients in each arm) demonstrated increased indirect allorecognition of mismatched donor MHC I and II peptides by recipient lymphocytes in BOS patients as compared to non-BOS controls. Recipient peripheral blood cells were cultured in the presence of mismatched donor HLA peptides (which had to be presented indirectly by MHC molecules on recipient APC), and proliferative responses and CD4 precursor frequencies were measured [21, 27–29]. These data show that indirect T cell alloreactivity takes place in BOS patients, but this observation is based on small numbers of subjects and does not prove causality between alloreactivity and BOS.

T Cell Phenotypes in BOS

Only a few manuscripts show an increase in overall T cell numbers in BOS. An analysis of peripheral blood cells showed increased numbers of activated cytotoxic CD8 T cells with elevation of granzyme B and decreased CD4:CD8 ratio in seven BOS vs. seven non-BOS patients [30]. BOS patients were also found to have increased CD8 T cells in their endobronchial biopsies but not in their BAL [31]. In fact, studies of BAL total T cells have in general failed to show differences between BOS and non-BOS. Compared to non-transplant patients, lung transplant recipients had increased numbers of CD8 T cells [31–34] and granzyme B [35, 36] in their BAL without a significant difference between BOS and stable patients. This points towards the concept that there is general local intrapulmonary lymphocytic inflammation post-transplant that may change the lung's response to subsequent stimuli but that BOS itself is not necessarily accompanied by a significant lymphocytic inflammatory response. Nevertheless, T cell inflammation may precede BOS, as suggested by the finding that acute rejection is a BOS risk factor, as discussed further below.

While total T cell numbers may not be markedly different, the T cell phenotype appears altered in BOS. A BAL study of 48 BOS and 50 non-BOS patients showed increased numbers of activated CD4 and CD8 T cells based on expression of CD25 [37]. Using CD69 as a marker of T cell activation, activated T cells were found to be increased in the blood, induced sputum, and BAL of 12 patients with evolving BOS in comparison with stable post-transplant patients [38]. Analysis of peripheral blood cells of 10 BOS patients compared to controls showed that activated CD4+ CD28– T cells were more numerous, produced more perforin and granzyme B enzymes, were more resistant to cyclosporine, and were associated with worse lung function and with death [39]. Based on this data, T cells isolated in patients with BOS do appear to be more active.

Th1 T cell polarization has been thought to be the predominant T cell phenotype in BOS given elevation of several Th1 cytokines in the serum [21, 38] and increased Th1 CD3 T cells in the blood, induced sputum, and BAL of BOS vs. stable patients [38]. In general, Th1 responses are considered to be the main orchestrators of organ rejection, with data showing that skewing away from Th1 towards Th2 polarization may be protective [40, 41]. However, more recent studies have found alloreactive Th2 cells to be deleterious in other transplant settings: Notably, it appears that CD8 T cells in fact block Th2 polarization, and in situations where CD8 T cells are impaired, Th2 CD4 T cells can cause rejection [42–44]. In lung transplantation, there are few data supporting a potential benefit of Th2 polarization: One group showed an association between BOS and decreased CCL17 levels [45] and reduced CCR4 on T cells [46]. CCL17 recruits Th2 cells, but also regulatory T cells, via the CCR4 receptor [47]. Based on another publication, while IL-13-positive Th2 cells were elevated in BOS patients compared to non-BOS patients, they were highest in those patients in whom BOS had stabilized vs. others whose lung function continued to deteriorate, implying a potential protective function of Th2 [38]. Conversely, other studies imply that Th2 may be detrimental and pro-fibrotic, with increased IL-13 receptor expression on myofibroblasts in human OB lesions [48] and elevated and biologically active IL-13 in BAL from BOS patients compared to stable controls [49].

Data regarding CD30, a T cell activation marker produced mostly by Th2 cells [50], remains inconclusive. Two early studies showed that elevated serum-soluble CD30 (sCD30) correlates with BOS [51, 52]. However, this was not replicated in later studies [53, 54], one of which actually showed a general decrease in sCD30 post-transplant, suggesting that improved immunosuppression decreased sCD30 without affecting development of BOS [54]. Based on the available data regarding T cell polarization in lung transplantation, it is likely that Th2 cells and their cytokines potentiate BOS, although the exact Th2/Th1 balance and the specific role of alloreactive T cells are not fully understood and likely vary according to the state of alloreactivity and immunosuppression.

While Th17 autoreactive T cells have been described in human BOS patients [55], alloreactive Th17 cells have only been studied in animal models of lung transplantation and will be discussed below.

Effect of Anti-T Cell Therapies on BOS

Responsiveness of BOS to immunosuppression has been described. Early studies are useful, since the baseline immunosuppression used in the 1990s was generally lower than in recent times. One such study showed that 9 of 10 patients had slowing of their FEV1 decline after treatment with methylprednisolone and anti-thymocyte globulin [56]. Withdrawal of azathioprine in seven lung transplant recipients who were rejection-free for 2 years led to development of BOS in four of them, but treatment with steroids and reinstitution of azathioprine did not help [57]. In more recent studies, positive responses to augmented immunosuppression have also been described. Total lymphoid irradiation slowed down progression of BOS in 27 patients [58] as well as in another cohort of six azithromycin-unresponsive patients [59]. Alemtuzumab, which causes profound CD4 T cell depletion, slowed down BOS progression in 7 of 10 BOS patients [60]. Induction with alemtuzumab has also been associated with reduced BOS (46 % vs. 54 % at 5 years) [61].

In spite of the positive reports mentioned above, the use of heavy immunosuppression, and the improved treatment of acute rejection, the incidence of BOS remains around 50 % at 5 years [62–64]. Despite alemtuzumab induction, BOS still occurred in 46 % of patients at 5 years [61]. Some have proposed that there may be potent pro-inflammatory pathways unresponsive to post-transplant immunosuppression, as demonstrated by persistently elevated numbers of T cells in the BAL of lung transplant recipients as compared to non-transplant controls [34–36]. T cell production of pro-inflammatory cytokines, including IFN-γ and IL-2, was also shown to be elevated in the blood and BAL post-lung transplant [65, 66].

HLA Mismatching and BOS

An indirect proof that alloreactivity is important for development of BOS is the demonstration that HLA mismatching predisposes to BOS. However, studies of HLA matching in lung transplantation have been hampered by the small numbers of patients with high-level matching, thus making comparisons difficult. Early database reviews did not identify an association between HLA matching and BOS [67]. Nevertheless, the most recent large study of the OPTN database (9,791 patients) did show that total HLA mismatches and HLA class I mismatches correlated with development of BOS and survival. HLA class II mismatches correlated with acute rejection but not with BOS or survival. The authors proposed that HLA class II, expressed on donor-derived APC that are present in the graft early after transplant, are important in mediating acute rejection. Later after transplant, donor APC are depleted, and recognition of HLA I mediates chronic rejection [68]. Several prior smaller studies also found a link between BOS and HLA mismatching. Most of these studies identified an association between BOS and HLA class I mismatches [69–73]. One study reports that HLA-DR (class II) mismatches increase the risk for BOS in a multivariate analysis of 102 patients [74], and another found a link between BOS and male donor-female recipient matching in 98 patients [75].

Effector Functions of the Alloimmune Response

The alloimmune T cell response triggers three main mechanisms of tissue injury: (1) direct CD8 T cell cytotoxicity, (2) CD4-mediated delayed type II hypersensitivity (DTH) reaction, and (3) potentiation of the B cell-mediated antibody response. In addition, the Th2 response may lead to immunoglobulin E generation and eosinophil recruitment, causing mucosal inflammation and airway hyperreactivity. Th17 cells, in turn, produce IL-17, which causes a strong pro-inflammatory reaction.

CD8 T Cell Cytotoxicity

The most commonly described mechanism of allograft rejection is cellular killing by cytotoxic CD8 T cells. Preexistent alloreactive CD8 T cells can respond directly to class I MHC expressed on donor cells. CD8 T cells that have been primed indirectly by foreign-alloantigen-self-MHC complexes generally should not recognize alloantigen in the context of allo-MHC [5, 76]. However, there have been reports of indirectly primed CD8 T cells being able to cause rejection [77]. Alloreactive CD4 T cells provide cytokine help and activation signals for priming of naïve CD8 T cells. Unlike other organ transplants, in mouse models of lung allograft rejection, CD8 T cells have been shown to cause rejection even in the absence of CD4 T cells, likely through alternate costimulatory pathways [78]. Activated CD8 T cells cause injury by attaching to target donor cells and releasing cytotoxic granules and enzymes (such as granzyme B) that cause donor cell apoptosis [5]. In an in vitro study, CD8 T cells primed with allogeneic airway epithelial cells caused subsequent lysis of those airway epithelial cells by binding to MHC class I and by secreting factors that further increased epithelial expression of MHC and Fas ligand (a pro-apoptotic molecule) [79].

CD4-Mediated Delayed Type II Hypersensitivity Type Reaction

CD4 T cells can be primed directly by MHC class II on donor cells or indirectly by alloantigen presented on recipient MHC class II. These specifically primed (usually Th1) CD4 T cells can then contribute to a nonspecific effector mechanism with secretion of IFN-γ, IL-2, TNF-α (alpha), and other cytokines that lead to recruitment of inflammatory leukocytes including macrophages and monocytes, and this can stimulate production of mediators of tissue injury such as reactive oxygen species, nitric oxide, and prostaglandins [5].

Alloreactive T Cells as Potentiators of the Antibody Response

Generation of donor-specific antibodies has been correlated with development of BOS [80] and is described in another chapter. The allogeneic CD4 T cell response is important for generation of antibody-mediated rejection [81]. During the humoral response, B cells process alloantigen and present it to CD4 T cells. CD4 T cells in turn provide cytokine help to B cells to produce antibodies specific to alloantigen. The humoral response can then lead to either antibody-mediated cellular cytotoxicity or complement fixation with endothelial activation and injury [82, 83].

Targets of Alloimmune Injury

The potent direct recognition of MHC class II alloantigen by recipient T cells and the associated tissue injury may be explained by increased MHC class II expression on donor lung cells. IFN-γ, the primary Th1 cytokine, has been shown to increase MHC class II expression on airway epithelial cells in vitro [79]. Several early, small studies demonstrated that patients with OB have increased MHC class II on vascular endothelium as well as on tracheal, bronchiolar, and alveolar epithelium [84–86]. In 80 transbronchial biopsies from lung transplant patients, increased MHC class II (HLA-DR) expression was found on epithelial and endothelial cells with increased expression of cathepsin E, which is an aspartic proteinase involved in antigen processing [87]. The authors proposed that epithelial cells themselves may be able to trigger delayed-type hypersensitivity reactions due to CD4 T cell direct recognition of the donor MHC II presenting allopeptide [87]. Another small study showed increased expression of costimulatory CD80 and CD86 molecules on bronchial epithelial cells obtained by bronchial brushings from BOS compared to non-BOS patients. This lends additional credence to the idea that epithelial cells may be able to directly activate alloreactive T cells [88].

Acute Cellular Rejection as a Risk Factor for BOS

Thirty-six percent of patients have at least one episode of acute rejection in the first year post-lung transplantation [89]. This staggering incidence of acute rejection is thought to be one of the reasons for subsequent predisposition to BOS. In fact, acute rejection has been found to be predictive of BOS in multiple cohorts comprising greater than 100 patients [71, 74, 90]. Even minimal grade A1 rejection was identified as a risk factor for BOS in cohorts of 128 patients [91] and 228 patients [92]. A single episode of A1 was a predictor of BOS in a study of 259 patients [93]. Furthermore, acute bronchiolar-based rejection, manifested as lymphocytic bronchiolitis, has been found to be an independent predictor of BOS with more severe B grade predicting increased BOS incidence [94].

There are good data that acute rejection is mediated by alloreactive T cells. BAL T cells show specific hyperreactivity to donor splenocytes during acute rejection [20], and augmented immunosuppression is relatively effective in treating episodes of acute rejection [95]. On pathology, acute rejection is characterized by infiltrates of T cells in the perivascular and peribronchial regions of the allograft [96]. Although both CD4 and CD8 T cells are present in the infiltrate, CD8 T cells have been found to predominate in several studies and may represent mediators of cytotoxic tissue injury [37, 97].

The general assumption is that alloreactive T cells cause repetitive injury during acute rejection and, thus, trigger mechanisms ultimately leading to OB. In fact, acute rejection appears to further enhance mechanisms of allorecognition by a self-perpetuating feedback loop. Increases in HLA-DR (class II) expression on pulmonary epithelial and endothelial cells have been shown during acute rejection ($n = 14$) [98]. Furthermore, class I HLA molecules are released into the BAL [99] as well as into the circulation during acute rejection [100]. Circulating soluble HLA in the latter study correlated with later development of BOS. The authors postulated that soluble HLA antigens serve as substrates for indirect presentation to alloreactive T cells and further potentiate the alloimmune response and subsequent injury [100].

Interactions of Alloimmune T Cells with Innate Immune Responses

In contrast to the adaptive immune system, the innate arm of the mammalian immune system has lesser specificity and generally no capacity for immunologic memory. Nevertheless, it interacts constantly with adaptive immune cells and responds to injury and infections within the allograft. The lung's constant exposure to the ambient external environment and inhaled or aspirated pathogens is quite unique and has been thought of as a major contributor to the high incidence of acute rejection and BOS. The altered, post-transplant innate immune responses and their relationship to BOS are described in another chapter. While innate immune mechanisms are altered post-lung transplant and are clearly sources of graft injury, this section will discuss whether and how innate immune activation actually potentiates alloimmune T cell responses. Innate immune cells are recruited to and activated in the allograft by ongoing damage due to ischemia-reperfusion injury at the time of transplant, acute rejection, infections, and environmental insults. In fact, endothelial damage from acute rejection has been shown to generate APC-recruiting chemokines. Activation of APC in turn leads to (1) upregulation of surface MHC expression and increased presentation of alloantigen to T cells, (2) upregulation of costimulatory molecules, (3) inhibition of Treg suppression, (4) production of cytokines for T cell differentiation, and (5) production of cytokines that further recruit lymphocytes [101, 102].

Innate Immunity Triggers are Associated with Rejection

Several nonspecific, injurious post-transplant events have been associated with acute and/or chronic lung allograft rejection, constituting indirect evidence that innate immunity can potentiate alloimmunity. Primary graft dysfunction was shown to be associated with generalized upregulation of inflammatory cytokines (CCL2, CXCL10, IL-1β, IL-2, IFN-γ, IL-12) as well as with increased generation of allo-specific antibodies and T cells, increased Th1, and increased predisposition to BOS [21, 103]. Gastroesophageal reflux in human lung transplant recipients has been associated with increased incidence of acute rejection [104] as well as BOS [105]. A small study of a miniature swine lung transplant model showed that GERD increased indirect allorecognition of MHC class I alloantigen [106]. In an orthotopic rat lung transplant model, gastric acid aspiration was found to increase acute rejection [107] as well as OB with increased CD3 T cell infiltration and Th1 cytokine elevation [108], although specific changes in T cell allorecognition were not evaluated. Sendai viral infection also worsened airway obliteration in allografts but not in syngeneic grafts in a model of orthotopic lung [109] as well as orthotopic tracheal [110] transplantation in rats.

APC and T Cell Alloreactivity

APC are generally thought to present processed antigen to lymphocytes in the lymph nodes. However, recent research indicates that antigen presentation by APC can occur directly in the lung [111]. A study of human lung biopsies has identified increased presence of intrapulmonary APC in patients with BOS [112]. Using the orthotopic mouse lung transplant model, decreased APC recruitment to the lung using CCR2-deficiency led to decreased indirect T cell allorecognition. However, acute rejection still occurred, indicating that direct mechanisms of allorecognition were sufficient to generate acute rejection [113]. Similarly, local alveolar macrophage depletion in a model of rat lung transplant led to decreased Th1 responses, but overall acute rejection pathology remained unchanged [114]. Therefore, it has been postulated that APC presence may be important for potentiation of indirect recognition and subsequent chronic rejection. In fact, in the tracheal transplant airway obliteration model, CCR2 blockade did not change lymphocyte infiltration but did decrease OB-like pathology [115]. Additionally, epithelial and endothelial cells have been shown to be capable of participating in the innate immune response: combined allotransplantation and viral infection stimulated production of IL-12p80 by the airway epithelium, which led to macrophage accumulation and increased obliteration in the heterotopic tracheal transplant mouse model [116]. Additional research is needed to determine to what extent APC participate in development of post-transplant OB.

Toll-Like Receptor Signaling

APC express germ-line encoded pattern recognition receptors (PRR) that recognize conserved pathogen-associated molecular patterns (PAMP). The best-described PRR are the Toll-like receptors (TLRs). TLR signaling, mostly through the adaptor protein MyD88, activates downstream transcription factors that lead to maturation and activation of APC and their migration to lymph nodes [101, 102]. TLR signaling was found to be important for priming of alloimmune T cells by DC activated by hyaluronan, an endogenous matrix product that was found to accumulate during skin transplant-related injury and was elevated in BAL of BOS patients [117].

In several animal models of organ transplantation, MyD88 has been found to be important for indirect antigen presentation by DC as well as for Th1 differentiation of alloreactive T cells; however, acute rejection occurred through direct allorecognition independent of TLR signaling [118–120]. TLR signaling has also been shown to block established tolerance in models of heart, skin, and bone marrow transplantation [121–123]. TLR signaling is thus thought to likely play a larger role in chronic rather than acute rejection, as demonstrated in an animal model of chronic kidney rejection [124].

TLR signaling has not been specifically studied in animal models of chronic lung rejection. Nevertheless, human genetic studies suggest that it may have an important role, perhaps through its potentiation of indirect allorecognition, by showing that polymorphisms in TLR4 and its adaptor protein CD14 changed not only the risk of acute rejection in lung and kidney transplantation but also the risk of BOS [125–127].

Regulatory T Cells and Transplantation Tolerance

The occasional observation of long-term allograft acceptance in the absence of immunosuppression has long fascinated the transplant community, and mechanisms and potential therapeutic applications of tolerance have been heavily investigated.

Multiple immune cells, including regulatory T cells, B cells, macrophages, myeloid-derived suppressor cells, tolerogenic DC, and mesenchymal stromal/stem cells, have been described as having the potential to assume a regulatory immunosuppressive phenotype. This section will focus on regulatory T cells.

Regulatory T Cells

The best-described regulatory T cells (Tregs) are CD4 T cells that express the FOXP3 transcription factor as well as CD25 and are therefore usually identified as CD4+CD25+FOXP3+ triple positive cells. CD45RA or CD45RO is also expressed by human Tregs. Natural Tregs are selected in the thymus and function to suppress anti-self responses. Induced Tregs are generated from CD4 T cells in the periphery by pro-tolerogenic signals. Tregs cause suppression by direct contact via their cytotoxic T-lymphocyte antigen 4 (CTLA4) directly binding to other cells. CTLA4 binds to APC and prevents them from activating other T cells. Tregs also produce suppressor cytokines, such as IL-10, that inhibit APC and transform other T cells into regulatory T cells. In addition, CD8, CD4–CD8–, NKT, and gamma-delta regulatory T cells have been described and implicated in transplantation tolerance [128]. Tregs have been shown to prevent or slow down rejection in many animal models [129].

Tregs in BOS

Several studies have described Treg deficiencies in patients with BOS vs. without BOS, and it has been postulated that Tregs protect against chronic lung allograft rejection. Studies that were conducted before the use of FOXP3 as a marker of Tregs showed increased CD4+CD25+CD69– regulatory T cells in the blood [38, 130, 131] and in the BAL [38] of stable patients as compared with BOS patients. In vitro, these regulatory T cells were hyporesponsive, suppressive of other autologous T cells, and produced IL-10 [130]. Increased CD4–CD8– CD30+ pro-tolerant T cells were measured upon peripheral blood stimulation by donor spleen cells in stable compared to BOS patients [132]. Other studies showed elevation of serum IL-10 with concurrently decreased Th1 cytokines [21] as well as increased IL-10 production by peripheral blood CD4 T cells [133] in BOS vs. non-BOS patients.

FOXP3+ Tregs have been described in more recent manuscripts. Compared to BOS patients, stable patients were found to have higher numbers of Tregs in their blood that specifically stimulated proliferation of IL-10-producing anti-collagen-V suppressive T cells. These studies suggested that Tregs participate in suppressing the autoimmune pathways that may be responsible for BOS, which are described in another chapter [134, 135]. A study of Tregs in the BAL showed that CCR7+CD45RA– CD4+CD25+FOXP3+Tregs were associated with protection against BOS, although overall numbers of Tregs were not found to correlate with outcomes [136]. In a larger cohort, Treg prevalence, measured as FOXP3+ cells as a percentage of CD4 T cells, was increased in the BAL but not in the blood of 14 stable vs. 6 BOS patients [137].

A mechanistic analysis of Tregs and tolerogenic DC was performed using co-cultures of monocyte-derived DC and autologous lymphocytes from BOS vs. stable patients. The stable patient cell cultures were characterized by less mature DC with decreased CD80 and CD83 expression as well as increased Tregs, higher IL-10 levels, increased CTLA4, and decreased CD28 costimulation molecules. This indicated that DC from stable recipients induced a tolerant T cell phenotype while DC from BOS patients induced a pro-inflammatory T cell phenotype. The tolerogenic in vitro effect of DC on T cells could be abolished using anti-CTLA4 blockade [138]. This is consistent with data from other transplant settings indicating that tolerogenic DC are involved in promoting tolerance [139].

While small studies in lung transplantation showed that the immunosuppressive regimen did not affect Treg prevalence [131, 140], data from other transplant scenarios indicate that individual agents can alter Tregs. Calcineurin inhibitors decrease the overall number of Tregs via inhibition of IL-2, which is necessary for Treg function. However, at least some studies show that calcineurin inhibitors preferentially decrease conventional T cells, leading to an increase in the Treg to effector T cell ratio [129]. Alemtuzumab anti-CD52 therapy was followed by a shift from myeloid to the more tolerogenic plasmacytoid DC phenotype [141, 142]. Furthermore, post-alemtuzumab immune reconstitution preferentially increased CD8+CD28− suppressive T cells [143]. Rapamycin has been reported to promote Tregs in vitro [144] and in vivo [145]. Nevertheless, the combined effect of immunosuppressive agents in lung transplantation remains poorly understood.

While much more remains to be learned about Tregs in lung transplantation and their effect on BOS development, these cells represent an interesting potential therapeutic strategy. In fact, administration of Tregs [146] and potentiation of Tregs by oral tolerance therapy to collagen V decreased BOS in rat tracheal transplant models [147]. Alloantigen-specific Tregs would theoretically constitute an ideal targeted immunosuppressive modality.

Animal Models of OB and Lessons Learned

In this section, we will discuss animal models of alloimmune T cell-dependent BOS. However, toxin-induced and antibody-induced animal models of OB have also been developed.

The Rodent Heterotopic Tracheal Transplant Model

Many lung transplant immunology paradigms are based on the heterotopic (meaning "out of place") tracheal transplant model in mice and rats. This model consists of implanting the trachea under the skin (and in some instances the omentum) of an allogeneic animal and is characterized by a triphasic time course with initial Th1-dominated lymphocytic infiltration [148, 149], subsequent epithelial loss, and finally fibrotic obliteration of the trachea [150]. The fact that this tracheal obliteration occurs only in the allografts and not in syngeneic controls has been an important piece of evidence that alloimmune T cells are key in the development of this post-transplant obliterative airway disease (OAD) [151]. Furthermore, RAG1-knockout mice that lack lymphocytes do not develop obliteration of a tracheal allograft [152]. Nevertheless, non-alloimmune mechanisms are thought to contribute to the OAD in this model. If the tracheal allograft stays implanted in an allogeneic recipient for 14 days and is then retransplanted into a syngeneic recipient, OAD progresses in spite of the lack of alloimmune stimuli [153]. Furthermore, an orthotopically transplanted trachea does not undergo the same level of obliteration, suggesting that the ischemic injury of the non-vascularized, heterotopically transplanted trachea is an important pro-fibrotic factor [154–156]. Unlike human BOS, OAD in heterotopically transplanted tracheas responds well to anti-T cell therapies, such as calcineurin inhibitors via IL-2 receptor blockade [157, 158] or rapamycin [159].

Direct vs. Indirect Allorecognition in the Heterotopic Tracheal Transplant Model

Heterotopic tracheal transplantation leads to an early CD8 T cell infiltration at 2 weeks, followed by a CD4-predominant T cell infiltration at about 6 weeks [151]. This supports the simplified idea that CD8 T cells cause acute rejection by direct recognition of MHC class I in the allograft, while CD4 T cells cause chronic injury via indirect allostimulation by recruited recipient APC. Further support for this paradigm is provided by experiments where CD4 T cells were more effective than CD8 T cells at causing rapid onset OAD, even though CD4 or CD8 T cells alone were both sufficient to cause OAD [152]. Additional evidence for the importance of indirect allorecognition in this model of OAD comes from a study in which tracheas from transgenic mice that expressed human antigens were used as donors. Human antigens cannot be recognized directly by mouse CD8 T cells. Therefore, OAD that developed in this setting had to be due to indirect recognition through alloantigen presentation by recipient APC [160, 161].

Conversely, other experiments support a role of direct allorecognition by CD8 T cells in OAD pathogenesis. To more specifically evaluate direct allorecognition by CD8 T cells in this model, the capacity of a recipient mouse to reject tracheas mismatched for a single minor histocompatibility antigen presented uniquely in the context of MHC class I on the donor trachea was analyzed. This antigen can be recognized only directly by CD8 T cells. Mice developed OAD, but disease onset was delayed compared to the usual timeline [162].

Ultimately, both the direct and indirect allorecognition routes appear to play a role in rodent allogeneic tracheal obliteration. A comprehensive analysis of the role of MHC class I and/or II deficiency in the donor and/or recipient confirmed that the direct allorecognition pathway was sufficient to cause OAD, but the indirect allorecognition pathway was a stronger factor. Furthermore, MHC class I molecules were stronger alloantigens than MHC class II [163]. Another study showed that a single MHC class I molecule mismatch or a single minor antigen mismatch was insufficient to lead to OAD in spite of T cell accumulation. However, a combination of these two mismatches led to OAD, demonstrating cooperation between directly alloreactive CD8 T cells and minor antigen-specific CD4 T cells [164].

Costimulatory Blockade in the Heterotopic Tracheal Transplant Model

T cell costimulatory blockade has been shown to reduce OAD in models of heterotopic tracheal transplantation. One method of costimulatory blockade employed was CTLA4-immunoglobulin transfection, which blocks the interaction between CD28 on T cells and B7 expressed on APC [165–167]. Another T cell costimulatory molecule that binds to B7 is ICOS, and anti-ICOS treatment also decreased OAD in this model [168]. Other experiments demonstrated the importance of the costimulatory pathway and the interaction between CD40 expressed on APC and CD40 ligand (CD40L) on T cells. This was achieved using CD40L-deficient mice [169] or anti-CD40L antibody treatment [170]. CD40L-knockout recipients had ineffective allospecific priming of CD8 T cells with surprisingly preserved CD8 T cell proliferation but reduction in OAD, suggesting uncoupling of cell proliferation from effector function of the T cells [171].

IL-10 in Tracheal Transplant Models

The suppressive cytokine IL-10 plays an important role in development of OAD in the heterotopic tracheal transplant model. IL-10 blockade worsened OAD in the rat heterotopic tracheal allograft, while recombinant IL-10 significantly decreased disease [172]. Recombinant viral expression of IL-10 in this model also decreased OAD [173, 174]. These findings were further corroborated by experiments with the intrapulmonary heterotopic tracheal transplant model (described below) where lentivirally delivered IL-10 also decreased OAD [175].

T Cell Recruitment in Tracheal Transplant Models

T cell recruitment via chemokine gradients has been shown to mediate OAD in rodent tracheal transplant models. Upon binding to a specific receptor, chemokine proteins mediate chemotaxis or directional movement of cells, usually toward sites of inflammation.

After heterotopic allogeneic transplantation of mouse tracheas, antibody blockade of either the chemokine the chemokine receptor CXCR3, or its ligands CXCL9 or CXCL10, led to reduction of OAD and decreased recruitment of CXCR3+

mononuclear cells [176]. This was supported with human data showing elevated CXCL9, CXCL10, and CXCL11 chemokines in the BAL at the time of acute rejection or BOS [176]. Additional human data show increased CXCR3 receptor expression on T cells in biopsies of acute rejection and OB. BAL T cells obtained during rejection were found to express CXCR3 and demonstrated chemotaxis to CXCL10, and BAL macrophages and epithelial cells stained positive for CXCL10 [177]. In a later mouse study that used both the heterotopic and orthotopic tracheal transplant models, CXCR3 knockout recipients had decreased OAD, but disease in CXCL9 or CXCL10 knockouts was unchanged, suggesting that CXCR3 expression on recruited lymphocytes is important but that the ligands are redundant and may compensate for each other [178].

The CCL5 chemokine and its receptors CCR1 and CCR5 were also studied. Combined blockade of CCR1 and CCR5 as well as treatment with anti-CCL5 reduced OAD [179, 180]. Other T cell recruitment pathways have been shown to mediate OAD in rodent tracheal transplantation including the leukotriene B4 pathway [181] and the adenosine-A2B receptor pathway [182]. Adenosine, generated by the effect of the enzyme CD73, appears to stimulate recruitment of T cells via the A2B receptor but may provide important negative regulation of T cell chemotaxis in transplant by binding to the A2A receptors on T cells. Blockade of the adenosine-A2A receptor pathway was shown to increase OAD while its potentiation reduced OAD in models of rodent tracheal transplantation [183, 184].

Studies in other transplant models have questioned the utility of single chemokine blockade as therapeutic strategies to reduce rejection [185–187]. Many other chemokines appear to be elevated post-lung transplant [188, 189] with redundant activities, and it remains unclear whether single or multi-chemokine blockade may become a therapeutic strategy in human transplantation.

The Orthotopic Tracheal Transplant Model

In mice and rats that undergo orthotopic tracheal transplantation (wherein the trachea is sutured in series or in parallel to the native trachea), concentric subepithelial fibrosis occurs in the allografts. However, epithelial destruction and airway obliteration are much less pronounced than in the heterotopic model, indicating that the epithelial injury in the heterotopic setting may be due to ischemia-reperfusion injury [154–156]. This model was used to investigate the role of Tregs with the finding that administration of exogenous Tregs decreased peritracheal fibrosis [146].

The Orthotopic Mouse Lung Transplant Model

The development of the orthotopic single left lung transplant model in mice has been an exciting advancement for the field of lung transplantation immunology

[190]. While technically challenging, the ability to use mouse reagents while studying the whole transplanted lung has yielded several new observations relevant to the field. However, the difficulty of generating OB, the ultimate killer in human lung transplantation, has been a source of major frustration. In spite of severe acute rejection, no OB lesions were seen at 1 month post-transplant with findings of normal epithelium and increased levels of anti-apoptotic protein Bcl-2. The hypothesis is that mouse epithelial cells are resistant to alloimmune injury alone and that other stimuli are necessary for development of OB, such as ischemia, as seen in the heterotopic tracheal transplant [191].

Nevertheless, two groups have now reported OB in the orthotopic mouse lung transplant model using strategies that in effect reduce the alloimmune signal. The first study employed a transplant across a minor MHC antigen mismatch, which generated OB lesions in about half of the mice at 21 days [192]. The second group used immunosuppression with cyclosporine and reported that OB lesions develop 3 months following major MHC antigen-mismatched transplantation in approximately 50 % of the animals [193]. In both cases, the OB lesions developed in the setting of severe rejection and cellular infiltration of the allograft, which is different from the human OB lungs where relative sparing of the interstitial and alveolar tissue is usually seen.

Th17 in OB

Development of OB in the minor-mismatched orthotopic mouse lung transplant model was found to be dependent on IL-17, and OB was significantly reduced by IL-17 neutralization. Allospecific and collagen V-specific IL-17-producing lymphocytes were identified as likely contributors to the inflammation, suggesting that concurrent alloimmune and autoimmune processes were generating a Th17 response [192]. The Th17 pathway was not measured in the OB model post-cyclosporine treatment [193]. IL-17-producing alloreactive T cells were evaluated in another study of the orthotopic mouse lung transplant model using T-bet-deficient mice with a strong polarization towards Th17. IL-17-producing CD8 T cells were identified as potentiators of acute rejection in T-bet-deficient mice and were found to be resistant to anti-CD154 costimulatory blockade [194] . These findings are consistent with the association of small airway fibrosis after BMT using T-bet-deficient donors and strong Th17 polarization [195]. In humans, IL-17 has been found to be elevated in the BAL of patients with acute rejection [196], and IL-17-dependent collagen V T cell reactivity was associated with BOS in another study [55]. These studies make Th17 and IL-17 exciting candidates as mediators of BOS, but additional confirmatory studies need to be done in both animals and humans to fully understand the relationship between these immune pathways and airway fibrosis and obliteration.

Location of Allorecognition in Animal Models of OB

Classically, APC are thought to circulate from the transplanted allograft to lymph nodes where they present alloantigen to T cells. In fact, in animal models of other solid organ transplants, acute rejection can be prevented by disrupting the lymphatic circulation [197]. However, in human lung transplantation, the lymphatic circulation is not surgically reconnected at the time of transplant, and access of APC to recipient pulmonary lymph nodes is likely limited. In studies of transplantation of the intestine, which has intrinsic lymphoid tissue similar to the lung, residual donor APC were found in the donor intestinal lymphoid organs and constituted a major source of alloreactive T cell priming [198].

In the case of lung transplantation, it has been hypothesized that allorecognition occurs in the lung itself. Abundant MHC class II-positive APC can be found in the lung post-transplant [112], and bronchus-associated lymphoid tissue (BALT) has been proposed as a site of intrapulmonary T cell priming. Rodent tracheal transplant models have been used to investigate this question. After heterotopic transplantation of the allogeneic mouse trachea, allospecific CD8 effector T cells traffic to the native lung, suggesting that the lung functions as an immunologic organ [199]. In another set of experiments, investigators transplanted a rat trachea inside the lung of an allogeneic recipient rat. This model has been shown to generate OAD inside the intrapulmonary tracheal allograft and not in isografts [200, 201] and has been proposed as a way to study alloimmunity in the context of the actual lung environment. De novo lymphoid tissue was found in the lungs containing allogeneic tracheas, and this lymphoid tissue was capable of maintaining the allospecific effector function of memory T cells after transplantation into another syngeneic rat. This suggested an important role of inducible BALT in generation and maintenance of allorecognition [202].

A more definitive study was performed using the orthotopic mouse lung transplant model. Using recipients that completely lacked all lymphatic tissue, acute rejection still developed, and clusters of recipient T cells and donor DC were identified within the lung allograft. This demonstrated that acute rejection can occur without secondary lymphoid organs and that allorecognition can take place in the lung itself [111]. This implies that the lung may be the actual site of activation of naïve allogeneic T cells immediately after transplant, making some refer to the lung as a giant "lymph node with alveoli" [203]. This makes the lung distinct from most other transplanted organs and may also explain the persistence of the indirect allorecognition pathway, whereby recipient APC infiltrate the lung and recognize donor antigen a long time after transplant.

The Orthotopic Rat Lung Transplant Model

The orthotopic left lung transplant has also been performed in the rat. The technique is easier given the larger size of the animals compared to mice, but reagents and transgenic tools in this species have always been limited. With cyclosporine immunosuppression, this model develops minimal OB [204]. In the setting of lesser immunosuppression, small airway obliteration has been achieved but is not identical to human OB, showing severe acute rejection and whole lung cellular infiltration in addition to the OB lesions, which are similar to the orthotopic mouse lung transplant OB pathology. In one study, OB was seen 2 months after rat orthotopic lung transplantation with delayed methylprednisolone treatment. This study showed that acute rejection predisposes to OB and decreased immunosuppression increases OB [205]. Another group increased allorecognition after orthotopic rat lung transplant by presensitizing with a donor skin transplant 1 week prior to lung transplant. With rapamycin treatment and initial treatment with cyclosporine, OB was seen at day 84, with significant Th1 cytokine upregulation and decreased FOXP3 expression [206]. Another study showed that early initiation of everolimus or mycophenolate mofetil prevented development of OB, but institution of immunosuppression once OB had developed was not effective in decreasing disease progression [207, 208]. These studies support the notion that allorecognition is important in triggering OB pathogenesis, but further progression of OB may be independent of alloimmune mechanisms. The orthotopic rat lung transplant model has also been useful to study the effect of environmental insults on the allograft, and relevant studies are outlined in the section on innate immunity above.

Other Animal Models of OB

Other OB models have been developed that support the role of alloimmunity in the pathogenesis of the disease but have not been used much to advance our understanding of the mechanisms underlying the pathogenesis of OB.

Pigs

Heterotopic subcutaneous transplantation of lung fragments has been performed in pigs and yields airway obliteration within 21 days, which can be delayed with immunosuppression [209–211]. The orthotopic lung transplantation in miniature swine has been a little more popular. OB lesions appear after tapering immunosuppression along with infiltration of predominantly CD8 T cells and increased expression of MHC class II on the bronchiolar epithelium and increased DC [212]. When inbred miniature swine became available, studies were performed using MHC-matched animals. Transplanting across minor antigen mismatch only led to OB in four animals with documentation of anti-donor T cell proliferation and preponderance of CD8 T cells in the lung [213]. Similar to the rodent orthotopic lung transplant, OB lesions are found amidst a completely destroyed and fibrotic lung with severe A4 rejection. Tacrolimus but not cyclosporine has been found to induce long-term tolerance of the orthotopic lung without OB in this miniature swine mismatched for minor antigens [214]. A higher mismatch status for the MHC molecules increased OB and made the disease resistant to tacrolimus [215]. This expensive animal model has not been widely used in the transplant world.

Human-Mouse Chimera

An interesting variation on the heterotopic models has been developed whereby human small airways were implanted subcutaneously into an immunodeficient mouse with concurrent infusion of allogeneic human leukocytes. This human-mouse chimeric airway transplant model showed development of T cell infiltration, anti-donor-specific human T cell expansion, and OB-like disease in the transplanted airways. However, a syngeneic control was not provided in this study [216].

Mouse Bone Marrow Transplantation

Murine allogeneic BMT has been shown to generate small airway obliteration after cyclophosphamide treatment at 2 months in one study [217] and peribronchiolar fibrosis using donor T-bet deficiency and Th17 polarization in another study [195]. These models also allow the study of allogeneic mechanisms and concurrent environmental exposures in the study of OB-like disease in the whole mouse lung.

These animal models of OB have allowed significant progress in our understanding of the disease and now offer a good arsenal of tools to study mechanisms of OB in the future. However, lung pathology in any of these models is not identical to human OB, in which alveolar and interstitial sparing stands in stark contrast to the fibrotic obliterated airways. Additional modifications of these animal systems will hopefully yield even better ways of modeling human disease.

New Directions

The number of lung transplants performed worldwide has been increasing over the last several decades. With improved therapies of primary graft dysfunction, acute rejection, and infection, BOS has become, even more than before, the ultimate obstacle preventing further progress in the therapeutic modality of lung transplantation. Embarrassingly, we are still uncertain as to whether specific immunosuppressive regimens may in fact potentiate mechanisms of BOS by decreasing Tregs or potentiating Th2 or Th17 responses. With the growth of many lung transplant programs, collaborative clinical studies need to be set up to study the effects of immunosuppression on various arms of the immune system and on BOS. With modern flow cytometric and immunological assays combined with methods to study immune processes in samples obtained directly from the lung itself, we can now obtain more relevant and definitive answers. Our knowledge of T cell alloreactivity in BOS is based mostly on very small studies performed in the 1990s. This topic should be revisited with a larger numbers of patients, more precise reagents to measure donor and third-party alloreactivity, and comparison of peripheral vs. intrapulmonary cells. This will enable us to determine the effects of specific medical regimens on T cell function and T cell subsets and correlate these processes with precisely defined outcomes.

Furthermore, progress made in animal modeling of the disease is an important factor in allowing us to dissect the mechanisms of OB. Models that lead to generation of OB in the whole orthotopic lung combined with improved reagents and modern immunological tools such as in vivo imaging of immune cells and capacity for genetic manipulation in individual cell subsets will allow us to advance the science. It will be important to better understand the crosstalk between various arms of the immune system: adaptive vs. innate, alloimmune vs. autoimmune, Th1 vs. Th17 or Th2, Tregs vs. other T cells or APC. The application of modern immunologic methods will also allow characterization of interactions between immune cells and lung structural cells that generate the fibrotic structures.

Finally, with the progressive increase in clinical activity, validation of animal findings in human subjects and clinical application of suggested therapies can now occur at a faster pace.

Conclusion

The fact that OB can develop in the absence of alloimmune stimuli suggests that there is a common pathway shared by the post-transplant and non-transplant OB that can progress in spite of alloimmunity. Nevertheless, alloimmunity is an important contributor to development of post-transplant OB as demonstrated in the many studies cited above. In the clinical arena we continue to struggle with the balance of under- and over-immunosuppression, and effective therapies for BOS remain elusive. Fortunately, with the recent development of new animal models of OB, with the renewed interest in OB by the basic science community, and with the identification of novel mechanisms of this disease, we have entered into a very exciting time in the field of lung transplantation. While our understanding of OB development remains terribly limited, I submit that new ideas for pathogenesis and treatment are now on the horizon. Further progress will rely on continued interaction and collaboration among institutions, among lung transplant centers, and among investigators conducting basic, clinical, and translational research to achieve a common goal of unraveling BOS enigmas.

Acknowledgments The author would like to thank Drs. Kymberly M. Gowdy, Scott M. Palmer, and Rebecca A. Shilling for their critical feedback on this manuscript, as well as Dr. David N. Howell for providing the OB pathology photomicrographs.

References

1. Hornick P, Rose M. Chronic rejection in the heart. Methods Mol Biol. 2006;333:131–44.
2. Wyatt JI. Liver transplant pathology—messages for the non-specialist. Histopathology. 2010;57(3):333–41.
3. Ponticelli C. Progression of renal damage in chronic rejection. Kidney Int Suppl. 2000;75:S62–70.
4. Snyder LD, Palmer SM. Immune mechanisms of lung allograft rejection. Semin Respir Crit Care Med. 2006;27(5):534–43.
5. Abbas AK, Lichtman AH, Pillai S. Cellular and molecular immunology. 6th ed. Philadelphia, PA: Elsevier; 2010.
6. Felix NJ, Allen PM. Specificity of T-cell alloreactivity. Nat Rev Immunol. 2007;7(12):942–53.
7. Sayegh MH, Carpenter CB. Role of indirect allorecognition in allograft rejection. Int Rev Immunol. 1996;13(3):221–9.
8. Bradley JA. Indirect T, cell recognition in allograft rejection. Int Rev Immunol. 1996;13(3):245–55.
9. Liu Z, Sun YK, Xi YP, Maffei A, Reed E, Harris P, et al. Contribution of direct and indirect recognition pathways to T cell alloreactivity. J Exp Med. 1993;177(6):1643–50.
10. Romaniuk A, Prop J, Petersen AH, Nieuwenhuis P, Wildevuur CR. Increased expression of class II major histocompatibility complex antigens in untreated and cyclosporine-treated rat lung allografts. J Heart Transplant. 1986;5(6):455–60.
11. Chang SC, Hsu HK, Perng RP, Shiao GM, Lin CY. Increased expression of MHC class II antigens in rejecting canine lung allografts. Transplantation. 1990;49(6):1158–63.
12. Burke CM, Glanville AR, Theodore J, Robin ED. Lung immunogenicity, rejection, and obliterative bronchiolitis. Chest. 1987;92(3):547–9.
13. Gokmen MR, Lombardi G, Lechler RI. The importance of the indirect pathway of allorecognition in clinical transplantation. Curr Opin Immunol. 2008;20(5):568–74.
14. D'Orsogna LJ, Roelen DL, Doxiadis II, Claas FH. Alloreactivity from human viral specific memory T-cells. Transpl Immunol. 2010;23(4):149–55.
15. Csencsits KL, Bishop DK. Contrasting alloreactive CD4+ and CD8+ T cells: there's more to it than MHC restriction. Am J Transplant. 2003;3(2):107–15.
16. Stewart S, Fishbein MC, Snell GI, Berry GJ, Boehler A, Burke MM, et al. Revision of the 1996 working formulation for the standardization of nomenclature in the diagnosis of lung rejection. J Heart Lung Transplant. 2007;26(12):1229–42.
17. Huisman C, van der Straaten HM, Canninga-van Dijk MR, Fijnheer R, Verdonck LF. Pulmonary complications after T-cell-depleted allogeneic stem cell transplantation: low incidence and strong association with acute graft-versus-host disease. Bone Marrow Transplant. 2006;38(8):561–6.
18. Griffith BP, Paradis IL, Zeevi A, Rabinowich H, Yousem SA, Duquesnoy RJ, et al. Immunologically mediated disease of the airways after pulmonary transplantation. Ann Surg. 1988;208(3):371–8.
19. Reinsmoen NL, Bolman RM, Savik K, Butters K, Matas AJ, Hertz MI. Improved long-term graft outcome in lung transplant recipients who have donor antigen-specific hyporeactivity. J Heart Lung Transplant. 1994;13(1 Pt 1):30–6; discussion 6–7.
20. Rabinowich H, Zeevi A, Paradis IL, Yousem SA, Dauber JH, Kormos R, et al. Proliferative responses of bronchoalveolar lavage lymphocytes from heart-lung transplant patients. Transplantation. 1990;49(1):115–21.
21. Bharat A, Narayanan K, Street T, Fields RC, Steward N, Aloush A, et al. Early posttransplant inflammation promotes the development of alloimmunity and chronic human lung allograft rejection. Transplantation. 2007;83(2):150–8.

22. de Haan A, van der Gun I, Hepkema BG, de Boer WJ, van der Bij W, de Leij LF, et al. Decreased donor-specific cytotoxic T cell precursor frequencies one year after clinical lung transplantation do not reflect transplantation tolerance: a comparison of lung transplant recipients with or without bronchiolitis obliterans syndrome. Transplantation. 2000;69(7):1434–9.
23. Goulmy E, Stijnen T, Groenewoud AF, Persijn GG, Blokland E, Pool J, et al. Renal transplant patients monitored by the cell-mediated lympholysis assay. Evaluation of its clinical value. Transplantation. 1989;48(4):559–63.
24. Duncan SR, Valentine V, Roglic M, Elias DJ, Pekny KW, Theodore J, et al. T cell receptor biases and clonal proliferations among lung transplant recipients with obliterative bronchiolitis. J Clin Invest. 1996;97(11):2642–50.
25. Duncan SR, Leonard C, Theodore J, Lega M, Girgis RE, Rosen GD, et al. Oligoclonal CD4(+) T cell expansions in lung transplant recipients with obliterative bronchiolitis. Am J Respir Crit Care Med. 2002;165(10):1439–44.
26. Stanford RE, Ahmed S, Hodson M, Banner NR, Rose ML. A role for indirect allorecognition in lung transplant recipients with obliterative bronchiolitis. Am J Transplant. 2003;3(6):736–42.
27. SivaSai KS, Smith MA, Poindexter NJ, Sundaresan SR, Trulock EP, Lynch JP, et al. Indirect recognition of donor HLA class I peptides in lung transplant recipients with bronchiolitis obliterans syndrome. Transplantation. 1999;67(8):1094–8.
28. Reznik SI, Jaramillo A, SivaSai KS, Womer KL, Sayegh MH, Trulock EP, et al. Indirect allorecognition of mismatched donor HLA class II peptides in lung transplant recipients with bronchiolitis obliterans syndrome. Am J Transplant. 2001;1(3):228–35.
29. Lu KC, Jaramillo A, Mendeloff EN, Huddleston CB, Sweet SC, Patterson GA, et al. Concomitant allorecognition of mismatched donor HLA class I- and class II-derived peptides in pediatric lung transplant recipients with bronchiolitis obliterans syndrome. J Heart Lung Transplant. 2003;22(1):35–43.
30. Fattal-German M, Frachon I, Cerrina J, Ladurie FL, Lecerf F, Dartevelle P, et al. Particular phenotypic profile of blood lymphocytes during obliterative bronchiolitis syndrome following lung transplantation. Transpl Immunol. 1994;2(3):243–51.
31. Zheng L, Orsida B, Whitford H, Levvey B, Ward C, Walters EH, et al. Longitudinal comparisons of lymphocytes and subtypes between airway wall and bronchoalveolar lavage after human lung transplantation. Transplantation. 2005;80(2):185–92.
32. Ward C, Snell GI, Zheng L, Orsida B, Whitford H, Williams TJ, et al. Endobronchial biopsy and bronchoalveolar lavage in stable lung transplant recipients and chronic rejection. Am J Respir Crit Care Med. 1998;158(1):84–91.
33. Ward C, Whitford H, Snell G, Bao H, Zheng L, Reid D, et al. Bronchoalveolar lavage macrophage and lymphocyte phenotypes in lung transplant recipients. J Heart Lung Transplant. 2001;20(10):1064–74.
34. Hodge G, Hodge S, Chambers D, Reynolds PN, Holmes M. Bronchiolitis obliterans syndrome is associated with absence of suppression of peripheral blood Th1 proinflammatory cytokines. Transplantation. 2009;88(2):211–8.
35. Hodge S, Hodge G, Ahern J, Liew CL, Hopkins P, Chambers DC, et al. Increased levels of T cell granzyme b in bronchiolitis obliterans syndrome are not suppressed adequately by current immunosuppressive regimens. Clin Exp Immunol. 2009;158(2):230–6.
36. Hodge G, Hodge S, Li-Liew C, Chambers D, Hopkins P, Reynolds PN, et al. Time post-lung transplant correlates with increasing peripheral blood T cell granzyme B and proinflammatory cytokines. Clin Exp Immunol. 2010;161(3):584–90.
37. Slebos DJ, Postma DS, Koeter GH, Van Der Bij W, Boezen M, Kauffman HF. Bronchoalveolar lavage fluid characteristics in acute and chronic lung transplant rejection. J Heart Lung Transplant. 2004;23(5):532–40.
38. Mamessier E, Lorec AM, Thomas P, Badier M, Magnan A, Reynaud-Gaubert M. T regulatory cells in stable posttransplant bronchiolitis obliterans syndrome. Transplantation. 2007;84(7):908–16.

39. Studer SM, George MP, Zhu X, Song Y, Valentine VG, Stoner MW, et al. CD28 down-regulation on CD4 T cells is a marker for graft dysfunction in lung transplant recipients. Am J Respir Crit Care Med. 2008;178(7):765–73.
40. Huurman VA, Velthuis JH, Hilbrands R, Tree TI, Gillard P, van der Meer-Prins PM, et al. Allograft-specific cytokine profiles associate with clinical outcome after islet cell transplantation. Am J Transplant. 2009;9(2):382–8.
41. Hildebrandt GC, Choi SW, Mueller G, Olkiewicz KM, Moore BB, Cooke KR. The absence of donor-derived IL-13 exacerbates the severity of acute graft-versus-host disease following allogeneic bone marrow transplantation. Pediatr Blood Cancer. 2008;50(4):911–4.
42. Laffont S, Coudert JD, Garidou L, Delpy L, Wiedemann A, Demur C, et al. CD8+ T-cell-mediated killing of donor dendritic cells prevents alloreactive T helper type-2 responses in vivo. Blood. 2006;108(7):2257–64.
43. VanBuskirk AM, Wakely ME, Orosz CG. Transfusion of polarized TH2-like cell populations into SCID mouse cardiac allograft recipients results in acute allograft rejection. Transplantation. 1996;62(2):229–38.
44. Bagley J, Sawada T, Wu Y, Iacomini J. A critical role for interleukin 4 in activating alloreactive CD4 T cells. Nat Immunol. 2000;1(3):257–61.
45. Paantjens AW, Kwakkel-van Erp JM, van Ginkel WG, van Kessel DA, van den Bosch JM, van de Graaf EA, et al. Serum thymus and activation regulated chemokine levels post-lung transplantation as a predictor for the bronchiolitis obliterans syndrome. Clin Exp Immunol. 2008;154(2):202–8.
46. Paantjens AW, van de Graaf EA, Kwakkel-van Erp JM, Hoefnagel T, van Kessel DA, van den Bosch JM, et al. Lung transplantation affects expression of the chemokine receptor type 4 on specific T cell subsets. Clin Exp Immunol. 2011;166(1):103–9.
47. Iellem A, Mariani M, Lang R, Recalde H, Panina-Bordignon P, Sinigaglia F, et al. Unique chemotactic response profile and specific expression of chemokine receptors CCR4 and CCR8 by CD4(+)CD25(+) regulatory T cells. J Exp Med. 2001;194(6):847–53.
48. Lama VN, Harada H, Badri LN, Flint A, Hogaboam CM, McKenzie A, et al. Obligatory role for interleukin-13 in obstructive lesion development in airway allografts. Am J Pathol. 2006;169(1):47–60.
49. Keane MP, Gomperts BN, Weigt S, Xue YY, Burdick MD, Nakamura H, et al. IL-13 is pivotal in the fibro-obliterative process of bronchiolitis obliterans syndrome. J Immunol. 2007;178(1):511–9.
50. Pellegrini P, Berghella AM, Contasta I, Adorno D. CD30 antigen: not a physiological marker for TH2 cells but an important costimulator molecule in the regulation of the balance between TH1/TH2 response. Transpl Immunol. 2003;12(1):49–61.
51. Fields RC, Bharat A, Steward N, Aloush A, Meyers BF, Trulock EP, et al. Elevated soluble CD30 correlates with development of bronchiolitis obliterans syndrome following lung transplantation. Transplantation. 2006;82(12):1596–601.
52. Golocheikine AS, Saini D, Ramachandran S, Trulock EP, Patterson A, Mohanakumar T. Soluble CD30 levels as a diagnostic marker for bronchiolitis obliterans syndrome following human lung transplantation. Transpl Immunol. 2008;18(3):260–3.
53. Bauwens AM, van de Graaf EA, van Ginkel WG, van Kessel DA, Otten HG. Pre-transplant soluble CD30 is associated with bronchiolitis obliterans syndrome after lung transplantation. J Heart Lung Transplant. 2006;25(4):416–9.
54. Kwakkel-van Erp JM, Otten HG, Paantjens AW, van Kessel DA, van Ginkel WG, van den Bosch JM, et al. Soluble CD30 measured after lung transplantation does not predict bronchiolitis obliterans syndrome in a tacrolimus/mycophenolate mofetil-based immunosuppressive regimen. J Heart Lung Transplant. 2008;27(10):1172–5.
55. Burlingham WJ, Love RB, Jankowska-Gan E, Haynes LD, Xu Q, Bobadilla JL, et al. IL-17-dependent cellular immunity to collagen type V predisposes to obliterative bronchiolitis in human lung transplants. J Clin Invest. 2007;117(11):3498–506.
56. Snell GI, Esmore DS, Williams TJ. Cytolytic therapy for the bronchiolitis obliterans syndrome complicating lung transplantation. Chest. 1996;109(4):874–8.

57. Hoffmeyer F, Hoeper MM, Spiekerkotter E, Harringer W, Haverich A, Fabel H, et al. Azathioprine withdrawal in stable lung and heart/lung recipients receiving cyclosporine-based immunosuppression. Transplantation. 2000;70(3):522–5.
58. Fisher AJ, Rutherford RM, Bozzino J, Parry G, Dark JH, Corris PA. The safety and efficacy of total lymphoid irradiation in progressive bronchiolitis obliterans syndrome after lung transplantation. Am J Transplant. 2005;5(3):537–43.
59. Verleden GM, Lievens Y, Dupont LJ, Van Raemdonck DE, De Vleeschauwer SI, Vos R, et al. Efficacy of total lymphoid irradiation in azithromycin nonresponsive chronic allograft rejection after lung transplantation. Transplant Proc. 2009;41(5):1816–20.
60. Reams BD, Musselwhite LW, Zaas DW, Steele MP, Garantziotis S, Eu PC, et al. Alemtuzumab in the treatment of refractory acute rejection and bronchiolitis obliterans syndrome after human lung transplantation. Am J Transplant. 2007;7(12):2802–8.
61. Shyu S, Dew MA, Pilewski JM, DeVito Dabbs AJ, Zaldonis DB, Studer SM, et al. Five-year outcomes with alemtuzumab induction after lung transplantation. J Heart Lung Transplant. 2011;30(7):743–54.
62. Snell GI, Westall GP. Immunosuppression for lung transplantation: evidence to date. Drugs. 2007;67(11):1531–9.
63. Hopkins PM, McNeil K. Evidence for immunosuppression in lung transplantation. Curr Opin Organ Transplant. 2008;13(5):477–83.
64. Hartwig MG, Snyder LD, Appel III JZ, Cantu III E, Lin SS, Palmer SM, et al. Rabbit anti-thymocyte globulin induction therapy does not prolong survival after lung transplantation. J Heart Lung Transplant. 2008;27(5):547–53.
65. Hodge G, Hodge S, Reynolds P, Holmes M. Intracellular cytokines in blood T cells in lung transplant patients—a more relevant indicator of immunosuppression than drug levels. Clin Exp Immunol. 2005;139(1):159–64.
66. Hodge G, Hodge S, Reynolds PN, Holmes M. Increased intracellular pro- and anti-inflammatory cytokines in bronchoalveolar lavage T cells of stable lung transplant patients. Transplantation. 2005;80(8):1040–5.
67. Quantz MA, Bennett LE, Meyer DM, Novick RJ. Does human leukocyte antigen matching influence the outcome of lung transplantation? An analysis of 3,549 lung transplantations. J Heart Lung Transplant. 2000;19(5):473–9.
68. Peltz M, Edwards LB, Jessen ME, Torres F, Meyer DM. HLA mismatches influence lung transplant recipient survival, bronchiolitis obliterans and rejection: implications for donor lung allocation. J Heart Lung Transplant. 2011;30(4):426–34.
69. Harjula AL, Baldwin JC, Glanville AR, Tazelaar H, Oyer PE, Stinson EB, et al. Human leukocyte antigen compatibility in heart-lung transplantation. J Heart Transplant. 1987;6(3):162–6.
70. Sundaresan S, Mohanakumar T, Smith MA, Trulock EP, Lynch J, Phelan D, et al. HLA-A locus mismatches and development of antibodies to HLA after lung transplantation correlate with the development of bronchiolitis obliterans syndrome. Transplantation. 1998;65(5):648–53.
71. Schulman LL, Weinberg AD, McGregor CC, Suciu-Foca NM, Itescu S. Influence of donor and recipient HLA locus mismatching on development of obliterative bronchiolitis after lung transplantation. Am J Respir Crit Care Med. 2001;163(2):437–42.
72. Chalermskulrat W, Neuringer IP, Schmitz JL, Catellier DJ, Gurka MJ, Randell SH, et al. Human leukocyte antigen mismatches predispose to the severity of bronchiolitis obliterans syndrome after lung transplantation. Chest. 2003;123(6):1825–31.
73. Brugiere O, Thabut G, Suberbielle C, Reynaud-Gaubert M, Thomas P, Pison C, et al. Relative impact of human leukocyte antigen mismatching and graft ischemic time after lung transplantation. J Heart Lung Transplant. 2008;27(6):628–34.
74. van den Berg JW, Hepkema BG, Geertsma A, Koeter GH, Postma DS, de Boer WJ, et al. Long-term outcome of lung transplantation is predicted by the number of HLA-DR mismatches. Transplantation. 2001;71(3):368–73.

75. Roberts DH, Wain JC, Chang Y, Ginns LC. Donor-recipient gender mismatch in lung transplantation: impact on obliterative bronchiolitis and survival. J Heart Lung Transplant. 2004;23(11):1252–9.
76. Valujskikh A, Zhang Q, Heeger PS. CD8 T cells specific for a donor-derived, self-restricted transplant antigen are nonpathogenic bystanders after vascularized heart transplantation in mice. J Immunol. 2006;176(4):2190–6.
77. Lee RS, Grusby MJ, Glimcher LH, Winn HJ, Auchincloss Jr H. Indirect recognition by helper cells can induce donor-specific cytotoxic T lymphocytes in vivo. J Exp Med. 1994;179(3):865–72.
78. Gelman AE, Okazaki M, Lai J, Kornfeld CG, Kreisel FH, Richardson SB, et al. CD4+ T lymphocytes are not necessary for the acute rejection of vascularized mouse lung transplants. J Immunol. 2008;180(7):4754–62.
79. Smith CR, Jaramillo A, Duffy BF, Mohanakumar T. Airway epithelial cell damage mediated by antigen-specific T cells: implications in lung allograft rejection. Hum Immunol. 2000;61(10):985–92.
80. Palmer SM, Davis RD, Hadjiliadis D, Hertz MI, Howell DN, Ward FE, et al. Development of an antibody specific to major histocompatibility antigens detectable by flow cytometry after lung transplant is associated with bronchiolitis obliterans syndrome. Transplantation. 2002;74(6):799–804.
81. Bradley JA, Mowat AM, Bolton EM. Processed MHC class I alloantigen as the stimulus for CD4+ T-cell dependent antibody-mediated graft rejection. Immunol Today. 1992;13(11):434–8.
82. Steele DJ, Laufer TM, Smiley ST, Ando Y, Grusby MJ, Glimcher LH, et al. Two levels of help for B cell alloantibody production. J Exp Med. 1996;183(2):699–703.
83. Sawyer GJ, Dalchau R, Fabre JW. Indirect T cell allorecognition: a cyclosporin A resistant pathway for T cell help for antibody production to donor MHC antigens. Transpl Immunol. 1993;1(1):77–81.
84. Taylor PM, Rose ML, Yacoub MH. Expression of MHC antigens in normal human lungs and transplanted lungs with obliterative bronchiolitis. Transplantation. 1989;48(3):506–10.
85. Yousem SA, Curley JM, Dauber J, Paradis I, Rabinowich H, Zeevi A, et al. HLA-class II antigen expression in human heart-lung allografts. Transplantation. 1990;49(5):991–5.
86. Milne DS, Gascoigne AD, Wilkes J, Sviland L, Ashcroft T, Malcolm AJ, et al. MHC class II and ICAM-1 expression and lymphocyte subsets in transbronchial biopsies from lung transplant recipients. Transplantation. 1994;57(12):1762–6.
87. Arbustini E, Morbini P, Diegoli M, Grasso M, Fasani R, Vitulo P, et al. Coexpression of aspartic proteinases and human leukocyte antigen-DR in human transplanted lung. Am J Pathol. 1994;145(2):310–21.
88. Elssner A, Jaumann F, Wolf WP, Schwaiblmair M, Behr J, Furst H, et al. Bronchial epithelial cell B7-1 and B7-2 mRNA expression after lung transplantation: a role in allograft rejection? Eur Respir J. 2002;20(1):165–9.
89. Christie JD, Edwards LB, Kucheryavaya AY, Aurora P, Dobbels F, Kirk R, et al. The Registry of the International Society for Heart and Lung Transplantation: twenty-seventh official adult lung and heart-lung transplant report—2010. J Heart Lung Transplant. 2010;29(10):1104–18.
90. Burton CM, Iversen M, Carlsen J, Mortensen J, Andersen CB, Steinbruchel D, et al. Acute cellular rejection is a risk factor for bronchiolitis obliterans syndrome independent of post-transplant baseline FEV1. J Heart Lung Transplant. 2009;28(9):888–93.
91. Hopkins PM, Aboyoun CL, Chhajed PN, Malouf MA, Plit ML, Rainer SP, et al. Association of minimal rejection in lung transplant recipients with obliterative bronchiolitis. Am J Respir Crit Care Med. 2004;170(9):1022–6.
92. Khalifah AP, Hachem RR, Chakinala MM, Yusen RD, Aloush A, Patterson GA, et al. Minimal acute rejection after lung transplantation: a risk for bronchiolitis obliterans syndrome. Am J Transplant. 2005;5(8):2022–30.

93. Hachem RR, Khalifah AP, Chakinala MM, Yusen RD, Aloush AA, Mohanakumar T, et al. The significance of a single episode of minimal acute rejection after lung transplantation. Transplantation. 2005;80(10):1406–13.
94. Glanville AR, Aboyoun CL, Havryk A, Plit M, Rainer S, Malouf MA. Severity of lymphocytic bronchiolitis predicts long-term outcome after lung transplantation. Am J Respir Crit Care Med. 2008;177(9):1033–40.
95. Floreth T, Bhorade SM, Ahya VN. Conventional and novel approaches to immunosuppression. Clin Chest Med. 2011;32(2):265–77.
96. Martinu T, Pavlisko EN, Chen DF, Palmer SM. Acute allograft rejection: cellular and humoral processes. Clin Chest Med. 2011;32(2):295–310.
97. Donnenberg VS, Burckart GJ, Zeevi A, Griffith BP, Iacono A, McCurry KR, et al. P-glycoprotein activity is decreased in CD4+ but not CD8+ lung allograft-infiltrating T cells during acute cellular rejection. Transplantation. 2004;77(11):1699–706.
98. Hasegawa S, Ockner DM, Ritter JH, Patterson GA, Trulock EP, Cooper JD, et al. Expression of class II major histocompatibility complex antigens (HLA-DR) and lymphocyte subset immunotyping in chronic pulmonary transplant rejection. Arch Pathol Lab Med. 1995;119(5):432–9.
99. Rizzo M, Sundaresan S, Lynch J, Trulock EP, Cooper J, Patterson GA, et al. Increased concentration of soluble human leukocyte antigen class I levels in the bronchoalveolar lavage of human pulmonary allografts. J Heart Lung Transplant. 1997;16(11):1135–40.
100. DeVito-Haynes LD, Jankowska-Gan E, Heisey DM, Cornwell RD, Meyer KC, Love RB, et al. Soluble HLA class I in epithelial lining fluid of lung transplants: associations with graft outcome. Hum Immunol. 1997;52(2):95–108.
101. Oberbarnscheidt MH, Zecher D, Lakkis FG. The innate immune system in transplantation. Semin Immunol. 2011;23(4):264–72.
102. Goldstein DR, Palmer SM. Role of Toll-like receptor-driven innate immunity in thoracic organ transplantation. J Heart Lung Transplant. 2005;24(11):1721–9.
103. Bharat A, Kuo E, Steward N, Aloush A, Hachem R, Trulock EP, et al. Immunological link between primary graft dysfunction and chronic lung allograft rejection. Ann Thorac Surg. 2008;86(1):189–95; discussion 96–7.
104. Shah N, Force SD, Mitchell PO, Lin E, Lawrence EC, Easley K, et al. Gastroesophageal reflux disease is associated with an increased rate of acute rejection in lung transplant allografts. Transplant Proc. 2010;42(7):2702–6.
105. Cantu E III, Appel JZ III, Hartwig MG, Woreta H, Green C, Messier R, et al. J. Maxwell Chamberlain Memorial Paper. Early fundoplication prevents chronic allograft dysfunction in patients with gastroesophageal reflux disease. Ann Thorac Surg. 2004;78(4):1142–51; discussion 1142–51.
106. Meltzer AJ, Weiss MJ, Veillette GR, Sahara H, Ng CY, Cochrane ME, et al. Repetitive gastric aspiration leads to augmented indirect allorecognition after lung transplantation in miniature swine. Transplantation. 2008;86(12):1824–9.
107. Hartwig MG, Appel JZ, Li B, Hsieh CC, Yoon YH, Lin SS, et al. Chronic aspiration of gastric fluid accelerates pulmonary allograft dysfunction in a rat model of lung transplantation. J Thorac Cardiovasc Surg. 2006;131(1):209–17.
108. Li B, Hartwig MG, Appel JZ, Bush EL, Balsara KR, Holzknecht ZE, et al. Chronic aspiration of gastric fluid induces the development of obliterative bronchiolitis in rat lung transplants. Am J Transplant. 2008;8(8):1614–21.
109. Winter JB, Gouw AS, Groen M, Wildevuur C, Prop J. Respiratory viral infections aggravate airway damage caused by chronic rejection in rat lung allografts. Transplantation. 1994;57(3):418–22.
110. Kuo E, Bharat A, Goers T, Chapman W, Yan L, Street T, et al. Respiratory viral infection in obliterative airway disease after orthotopic tracheal transplantation. Ann Thorac Surg. 2006;82(3):1043–50.

111. Gelman AE, Li W, Richardson SB, Zinselmeyer BH, Lai J, Okazaki M, et al. Cutting edge: acute lung allograft rejection is independent of secondary lymphoid organs. J Immunol. 2009;182(7):3969–73.
112. Leonard CT, Soccal PM, Singer L, Berry GJ, Theodore J, Holt PG, et al. Dendritic cells and macrophages in lung allografts: a role in chronic rejection? Am J Respir Crit Care Med. 2000;161(4 Pt 1):1349–54.
113. Gelman AE, Okazaki M, Sugimoto S, Li W, Kornfeld CG, Lai J, et al. CCR2 regulates monocyte recruitment as well as CD4 T1 allorecognition after lung transplantation. Am J Transplant. 2010;10(5):1189–99.
114. Sekine Y, Bowen LK, Heidler KM, Van Rooijen N, Brown JW, Cummings OW, et al. Role of passenger leukocytes in allograft rejection: effect of depletion of donor alveolar macrophages on the local production of TNF-alpha, T helper 1/T helper 2 cytokines, IgG subclasses, and pathology in a rat model of lung transplantation. J Immunol. 1997;159(8):4084–93.
115. Belperio JA, Keane MP, Burdick MD, Lynch III JP, Xue YY, Berlin A, et al. Critical role for the chemokine MCP-1/CCR2 in the pathogenesis of bronchiolitis obliterans syndrome. J Clin Invest. 2001;108(4):547–56.
116. Mikols CL, Yan L, Norris JY, Russell TD, Khalifah AP, Hachem RR, et al. IL-12 p80 is an innate epithelial cell effector that mediates chronic allograft dysfunction. Am J Respir Crit Care Med. 2006;174(4):461–70.
117. Tesar BM, Jiang D, Liang J, Palmer SM, Noble PW, Goldstein DR. The role of hyaluronan degradation products as innate alloimmune agonists. Am J Transplant. 2006;6(11):2622–35.
118. Goldstein DR, Tesar BM, Akira S, Lakkis FG. Critical role of the Toll-like receptor signal adaptor protein MyD88 in acute allograft rejection. J Clin Invest. 2003;111(10):1571–8.
119. McKay D, Shigeoka A, Rubinstein M, Surh C, Sprent J. Simultaneous deletion of MyD88 and Trif delays major histocompatibility and minor antigen mismatch allograft rejection. Eur J Immunol. 2006;36(8):1994–2002.
120. Tesar BM, Zhang J, Li Q, Goldstein DR. TH1 immune responses to fully MHC mismatched allografts are diminished in the absence of MyD88, a Toll-like receptor signal adaptor protein. Am J Transplant. 2004;4(9):1429–39.
121. Chen L, Wang T, Zhou P, Ma L, Yin D, Shen J, et al. TLR engagement prevents transplantation tolerance. Am J Transplant. 2006;6(10):2282–91.
122. Walker WE, Nasr IW, Camirand G, Tesar BM, Booth CJ, Goldstein DR. Absence of innate MyD88 signaling promotes inducible allograft acceptance. J Immunol. 2006;177(8):5307–16.
123. Miller DM, Thornley TB, Pearson T, Kruger AJ, Yamazaki M, Shultz LD, et al. TLR agonists prevent the establishment of allogeneic hematopoietic chimerism in mice treated with costimulation blockade. J Immunol. 2009;182(9):5547–59.
124. Wang S, Schmaderer C, Kiss E, Schmidt C, Bonrouhi M, Porubsky S, et al. Recipient Toll-like receptors contribute to chronic graft dysfunction by both MyD88- and TRIF-dependent signaling. Dis Model Mech. 2010;3(1–2):92–103.
125. Palmer SM, Burch LH, Mir S, Smith SR, Kuo PC, Herczyk WF, et al. Donor polymorphisms in Toll-like receptor-4 influence the development of rejection after renal transplantation. Clin Transplant. 2006;20(1):30–6.
126. Palmer SM, Klimecki W, Yu L, Reinsmoen NL, Snyder LD, Ganous TM, et al. Genetic regulation of rejection and survival following human lung transplantation by the innate immune receptor CD14. Am J Transplant. 2007;7(3):693–9.
127. Palmer SM, Burch LH, Trindade AJ, Davis RD, Herczyk WF, Reinsmoen NL, et al. Innate immunity influences long-term outcomes after human lung transplant. Am J Respir Crit Care Med. 2005;171(7):780–5.
128. Wood KJ, Bushell A, Hester J. Regulatory immune cells in transplantation. Nat Rev Immunol. 2012;12(6):417–30.
129. Tang Q, Bluestone JA, Kang SM. CD4(+)Foxp3(+) regulatory T cell therapy in transplantation. J Mol Cell Biol. 2012;4(1):11–21.

130. Meloni F, Vitulo P, Bianco AM, Paschetto E, Morosini M, Cascina A, et al. Regulatory CD4+CD25+ T cells in the peripheral blood of lung transplant recipients: correlation with transplant outcome. Transplantation. 2004;77(5):762–6.
131. Meloni F, Morosini M, Solari N, Bini F, Vitulo P, Arbustini E, et al. Peripheral CD4+ CD25+ Treg cell expansion in lung transplant recipients is not affected by calcineurin inhibitors. Int Immunopharmacol. 2006;6(13–14):2002–10.
132. Polster K, Walker A, Fildes J, Entwistle G, Yonan N, Hutchinson IV, et al. CD4-veCD8-ve CD30+ve T cells are detectable in human lung transplant patients and their proportion of the lymphocyte population after in vitro stimulation with donor spleen cells correlates with preservation of lung physiology. Transplant Proc. 2005;37(5):2257–60.
133. Bianco AM, Solari N, Miserere S, Pellegrini C, Vitulo P, Pozzi E, et al. The frequency of interleukin-10- and interleukin-5-secreting CD4+ T cells correlates to tolerance of transplanted lung. Transplant Proc. 2005;37(5):2255–6.
134. Bharat A, Fields RC, Steward N, Trulock EP, Patterson GA, Mohanakumar T. CD4+25+ regulatory T cells limit Th1-autoimmunity by inducing IL-10 producing T cells following human lung transplantation. Am J Transplant. 2006;6(8):1799–808.
135. Bharat A, Fields RC, Trulock EP, Patterson GA, Mohanakumar T. Induction of IL-10 suppressors in lung transplant patients by CD4+25+ regulatory T cells through CTLA-4 signaling. J Immunol. 2006;177(8):5631–8.
136. Gregson AL, Hoji A, Palchevskiy V, Hu S, Weigt SS, Liao E, et al. Protection against bronchiolitis obliterans syndrome is associated with allograft CCR7+ CD45RA- T regulatory cells. PLoS One. 2010;5(6):e11354.
137. Bhorade SM, Chen H, Molinero L, Liao C, Garrity ER, Vigneswaran WT, et al. Decreased percentage of CD4+FoxP3+ cells in bronchoalveolar lavage from lung transplant recipients correlates with development of bronchiolitis obliterans syndrome. Transplantation. 2010;90(5):540–6.
138. Botturi K, Lacoeuille Y, Thomas P, Boniface S, Reynaud-Gaubert M, Magnan A. CTLA-4-mediated regulatory phenotype of T-cells in tolerant lung recipients. Eur Respir J. 2008;31(6):1167–76.
139. Solari MG, Thomson AW. Human dendritic cells and transplant outcome. Transplantation. 2008;85(11):1513–22.
140. Meloni F, Cascina A, Miserere S, Perotti C, Vitulo P, Fietta AM. Peripheral CD4(+)CD25(+) TREG cell counts and the response to extracorporeal photopheresis in lung transplant recipients. Transplant Proc. 2007;39(1):213–7.
141. Kirsch BM, Haidinger M, Zeyda M, Bohmig GA, Tombinsky J, Muhlbacher F, et al. Alemtuzumab (Campath-1H) induction therapy and dendritic cells: impact on peripheral dendritic cell repertoire in renal allograft recipients. Transpl Immunol. 2006;16(3–4):254–7.
142. Trzonkowski P, Zilvetti M, Friend P, Wood KJ. Recipient memory-like lymphocytes remain unresponsive to graft antigens after CAMPATH-1H induction with reduced maintenance immunosuppression. Transplantation. 2006;82(10):1342–51.
143. Trzonkowski P, Zilvetti M, Chapman S, Wieckiewicz J, Sutherland A, Friend P, et al. Homeostatic repopulation by CD28-CD8+ T cells in alemtuzumab-depleted kidney transplant recipients treated with reduced immunosuppression. Am J Transplant. 2008;8(2):338–47.
144. Kopf H, de la Rosa GM, Howard OM, Chen X. Rapamycin inhibits differentiation of Th17 cells and promotes generation of FoxP3+ T regulatory cells. Int Immunopharmacol. 2007;7(13):1819–24.
145. Shin HJ, Baker J, Leveson-Gower DB, Smith AT, Sega EI, Negrin RS. Rapamycin and IL-2 reduce lethal acute graft-versus-host disease associated with increased expansion of donor type CD4+CD25+Foxp3+ regulatory T cells. Blood. 2011;118(8):2342–50.
146. Shi Q, Cao H, Liu J, Zhou X, Lan Q, Zheng S, et al. CD4+ Foxp3+ regulatory T cells induced by TGF-beta, IL-2 and all-trans retinoic acid attenuate obliterative bronchiolitis in rat trachea transplantation. Int Immunopharmacol. 2011;11(11):1887–94.

147. Yasufuku K, Heidler KM, Woods KA, Smith Jr GN, Cummings OW, Fujisawa T, et al. Prevention of bronchiolitis obliterans in rat lung allografts by type V collagen-induced oral tolerance. Transplantation. 2002;73(4):500–5.
148. Boehler A, Bai XH, Liu M, Cassivi S, Chamberlain D, Slutsky AS, et al. Upregulation of T-helper 1 cytokines and chemokine expression in post-transplant airway obliteration. Am J Respir Crit Care Med. 1999;159(6):1910–7.
149. Neuringer IP, Walsh SP, Mannon RB, Gabriel S, Aris RM. Enhanced T cell cytokine gene expression in mouse airway obliterative bronchiolitis. Transplantation. 2000;69(3):399–405.
150. Boehler A, Chamberlain D, Kesten S, Slutsky AS, Liu M, Keshavjee S. Lymphocytic airway infiltration as a precursor to fibrous obliteration in a rat model of bronchiolitis obliterans. Transplantation. 1997;64(2):311–7.
151. Neuringer IP, Mannon RB, Coffman TM, Parsons M, Burns K, Yankaskas JR, et al. Immune cells in a mouse airway model of obliterative bronchiolitis. Am J Respir Cell Mol Biol. 1998;19(3):379–86.
152. Higuchi T, Jaramillo A, Kaleem Z, Patterson GA, Mohanakumar T. Different kinetics of obliterative airway disease development in heterotopic murine tracheal allografts induced by CD4+ and CD8+ T cells. Transplantation. 2002;74(5):646–51.
153. King MB, Pedtke AC, Levrey-Hadden HL, Hertz MI. Obliterative airway disease progresses in heterotopic airway allografts without persistent alloimmune stimulus. Transplantation. 2002;74(4):557–62.
154. Harada H, Lama VN, Badri LN, Ohtsuka T, Petrovic-Djergovic D, Liao H, et al. Early growth response gene-1 promotes airway allograft rejection. Am J Physiol. 2007;293(1):L124–30.
155. Minamoto K, Harada H, Lama VN, Fedarau MA, Pinsky DJ. Reciprocal regulation of airway rejection by the inducible gas-forming enzymes heme oxygenase and nitric oxide synthase. J Exp Med. 2005;202(2):283–94.
156. Minamoto K, Pinsky DJ. Recipient iNOS but not eNOS deficiency reduces luminal narrowing in tracheal allografts. J Exp Med. 2002;196(10):1321–33.
157. Hollmen M, Tikkanen JM, Nykanen AI, Koskinen PK, Lemstrom KB. Tacrolimus treatment effectively inhibits progression of obliterative airway disease even at later stages of disease development. J Heart Lung Transplant. 2008;27(8):856–64.
158. Gu Y, Takao M, Kai M, Lu L, Shimamoto A, Onoda K, et al. The role of cyclosporine A and interleukin-2 in obliterative airway disease in a rat tracheal transplant model. Ann Thorac Cardiovasc Surg. 2000;6(4):224–31.
159. Fahrni JA, Berry GJ, Morris RE, Rosen GD. Rapamycin inhibits development of obliterative airway disease in a murine heterotopic airway transplant model. Transplantation. 1997;63(4):533–7.
160. Smith MA, Jaramillo A, SivaSai KS, Naziruddin B, Kaleem Z, Patterson GA, et al. Indirect recognition and antibody production against a single mismatched HLA-A2-transgenic molecule precede the development of obliterative airway disease in murine heterotopic tracheal allografts. Transplantation. 2002;73(2):186–93.
161. Qu N, de Haan A, Harmsen MC, Kroese FG, de Leij LF, Prop J. Specific immune responses against airway epithelial cells in a transgenic mouse-trachea transplantation model for obliterative airway disease. Transplantation. 2003;76(7):1022–8.
162. Higuchi T, Maruyama T, Jaramillo A, Mohanakumar T. Induction of obliterative airway disease in murine tracheal allografts by CD8+ CTLs recognizing a single minor histocompatibility antigen. J Immunol. 2005;174(4):1871–8.
163. Chalermskulrat W, Neuringer IP, Brickey WJ, Felix NJ, Randell SH, Ting JP, et al. Hierarchical contributions of allorecognition pathways in chronic lung rejection. Am J Respir Crit Care Med. 2003;167(7):999–1007.
164. Richards DM, Dalheimer SL, Ehst BD, Vanasek TL, Jenkins MK, Hertz MI, et al. Indirect minor histocompatibility antigen presentation by allograft recipient cells in the draining lymph node leads to the activation and clonal expansion of CD4+ T cells that cause obliterative airways disease. J Immunol. 2004;172(6):3469–79.

165. Kita Y, Suzuki K, Nogimura H, Takahashi T, Kazui T. CTLA4Ig-gene transfection inhibits obliterative airway disease in rats. Ann Thorac Surg. 2003;75(4):1123–7.
166. Konishi K, Inobe M, Yamada A, Murakami M, Todo S, Uede T. Combination treatment with FTY720 and CTLA4IgG preserves the respiratory epithelium and prevents obliterative disease in a murine airway model. J Heart Lung Transplant. 2002;21(6):692–700.
167. Tikkanen JM, Lemstrom KB, Koskinen PK. Blockade of CD28/B7-2 costimulation inhibits experimental obliterative bronchiolitis in rat tracheal allografts: suppression of helper T cell type1-dominated immune response. Am J Respir Crit Care Med. 2002;165(5):724–9.
168. KleinJan A, Willart MA, Kuipers H, Coyle AJ, Hoogsteden HC, Lambrecht BN. Inducible costimulator blockade prolongs airway luminal patency in a mouse model of obliterative bronchiolitis. Transplantation. 2008;86(10):1436–44.
169. Rumbley CA, Silver SJ, Phillips SM. Dependence of murine obstructive airway disease on CD40 ligand. Transplantation. 2001;72(10):1616–25.
170. Fernandez FG, McKane B, Marshbank S, Patterson GA, Mohanakumar T. Inhibition of obliterative airway disease development following heterotopic murine tracheal transplantation by costimulatory molecule blockade using anti-CD40 ligand alone or in combination with donor bone marrow. J Heart Lung Transplant. 2005;24(7 Suppl):S232–8.
171. Shah PD, West EE, Whitlock AB, Orens JB, McDyer JF. CD154 deficiency uncouples allograft CD8+ T-cell effector function from proliferation and inhibits murine airway obliteration. Am J Transplant. 2009;9(12):2697–706.
172. Naidu B, Krishnadasan B, Whyte RI, Warner RL, Ward PA, Mulligan MS. Regulatory role of IL-10 in experimental obliterative bronchiolitis in rats. Exp Mol Pathol. 2002;73(3):164–70.
173. Shoji F, Yonemitsu Y, Okano S, Yoshino I, Nakagawa K, Nakashima Y, et al. Airway-directed gene transfer of interleukin-10 using recombinant Sendai virus effectively prevents post-transplant fibrous airway obliteration in mice. Gene Ther. 2003;10(3):213–8.
174. Boehler A, Chamberlain D, Xing Z, Slutsky AS, Jordana M, Gauldie J, et al. Adenovirus-mediated interleukin-10 gene transfer inhibits post-transplant fibrous airway obliteration in an animal model of bronchiolitis obliterans. Hum Gene Ther. 1998;9(4):541–51.
175. Hirayama S, Sato M, Liu M, Loisel-Meyer S, Yeung JC, Wagnetz D, et al. Local long-term expression of lentivirally delivered IL-10 in the lung attenuates obliteration of intrapulmonary allograft airways. Hum Gene Ther. 2011;22(11):1453–60.
176. Belperio JA, Keane MP, Burdick MD, Lynch III JP, Xue YY, Li K, et al. Critical role for CXCR3 chemokine biology in the pathogenesis of bronchiolitis obliterans syndrome. J Immunol. 2002;169(2):1037–49.
177. Agostini C, Calabrese F, Rea F, Facco M, Tosoni A, Loy M, et al. Cxcr3 and its ligand CXCL10 are expressed by inflammatory cells infiltrating lung allografts and mediate chemotaxis of T cells at sites of rejection. Am J Pathol. 2001;158(5):1703–11.
178. Medoff BD, Wain JC, Seung E, Jackobek R, Means TK, Ginns LC, et al. CXCR3 and its ligands in a murine model of obliterative bronchiolitis: regulation and function. J Immunol. 2006;176(11):7087–95.
179. Uchida O, Kajiwara N, Hayashi A, Miyajima K, Nagatsuka T, Hayashi H, et al. Met-RANTES ameliorates fibrous airway obliteration and decreases ERK expression in a murine model of bronchiolitis obliterans. Ann Thorac Cardiovasc Surg. 2007;13(2):82–6.
180. Suga M, Maclean AA, Keshavjee S, Fischer S, Moreira JM, Liu M. RANTES plays an important role in the evolution of allograft transplant-induced fibrous airway obliteration. Am J Respir Crit Care Med. 2000;162(5):1940–8.
181. Medoff BD, Seung E, Wain JC, Means TK, Campanella GS, Islam SA, et al. BLT1-mediated T cell trafficking is critical for rejection and obliterative bronchiolitis after lung transplantation. J Exp Med. 2005;202(1):97–110.
182. Zhao Y, LaPar DJ, Steidle J, Emaminia A, Kron IL, Ailawadi G, et al. Adenosine signaling via the adenosine 2B receptor is involved in bronchiolitis obliterans development. J Heart Lung Transplant. 2010;29(12):1405–14.
183. Lau CL, Zhao Y, Kron IL, Stoler MH, Laubach VE, Ailawadi G, et al. The role of adenosine A2A receptor signaling in bronchiolitis obliterans. Ann Thorac Surg. 2009;88(4):1071–8.

184. Ohtsuka T, Changelian PS, Bouis D, Noon K, Harada H, Lama VN, et al. Ecto-5′-nucleotidase (CD73) attenuates allograft airway rejection through adenosine 2A receptor stimulation. J Immunol. 2010;185(2):1321–9.
185. Kwun J, Hazinedaroglu SM, Schadde E, Kayaoglu HA, Fechner J, Hu HZ, et al. Unaltered graft survival and intragraft lymphocytes infiltration in the cardiac allograft of Cxcr3–/– mouse recipients. Am J Transplant. 2008;8(8):1593–603.
186. Zerwes HG, Li J, Kovarik J, Streiff M, Hofmann M, Roth L, et al. The chemokine receptor Cxcr3 is not essential for acute cardiac allograft rejection in mice and rats. Am J Transplant. 2008;8(8):1604–13.
187. Martinu T, Kinnier CV, Gowdy KM, Kelly FL, Snyder LD, Jiang D, et al. Innate immune activation potentiates alloimmune lung disease independent of chemokine (C-X-C motif) receptor 3. J Heart Lung Transplant. 2011;30(6):717–25.
188. Mamessier E, Milhe F, Badier M, Thomas P, Magnan A, Reynaud-Gaubert M. Comparison of induced sputum and bronchoalveolar lavage in lung transplant recipients. J Heart Lung Transplant. 2006;25(5):523–32.
189. Meloni F, Solari N, Miserere S, Morosini M, Cascina A, Klersy C, et al. Chemokine redundancy in BOS pathogenesis. A possible role also for the CC chemokines: MIP3-beta, MIP3-alpha, MDC and their specific receptors. Transpl Immunol. 2008;18(3):275–80.
190. Krupnick AS, Lin X, Li W, Okazaki M, Lai J, Sugimoto S, et al. Orthotopic mouse lung transplantation as experimental methodology to study transplant and tumor biology. Nat Protoc. 2009;4(1):86–93.
191. Okazaki M, Gelman AE, Tietjens JR, Ibricevic A, Kornfeld CG, Huang HJ, et al. Maintenance of airway epithelium in acutely rejected orthotopic vascularized mouse lung transplants. Am J Respir Cell Mol Biol. 2007;37(6):625–30.
192. Fan L, Benson HL, Vittal R, Mickler EA, Presson R, Fisher AJ, et al. Neutralizing IL-17 prevents obliterative bronchiolitis in murine orthotopic lung transplantation. Am J Transplant. 2011;11(5):911–22.
193. De Vleeschauwer S, Jungraithmayr W, Wauters S, Willems S, Rinaldi M, Vaneylen A, et al. Chronic rejection pathology after orthotopic lung transplantation in mice: the development of a murine BOS model and its drawbacks. PLoS One. 2012;7(1):e29802.
194. Lendermon EA, Dood-o JM, Miller HL, Zhong Q, McDyer JF. T-bet deficiency in mouse orthotopic lung transplant. J Heart Lung Transplant. 2012;31(4S):S30 (published in abstract form).
195. Gowdy KM, Nugent JL, Martinu T, Potts E, Snyder LD, Foster WM, et al. Protective role of T-bet and Th1 cytokines in pulmonary graft-versus-host disease and peribronchiolar fibrosis. Am J Respir Cell Mol Biol. 2012;46(2):249–56.
196. Vanaudenaerde BM, Dupont LJ, Wuyts WA, Verbeken EK, Meyts I, Bullens DM, et al. The role of interleukin-17 during acute rejection after lung transplantation. Eur Respir J. 2006;27(4):779–87.
197. Ng YH, Chalasani G. Role of secondary lymphoid tissues in primary and memory T-cell responses to a transplanted organ. Transplant Rev (Orlando). 2010;24(1):32–41.
198. Wang J, Dong Y, Sun JZ, Taylor RT, Guo C, Alegre ML, et al. Donor lymphoid organs are a major site of alloreactive T-cell priming following intestinal transplantation. Am J Transplant. 2006;6(11):2563–71.
199. West EE, Lavoie TL, Orens JB, Chen ES, Ye SQ, Finkelman FD, et al. Pluripotent allospecific CD8+ effector T cells traffic to lung in murine obliterative airway disease. Am J Respir Cell Mol Biol. 2006;34(1):108–18.
200. Dutly AE, Andrade CF, Verkaik R, Kugathasan L, Trogadis J, Liu M, et al. A novel model for post-transplant obliterative airway disease reveals angiogenesis from the pulmonary circulation. Am J Transplant. 2005;5(2):248–54.
201. Sato M, Liu M, Anraku M, Ogura T, D'Cruz G, Alman BA, et al. Allograft airway fibrosis in the pulmonary milieu: a disorder of tissue remodeling. Am J Transplant. 2008;8(3):517–28.
202. Sato M, Hirayama S, Hwang DM, Lara-Guerra H, Wagnetz D, Waddell TK, et al. The role of intrapulmonary de novo lymphoid tissue in obliterative bronchiolitis after lung transplantation. J Immunol. 2009;182(11):7307–16.

203. Shilling RA, Wilkes DS. Immunobiology of chronic lung allograft dysfunction: new insights from the bench and beyond. Am J Transplant. 2009;9(8):1714–8.
204. Lee AG, Wagner FM, Giaid A, Chen MF, Hamid Q, Serrick C, et al. Immunohistochemical characterization of inflammatory and proliferative events during chronic rejection in rat lung allografts. Transplantation. 1997;64(3):465–71.
205. Hirt SW, You XM, Moller F, Boeke K, Starke M, Spranger U, et al. Development of obliterative bronchiolitis after allogeneic rat lung transplantation: implication of acute rejection and the time point of treatment. J Heart Lung Transplant. 1999;18(6):542–8.
206. Jungraithmayr W, Vogt P, Inci I, Hillinger S, Arni S, Korom S, et al. A model of chronic lung allograft rejection in the rat. Eur Respir J. 2010;35(6):1354–63.
207. von Suesskind-Schwendi M, Brunner E, Hirt SW, Diez C, Ruemmele P, Puehler T, et al. Suppression of bronchiolitis obliterans in allogeneic rat lung transplantation—effectiveness of everolimus. Exp Toxicol Pathol. 2013;65(4):383–9.
208. von Suesskind-Schwendi M, Hirt SW, Diez C, Ruemmele P, Puehler T, Schmid C, et al. Impact of the severity of acute rejection in the early phase after rat lung transplantation on the effectiveness of mycophenolate mofetil to treat chronic allograft rejection. Eur J Cardiothorac Surg. 2012;42(1):142–8.
209. Uusitalo MH, Salminen US, Ikonen TS, Taskinen EI, Lautenschlager IT, Maasilta PK, et al. Alloimmune injury preceding airway obliteration in porcine heterotopic lung implants: a histologic and immunohistologic study. Transplantation. 1999;68(7):970–5.
210. Salminen US, Ikonen T, Uusitalo M, Taskinen E, Korpela A, Maasilta P, et al. Obliterative lesions in small airways in an immunosuppressed porcine heterotopic bronchial allograft model. Transpl Int. 1998;11 Suppl 1:S515–8.
211. Salminen US, Alho H, Taskinen E, Maasilta P, Ikonen T, Harjula AL. Effects of rapamycin analogue SDZ RAD on obliterative lesions in a porcine heterotopic bronchial allograft model. Transplant Proc. 1998;30(5):2204–5.
212. al-Dossari GA, Kshettry VR, Jessurun J, Bolman RM III. Experimental large-animal model of obliterative bronchiolitis after lung transplantation. Ann Thorac Surg. 1994;58(1):34–9; discussion 9–40.
213. Allan JS, Wain JC, Schwarze ML, Houser SL, Benjamin LC, Madsen JC, et al. Modeling chronic lung allograft rejection in miniature swine. Transplantation. 2002;73(3):447–53.
214. Shoji T, Muniappan A, Guenther DA, Wain JC, Houser SL, Hoerbelt R, et al. Long-term acceptance of porcine pulmonary allografts without chronic rejection. Transplant Proc. 2005;37(1):72–4.
215. Shoji T, Sahara H, Muniappan A, Guenther DA, Houser SL, Pujara AC, et al. An MHC class II disparity raises the threshold for tolerance induction in pulmonary allografts in miniature swine. Transplant Proc. 2006;38(10):3268–70.
216. Xue J, Zhu X, George MP, Myerburg MM, Stoner MW, Pilewski JW, et al. A human-mouse chimeric model of obliterative bronchiolitis after lung transplantation. Am J Pathol. 2011;179(2):745–53.
217. Panoskaltsis-Mortari A, Tram KV, Price AP, Wendt CH, Blazar BR. A new murine model for bronchiolitis obliterans post-bone marrow transplant. Am J Respir Crit Care Med. 2007;176(7):713–23.

Chapter 7
Antibody-Mediated Rejection and the Bronchiolitis Obliterans Syndrome

Henry W. Ainge-Allen and Allan R. Glanville

Abstract Why do apparently healthy, noninfected lungs fail after successful lung transplantation? Is there a unifying cause or do many insults and injuries lead to a stereotypic allograft response exacerbated by regional ischemia of the terminal bronchioles so that fibrogenesis dominates the histopathological result? These are basic questions that have troubled the lung transplant clinician since the first successful lung transplants were performed in the early 1980s. Perhaps we are closer to an understanding now, and the answer hinges, of course, on the concept of self and nonself and the recognition of the dichotomy that allows clonal expansion of B lymphocytes to mature into plasma cells that manufacture quantities of antibodies with allograft specificity ["the shock troops" of antibody-mediated rejection (AMR)]. The process is typically stealthy, however, and tends to remain clandestine until it is almost too late to undo or reverse the damage. If one does not seek, one will not find evidence that allograft damage is occurring due to AMR, and, as always, the tools that can be used to detect AMR are critical. We now have the tools, and the findings are quite overwhelming in their complexity. Therefore, some simplification is mandated. Hence, this chapter will attempt to clearly and succinctly explain how our understanding of the role and importance of antibodies to components of the pulmonary allograft has grown to the point where a seminal consensus can be reached about histopathological diagnosis that will help forge therapeutic endeavors with a novel uniformity of descriptive language, from whence adequate trials examining therapeutic efficacy will surely spring.

Keywords Antibodies • Capillaritis • Rejection • Chronic lung allograft dysfunction • Bronchiolitis obliterans syndrome

---

H.W. Ainge-Allen, M.D., Ph.D. • A.R. Glanville, M.B.B.S., M.D., F.R.A.C.P. (✉)
Lung Transplant Unit, St. Vincent's Hospital, Victoria Street,
Darlinghurst, Sydney, NSW 2010, Australia
e-mail: henryaingeallen@gmail.com; aglanville@stvincents.com.au

K.C. Meyer and A.R. Glanville (eds.), *Bronchiolitis Obliterans Syndrome in Lung Transplantation*, Respiratory Medicine 8, DOI 10.1007/978-1-4614-7636-8_7,

Introduction

The nature of antibody-mediated rejection (AMR) after solid organ transplantation (SOT) remains a topic of debate among pathologists, immunologists, and clinicians and represents one of the great frontiers of research in transplantation medicine. While AMR is well recognized as a cause of acute graft loss in the immediate postoperative period, it is perhaps the ultimate cause of graft loss in the long term as well. In fact, there is a strong belief that pulmonary AMR is implicated in the pathogenesis of refractory "chronic rejection" after lung transplantation (LTX) and can manifest itself as the bronchiolitis obliterans syndrome (BOS). AMR is thought to be the major cause of late graft loss after kidney transplantation [1], and it would be naïve to surmise that the same factors would not be operational after LTX and capable of leading to chronic lung allograft dysfunction (CLAD).

AMR is driven by the humoral or B-cell arm of the immune system as opposed to T-cell-mediated rejection, which is often referred to as "cellular rejection" [2]. In AMR, the recipient's immune system recognizes the extracellular peptides on the cells of the donor organ as nonself and produces antibodies against them. The binding of these antibodies to the donor organ results in an inflammatory process that includes complement-mediated cell lysis [3] and antibody-dependent cell-mediated cytotoxicity [4]. In this chapter, our discussion surrounding AMR will focus on the antigens that elicit an antibody response and the extent to which they each contribute to graft dysfunction rather than the basic concepts of AMR.

AMR in SOT refers broadly to the formation of a circulating antibody to the donor organ; however, it has been described primarily in the setting of the formation of donor-specific antibodies (DSA) against mismatched human leukocyte antigens (HLA). While the potential for antibodies against additional targets has been raised in recent years, AMR in common parlance refers primarily to these anti-HLA DSA. The HLA represents the major histocompatibility complex (MHC) in humans, which are the most polymorphic genes known, with more than 200 alleles of class I and class II HLA genes that are codominantly expressed, such that most individuals are heterozygous at each gene locus. Six different HLA subtypes are expressed on cell surfaces, three class I (A, B, C) and three class II (Dp, Dq, Dr). With codominant expression, individuals may code for a maximum of 12 different HLA gene products [5]. As such, the probability of random complete matching of donors and recipients in the setting of lungs is diminishingly small. We will explore the various diagnostic tests utilized in the detection of anti-HLA DSA and other antibodies later in the chapter.

The effects of DSA have been documented most comprehensively in class I HLA. HLA class I molecules are constitutively expressed on all nucleated cells in the body, although to varying degrees, and hematopoietic cells express the greatest amount. HLA class II molecules are expressed constitutively on the surface of some hematopoietic cells and thymic stromal cells; however, they can be expressed by other cells following exposure to the cytokine, interferon-γ(gamma), and on bronchial epithelia [6]. Interferon-γ, an inflammatory mediator, is released from T helper

Table 7.1 Stages of antibody-mediated rejection

Stage	Circulating antibody[a]	Biopsy specimen	Graft dysfunction
Stage I	Yes	Normal	No
Stage II	Yes	Normal C4D positive	No
Stage III	Yes	Abnormal C4D positive	No
Stage IV	Yes	Abnormal C4D positive	Yes

[a]Presence of circulating antibody to human leukocyte antigen or other donor antigens

cells, cytotoxic T cells, and natural killer cells during an inflammatory response [7]. There is growing evidence that DSA against class II HLA can result in AMR, which is supported by the expression of HLA class II molecules in the donor organ. This aspect of AMR will be explored later in the chapter.

The initiation of the classical pathway of the complement cascade by antibodies at the donor organ interface is a central event in the process of AMR. This consists of a series of enzyme cleavage reactions following the binding of C1q to the antigen–antibody complex that result in pathogen opsonization and peptide-mediated local inflammation. During this process, complement breakdown products are deposited on the endothelium and on the basement membranes of inflamed tissue [3]. Most significant from the standpoint of AMR is C4d, a breakdown product of activated C4b, which is deposited in the donor graft during AMR. C4d deposition is one of the best known markers for AMR, and positive staining for C4d in a graft biopsy concurrently with the detection of a circulating DSA is considered diagnostic of AMR [2].

Staging of AMR varies slightly from organ to organ (Table 7.1). In the kidney, AMR is a well-established phenomenon, and staging follows the 2005 Banff diagnostic criteria [2]. The general principles of staging, however, remain constant. Staging is dependent on the presence or absence of clinical graft dysfunction, histopathological changes, positive C4D staining, and circulating antibody, irrespective of whether the antibody specificity is anti-HLA or to an alternate donor antigen. These criteria are summarized below.

The presence of positive C4D staining in the absence of a detectable antibody is suspicious for AMR, but this is not included within the renal diagnostic criteria [1]. However, building evidence suggests that autoantibodies may play a significant role in AMR of the pulmonary allograft.

AMR has varied clinical presentations that extend beyond the realm of chronic graft dysfunction. These presentations appear to be dependent upon the mechanism of antibody production, the strength of the antibody response, and the timing of the AMR relative to transplantation. Hyperacute rejection (within the first 24 h) can result from high titers of pre-transplant antibodies, particularly anti-HLA DSA in the so-called "sensitized patient." This process is rapidly progressive and usually results in graft loss. Acute AMR may occur within the first week due to an anamnestic response that leads to a vigorous increase of a previously low-level or even undetectable pre-transplant antibody. Clinically, this is similar to hyperacute rejection and leads to rapid graft loss. In less severe cases, which sometimes occur in patients who were desensitized prior to transplantation, the graft is not lost, but long-term graft damage frequently occurs due to the acute event [8].

Recipients who are not pre-sensitized to donor antibodies can develop a de novo DSA response resulting in AMR. When this occurs acutely in the weeks and months after transplantation, it is typically aggressive, but it may be responsive to treatment. The development of late de novo AMR is often indolent, with a lengthy silent period that eventually manifests clinically as slowly progressive graft dysfunction [8]. It is suspected that this late-onset AMR plays a large part in chronic rejection processes and graft dysfunction. The extent to which these processes contribute to BOS after lung transplantation remains a focus for research.

There is also an emerging body of evidence to support the concept of non-HLA AMR as a potential cause of BOS. The lung allograft sustains injuries from a variety of sources that include ischemia reperfusion injury, alloimmunity, and external pathogens. Individually, collectively, and severally, these can lead to the release of inflammatory mediators and growth factors, thereby producing an environment that is conducive not only to alloimmune processes but autoimmune processes as well. While multiple autoantigens have been suggested as potential targets for this process, the two for which the strongest research evidence exists are collagen type V (Col-V) and K-α(alpha)1 tubulin. K-α1 tubulin is an antigen expressed on the surface of airway epithelial cells (AEC) [9]. Col-V is a minor collagen, intercalated within fibrils of collagen type I, and Col-V is considered a sequestered antigen in the normal lung due to its location within peribronchial and perivascular spaces. When the transplanted lung becomes inflamed, however, this antigen can be exposed and become a target for both cellular [10] and humoral immune responses [11].

AMR in Other SOT

AMR remains an area of research interest after lung transplantation and is beginning to assume a greater clinical relevance in day-to-day practice. Indeed, it is already recognized as a core clinical problem in transplantation of other solid organs. This relative paucity of data is largely due to the fact that we do not yet have large, long-term studies that focus on AMR in lung transplantation. Not surprisingly, the bulk of evidence for AMR comes from transplantation of the kidney, the organ in which it was first described. Williams et al. reported on hyperacute rejection in seven renal transplant recipients with preexisting circulating anti-HLA antibodies in 1968 [12]. Since that initial report, AMR has been shown convincingly to cause hyperacute, acute, and chronic rejection in the kidney as well as other solid organs [13]. The depth of evidence for AMR in renal transplantation relies on the numerical superiority of renal transplants that have been performed around the world. A total of 17,682 renal transplants in the United States in 2009 alone, which was 3 times the next most common transplanted organ and more than tenfold the number of lung transplants performed over the same period [14].

Though the strongest evidence for AMR lies in the settings of hyperacute and acute rejection, we will focus our discussions on the evidence that AMR represents a cause of chronic rejection and graft dysfunction in SOT, as this provides the most accurate parallel to CLAD in lung transplantation. The first evidence for the role of AMR in chronic rejection came in 1969, when Morris et al. detected HLA antibodies in 11/29 (38 %) of patients who had rejected their renal transplant after a minimum of 2 months post-transplant [15], and this percentage steadily rose with the development of more sophisticated investigations. In 2002, Lee et al. [16] reported that HLA antibodies were detected by enzyme-linked immunosorbent assay (ELISA) both pre- and post-transplantation for all 29 recipients who subsequently developed chronic rejection. This stood in contrast to an 11 % rate of HLA antibody detection in those who did not develop chronic rejection ($n=129$, $p<0.01$). However, a significant difference in graft survival times between those who did vs. those who did not develop HLA antibodies was not observed, and similar findings have been reflected in subsequent reports [17–20]. It was noted in some studies that class II HLA antibodies in particular were present prior to the onset of chronic rejection [18, 20].

More recently, anti-HLA DSA have been utilized to predict AMR. In 2003 Worthington et al. [21] reported on a study group in which 50.9 % of patients who progressed to graft failure within the 5-year follow-up period ($n=112$) demonstrated evidence of de novo DSA by ELISA as compared to 1.6 % in the control group ($n=123$). While this was highly significant ($p<0.01$), the antibodies were not detected in 36 % until after the onset of graft failure, and these results have been supported by subsequent work [19, 22]. The detection of DSA does not necessarily represent a timely or sensitive screening method for the prediction of chronic graft dysfunction in isolation, which is potentially due to adsorption of circulating antibodies by the graft. However, when the presence of de novo DSA is combined with other criteria that define clinical AMR, the combination provides a more accurate clinical picture.

C4d staining of grafts, a recognized part of the diagnostic criteria for AMR in renal transplantation, was initially demonstrated as an independent marker for acute rejection [2, 23]. In a retrospective review of 265 patients, Nickeleit et al. [24] did not find an association between C4d staining alone and chronic rejection. Subsequent studies have supported this [25]; however, when C4d is used in conjunction with other markers like DSA or transplant glomerulopathy, it is highly predictive of graft loss. Similar results have been published in the heart transplant literature. Rodriguez et al. [26] reported in 2005 that C4d deposition was detected in 16 patients from a consecutive series of 165 recipients who underwent right ventricular endomyocardial, biopsies but only 5 of the 16 recipients went on to develop AMR as determined by the combination of immunofluorescence criteria and clinical graft dysfunction. Of these five, three had circulating DSA by flow cytometry.

In 2009 Einecke et al. [19] reported on one of the major problems with the current diagnostic criteria for AMR. While 17 of 27 kidney failures after 1 year could be attributed to AMR if defined by microcirculation changes on biopsy and anti-HLA DSA, only seven fit the current definition for clinical AMR due to the requirements for positive C4d staining ($n = 173$). By multivariate analysis, C4d staining was not a significant factor. Indeed, there is a subset of recipients with DSA who develop AMR in the absence of C4d staining, and evidence indicates that C4d, though it represents an excellent marker for acute graft rejection, is less sensitive in predicting chronic rejection.

Though DSA antibodies have more of a role in the hyperacute and acute setting, it is worth briefly mentioning the impact of recipient pre-sensitization to DSA on graft loss. In 2008 Lefaucheur et al. [27] analyzed the significance of pre-sensitization with DSA prior to transplantation and found an 8-year graft survival of 67.95 % in those with preformed DSA vs. 77.3 % in those without preformed DSA ($p = 0.03$). The incidence of AMR in those with pre-transplant DSA was 34.9 %, and these recipients had an 8-year graft survival of 43.6 %. Although the episodes of AMR associated with graft dysfunction occurred mainly in the acute setting with a median onset at 16 days post-transplant, the group continued to experience more graft loss out to 8 years.

Pulmonary AMR

Given that AMR represents a major cause of progressive chronic allograft dysfunction in other solid organ transplants, it seems intuitive that it plays a role after lung transplantation, where CLAD predominantly manifests as BOS. In 1998 two retrospective analyses demonstrated that the development of antibodies to HLA after transplantation correlated significantly with BOS ($p = 0.02$) [28]. Work by Sundaresan et al. determined that HLA antibodies were a significant predictor of BOS by both univariate and multivariate analysis [29].

While this fits with the putative process of AMR in other SOT, at present there are only limited data on the effects of DSA as a marker of AMR after lung transplantation. No studies have a follow-up of greater than 2 years. To our knowledge, no studies in LTX have yet examined the impact of pre-sensitization with DSA. In 2010 Hachem et al. [30] reported on a protocol change at their institute in which they preemptively treated patients who developed de novo DSA with intravenous gammaglobulin and rituximab (the specifics of therapy for AMR will be discussed later in the chapter). Given the nature of the therapy, it is not surprising that they did not detect an association between the treatment arm and BOS ($n = 116$), although there was an association between those who had persistent DSA after treatment and the development of BOS ($p = 0.03$). Four patients who did not receive treatment due to concurrent critical illness all died within 30 days.

The strong evidence from other SOT [17, 19, 21] makes it unlikely that a prospective, placebo-controlled study will provide a direct comparison between patients with untreated DSA and DSA negative patients due to ethical concerns. However, it is possible that studies with longer follow-up periods may elicit further information. A study by Worthington et al. in renal transplant recipients found that the mean time from antibody production to graft failure was 996.9 days [21], while the longest follow-up period in a study directly investigating DSA in LTX was 2 years by Hachem et al. [30]. The LTX literature may simply not yet have reports for which the duration of follow-up time required to demonstrate the full effects *of* de novo DSA is adequate.

One of the most salient points of evidence from other SOT is that the detection of anti-HLA DSA represents a more sensitive predictor of chronic graft dysfunction when it is used in conjunction with C4d staining of the graft [25, 26]. In 2003 Magro et al. [31] reported that C4d deposition in septal capillaries corresponded to morphological evidence of AMR as defined by septal capillary necrosis in 30 of 33 cases, with higher deposition patterns corresponding to more marked capillary necrosis and absent or limited deposition demonstrating minimal or no necrosis. Additionally, all patients with symptomatic acute rejection showed histopathological evidence compatible with AMR, and patients with BOS were found to have deposits of C4d and other immunoreactants in the bronchial wall. However, the only statistically significant finding for BOS was the deposition of C1q within the bronchial wall. They did not find any association with HLA antibodies as detected by panel-reactive antibodies (PRA), which led them to conclude that AMR after LTX was not HLA mediated. With the benefit of hindsight, it is arguable that more sensitive screens for HLA antibodies now available may have detected DSA in these cases. Alternatively, these cases may indeed have represented true non-HLA-mediated AMR.

Concurrent work by the same group [32] directly explored the involvement of humoral immunity as a potential cause of BOS. Fresh frozen tissue from 13 single-lung transplant recipients was analyzed for deposition of C1q, C4d, C5b-9, and IgG, IgM, and IgA. An indirect immunofluorescent assay was also conducted with patient serum against cytospins of the pulmonary endothelium. In each case, the tissue samples showed a microvascular injury syndrome involving the bronchial wall that was characterized by one or more of hemorrhage, fibrin deposition, and endothelial cell necrosis. Other features included bronchial epithelial and chondrocyte necrosis. The end-stage lesion was a thinned bronchial epithelial lining with mural fibrosis. Immunofluorescent analysis showed deposition of C1q, C3, C4d, C5b-9, and Ig in the bronchial epithelium, chondrocytes, basement membrane zone of the bronchial epithelium, and bronchial wall microvasculature. The indirect anti-endothelial cell antibody assay result was positive in all instances where it was tested. It was concluded that AMR may be involved in the pathogenesis of BOS and that the antigenic targets included the bronchial wall microvasculature, the bronchial epithelium, and chondrocytes.

While this intriguing body of work stands as direct evidence for an antibody-mediated process as a cause of BOS, at present there is a lack of consensus in the literature, with conflicting reports on the utility of C4d and other immunohistochemical markers in AMR. Wallace et al. [33] retrospectively stained transbronchial biopsies ($n = 68$) from recipients with acute cellular rejection, obliterative bronchiolitis, or diffuse alveolar damage for C4d and found a variable, focal, nonspecific staining pattern of C4d that was not consistent across the different diagnostic groups. Another study by the Pittsburgh group [34] reported that specific subendothelial C4d deposition was seen in 5 of 16 (31 %) patients with anti-HLA-Ab and was absent in 16 patients without anti-HLA-Ab ($p < 0.05$). Because only 4 of 15 of those who developed BOS demonstrated positive C4d staining, they concluded that C4d was not a sensitive marker for BOS. With no large studies on the utility of C4d to date, this clinical question remains unanswered. Perhaps the devil is in the detail, and the variability of conclusions reflects a lack of consensus criteria for C4d staining positivity. The Pathology Council Working Group of the International Society for Heart and Lung Transplantation (ISHLT) has just released their initial consensus statement on the pathological criteria of pulmonary AMR, which should address exactly this source of confounding and allow a greater uniformity of definition [35].

There is also an increasing body of evidence to support the relevance of non-HLA antibody targets for AMR as a potential cause of BOS. A study of LTX recipients with BOS who had no detectable anti-HLA antibodies by low-PRA, cytotoxicity, or ELISA used flow cytometry to test for the presence of non-HLA antibodies directed against AEC [9]. Twelve of 36 patients with BOS had antibodies that bound to AEC, while none of the controls did. They also noted acceleration of the fibroproliferation cascade when AEC were incubated with the patient sera, which is one of the major recognized pathways that leads to chronic allograft dysfunction. The target antigen was found to be K-α(alpha)1 tubulin on Western blot analysis.

Tiriveedhi et al. [11] examined a case series of 12 LTX recipients with collagen V (Col-V) antibodies who developed BOS and reported that, antibodies to the α(alpha)1 chain of the Col-V antibody were present at the time of BOS onset in the sera of all 12 patients, while antibodies to the α(alpha)2 chain were only present in two patients. They suggested that antibodies to the α1 chain were immunodominant and could potentially represent a cause of BOS. This was further supported by the detection by immunohistochemistry of Col α1 (V) antibodies on frozen sections of biopsies taken 6 months after the onset of BOS [11]. Col-V antibodies have also been implicated as a potential cause of primary graft dysfunction [36], a known risk factor for the subsequent development of BOS [37]. The role of autoantibodies against Col-V and K-α1 tubulin as risk factors for BOS certainly requires further investigation; however, there can be little doubt that anti-HLA antibodies alone represent only a portion of the spectrum of AMR. Further support for the concept has been provided by Hagedorn et al., who found that BOS grades could be differentiated by a profile of autoantibodies binding to 28 proteins or their peptides [38]. Fukami et al. reported that animals receiving anti-MHC class I, but not control antibodies, developed marked cellular infiltration around vessels and bronchiole of lung by day 15 followed by epithelial hyperplasia, fibrosis, and occlusion of the distal airways similar to chronic rejection following human lung transplantation. Lungs of mice receiving anti-MHC class I showed increased expression of chemokines, their receptors, and growth factors and induced IL-17 as well as de novo antibodies to self-antigens, K-α1 tubulin, and collagen V [39].

Taken together, these pieces of evidence provide strong support for the notion that there is an antibody-mediated process contributing to BOS. Whether that process is driven primarily by anti-HLA antibodies or a spectrum of antigenic targets in addition to HLA molecules remains to be determined, as does the total contribution of AMR to BOS. It is likely that different individuals will have different profiles that are dependent on factors such as HLA match, history of cellular rejection, graft infection, and gastric aspiration with the response modulated by genetic polymorphisms.

Screening for DSA

There is no consensus on the frequency of screening for anti-HLA antibodies before and after LTX despite the potential risk of graft dysfunction secondary to AMR [40]. Of course, the detection of anti-HLA antibodies alone is not synonymous with the presence of DSA, which represent the centerpiece of the immunological diagnosis of AMR. Prior to the development of the new technologies such as single-antigen bead assays (Luminex testing), screening for individual DSA was impractical, and tests for the presence of HLA antibodies could only play a surrogate role. However, it is now possible to test specifically for individual HLA antibodies and thereby detect the presence of true DSA.

Complement-dependent cytotoxicity (CDC) cross-matching was one of the initial techniques used to detect clinically relevant antibodies before transplantation in order to determine the viability of the graft for a specific donor-recipient match [41]. In this technique, separated donor B- and T-cell lymphocytes are incubated with the potential recipient's serum in the presence of complement. If death of the donor cells above control levels is detected, cytotoxic antibodies are considered to be present, and the presence of these antibodies is considered a contraindication to transplant [36]. This technique is time consuming, and can only be performed in LTX when donor cells are available before retrieval, due to the importance of minimizing the ischemic time. It also has a low sensitivity compared to newer techniques, and it is unable to detect low-level antibody titers, which can contribute to graft failure [42].

One of the limitations of the CDC cross-match is that anti-HLA antibodies may be present that adsorb to the target lymphocytes but do not activate complement and cause cell lysis. These monovalent antibodies are unable to affect the high-affinity, bivalent interactions with C1q required to activate the complement cascade and cause cell lysis. The addition of goat antihuman kappa light chain immunoglobulin (IgL) reagent (AHG) to the incubating serum allows these antibodies to cause direct cell lysis [43]. Therefore, the AHG-CDC has largely replaced the classical CDC cross-match [43].

Flow cytometry cross-matching was developed as a more sensitive screen for donor-reactive antibodies. This technique involves incubation of patient serum with donor lymphocytes that are then stained with fluorochrome-conjugated secondary antibodies that are typically anti-IgG. The presence of antibody can then be detected by the surface fluorescence of the antibodies. This allows for the detection of donor-reactive antibodies independent of complement fixation. Depending on the sample, flow cytometry can be 1–3 logs more sensitive than AHG-CDC cross-matching. Though these antibodies are present in a far lower titer, they are clinically significant. In a study of flow cytometry cross-match-positive CDC cross-match-negative kidney transplants, Piatosa et al. [44] found an absolute reduction in 5-year graft survival of 11.5 % vs. negative controls.

The panel-reactive antibody (PRA) allows for a surrogate measure of donor-reactive antibodies as part of the workup for transplant. By performing the tests outlined in our discussion of cross-matching on lymphocyte cell lines of people with known HLA types (see above), we are able to approximate the percentage of the population against whom the potential recipient has antibodies. This allows detection of people who have been hypersensitized to HLA antibodies, as may occur with pregnancy or multiple blood transfusions. The level of sensitivity depends on the number of patients whose lymphocytes are included in the panel, which varies from center to center. Shah investigated the clinical implications of pre-transplant PRA and found that graft loss was increased in the PRA-positive patients vs. PRA-negative ones with a hazard ratio of 1.01 ($p<0.01$) [40].

Solid-phase antibody techniques are the newest development in the detection of anti-HLA antibodies. In this technique, purified HLA antibodies bound to a solid matrix (e.g., beads) are used as the substrate to which the antibodies from the patient's serum can bind. These antibodies can then be detected either through ELISA or via flow cytometry [45]. A study of PRA in kidney transplants comparing AHG-CDC with solid-phase assays by ELISA and flow cytometry found concordance of the results in 83 % of samples ($n=264$). In the remaining 32 samples, 0 of 32 were positive by AHG-CDC, 20 of 32 were positive by ELISA, and 32 of 32 were positive by flow cytometry [46]. They concluded that flow cytometry was the most sensitive technique available, and subsequent studies have supported this finding.

The development of increasingly sensitive techniques for the detection of anti-HLA antibodies is driven, in part, by the understanding that the antibody levels detected do not necessarily correspond to their clinical effects. A study of flow PRA in kidney transplant recipients with negative AHG-CDC PRA found that those with a positive flow PRA were more likely to suffer an episode of rejection (36 %, 4/11) than those without (8 %, 3/36, $p<0.02$) [47]. This is not to suggest that noncomplement fixing antibodies detected by flow represent an absolute contraindication to transplant. Shah's retrospective review of 10,000 LTX from 1987 to 2005 found that though a positive PRA was associated with an increased 30-day (HR, 2.6) and overall mortality (HR 1.3) on multivariate analysis, when the cohort from 1998 to 2005 was analyzed alone, the effect was not seen. They concluded that the development of more sensitive screening techniques in this era has allowed for better management of the sensitized patient [40]. The presence of positive flow PRA indicates that the patient is at an increased risk of graft dysfunction and acute AMR, and, therefore, requires closer monitoring than those with negative flow PRA to achieve the best outcomes.

Single-antigen bead flow cytometry provides the ability to detect specific anti-HLA antibodies, which, when combined with donor HLA typing, directly informs us of the presence and level of DSA. The most well-known of these is the LUMINEX single-antigen bead assay, which operates by using beads coated with known individual HLA antigens such that flow cytometry can determine the individual HLA antigens to which the recipient's antibodies are binding. Currently, the mean fluorescence intensity (MFI) and standard deviation (SD) of the cutoff between positive and negative are set at 1,000 ± 500 [48, 49]. Though the single-antigen bead LUMINEX provides a quantitative measure, the MFIs do not have a clinical impact based on their level. Seemingly low MFIs may translate into AMR. Equally important, the majority of patients pre-sensitized with DSA detected by LUMINEX do not go on to have episodes of AMR [27, 48, 49]. The findings in those who develop de novo DSA are similar [19, 21, 22].

While it is evident that screening for DSA by LUMINEX prior to transplantation is worthwhile, at present there is no consensus on appropriate post-transplant screening intervals, which is not surprising given the valid questions regarding their clinical significance. The Pathology Council of the ISHLT encourages the development of site protocols for regular DSA surveillance and biopsy [50]. At our center, we screen potential recipients as part of the transplant workup, on the night of transplant, at regular intervals after transplant, and when clinically mandated by a drop in lung function.

Diagnosis

Though the Banff reports [2, 51] have provided diagnostic criteria for AMR in kidney transplantation since 2003, it is only recently that a consensus agreement has been reached by the Pathology Council of the ISHLT with the caveat that pulmonary AMR remains an area of investigation in which there are no large unifying studies [50]. Pragmatically, it has been agreed that the diagnosis of AMR requires the "triple-test" of clinical allograft dysfunction, circulating DSA, and pathological findings.

The classical histopathological findings of AMR comprise capillary injury with neutrophilic margination, defined by the Council as neutrophilic infiltrates within the interstitial capillaries and septae in the absence of karyorrhectic changes and fibrin accumulation. The histopathological findings in general represent nonspecific patterns of inflammation and injury, which can also be produced by a broad spectrum of disorders. Histopathologically, AMR should be considered a diagnosis of exclusion, and current recommendations state that reporting should use the terms "No evidence of AMR" or "Findings suggestive of AMR," thereby informing the treating physician of the need for serological studies, if such had not been conducted prior to the biopsy.

The list of histopathological indications for performing immunostaining is diverse (Table 7.2). C4d staining is reported as strong or weak. *Strong* C4d staining

Table 7.2 Histopathological indications for immunopathological evaluation

1. Neutrophilic capillaritis
2. Neutrophilic septal margination
3. High-grade acute cellular rejection (≥A3)
4. Persistent/recurrent acute cellular rejection (any A grade)
5. Acute lung injury pattern/diffuse alveolar damage
6. High-grade lymphocytic bronchiolitis (grade B2R)
7. Persistent low-grade lymphocytic bronchiolitis (grade B1R)
8. Obliterative bronchiolitis (grade C1)
9. Arteritis in the absence of infection or cellular rejection
10. Graft dysfunction without morphological explanation
11. Any histological findings in setting of de novo DSA

demonstrates continuous linear endothelial deposition that outlines the capillary vasculature in longitudinal sectioning and creates ringed or "doughnut" shapes in cross section. *Weak* staining has a fainter pattern that appears patchy or granular.

In light of the limited published data, the ISHLT has defined C4d positivity in lung allografts as being immunoreactivity in >50 % of the interstitial capillaries, including multifocal and diffuse staining. Focal staining (<50 %) is classified as negative, but should be included in reporting, as serological studies may be indicated. Recommended follow-up for positive C4d staining is 1 month after treatment has been completed, with continued staining until there is complete resolution with negative C4d staining follow-up biopsy specimens.

C4d positivity is required to achieve a clinical diagnosis of renal AMR [51], but there is a subset of LTX recipients who have been clinically diagnosed with AMR in the past despite being C4d-negative, in light of consistent histopathological findings and in the absence of an alternative diagnosis [34]. The ISHLT Pathology Council Working Group affirmed that the definitive diagnosis of pulmonary AMR requires the combination of clinical dysfunction, circulating DSA, and C4d immunoreactivity. Certainly AMR may present as an acute illness or simply with an otherwise unexplained drop in lung function that is potentially the harbinger of BOS. Pulmonary AMR can occur at any time and should always be considered as a potential cause in the differential diagnosis of allograft dysfunction [52]. DSA can be detected using the methods discussed earlier in the chapter, but single-antigen flow cytometry (LUMINEX) is the most sensitive technology utilized for this purpose and is becoming a widely used method for DSA detection [19, 30].

Management

The basic tenet of therapy for AMR is to remove circulating DSA from the patient's serum and prevent further production of DSA, which perhaps is a lofty goal. DSA are central to the pathogenesis of AMR, and it is likely that their removal prevents further damage to the graft. However, it should be emphasized that it is not the circulating antibody that does the damage; it is the antibody bound to the graft (a simple concept, but one best remembered). Nevertheless, the three treatment modalities in common usage in the treatment of AMR are therapeutic plasma exchange (plasmapheresis), intravenous immunoglobulin (IVIG), and the anti-CD20 monoclonal antibody, rituximab, and these are usually used in combination with each other. The ultimate therapeutic goal is maintenance of graft function, but measurements of circulating antibody are often used as a surrogate goal.

Plasmapheresis

Plasmapheresis is an extracorporeal treatment involving the removal of blood from the patient followed by separation of the plasma from the other blood products, after which the plasma is either filtered or replaced before the blood is returned to the patient's circulation. There are several forms of plasmapheresis. *Plasma exchange*, in which the plasma is discarded and substituted (usually with albumin); *double filtration plasmapheresis*, in which the separated plasma is filtered again into large and small molecular weight components with the large molecular weight component discarded and the low molecular weight component, which contains albumin but not the IgG, is returned to the circulation; and *immunoadsorption plasmapheresis*, in which the plasma is passed through an adsorption column such that antibodies are adsorbed depending on affinity for the membrane that it contains. Plasmapheresis can remove DSA from the patient's circulation more rapidly than other interventions, and it has the benefit of reducing complement levels in the blood for up to 48 h after it has been performed. One disadvantage of plasmapheresis is that it adds a level of immunosuppression that may not be desirable due to risk of infections. Also, antibody levels quickly rebound if it is used as monotherapy. Hence, it is commonly used with adjunctive therapies, particularly IVIG, which can be used in a lower dose when combined with plasmapheresis [1, 38].

Intravenous Immunoglobulin

Although high-dose IVIG (2 mg/kg IV that is often given in three divided doses on alternate days) has been recognized as an effective treatment for AMR, the mechanisms by which it induces desensitization remain unknown. There are several theories that have been proposed to explain the effect of IVIG. The benefits of IVIG were originally thought to be due to the neutralizing effects on circulating antibodies, but the benefit extends well beyond the half-life, suggesting that regulation of adaptive cellular immunity occurs. The likely mechanism for this is through the saturation of Fc receptors on the surface of a number of immune cell subsets. Some Fc receptors are known to have immunosuppressant effects, particularly via expression of FcgRIIb, which is induced in response to IVIG and can induce B-cell apoptosis. There is also some evidence that IVIG can inhibit T-cell activation as well as the actions of monocytes and macrophages. Although immunoglobulin is known to be a potent activator of the complement cascade, new data have shown that immunoglobulins can also act as inhibitor of this cascade via binding to complement and scavenging activated complement, thereby suppressing AMR. It is likely that the mechanisms by which IVIG lowers DSA and prevents recurrence are multiple [53].

Rituximab is a monoclonal antibody to CD20; a receptor expressed on the surface of immature B lymphocytes and B memory lymphocytes. Rituximab does not work by reducing circulating DSA but by reducing long-term production of DSA. As the antibody-secreting plasma cells do not express CD20 on their surface, rituximab has an indirect influence on the production of DSA by causing apoptosis of the immature B cells, which prevents clonal expansion of the DSA-producing cell line that is causing AMR. It is also possible that additional therapeutic benefit may come from modifications of cellular immunity as well as the effect on DSA production.

Therapy can be given either as desensitization therapy prior to transplantation to prevent AMR or when an episode of AMR is detected following the development of de novo DSA post-transplant. No evidence-based, standardized protocols for the treatment of AMR currently exist for any SOT. However, there is a clear need to establish best practice, which will likely constitute IVIG or IVIG/plasmapheresis as the standard of care. The efficacy of novel therapeutics also needs to be assessed following standardization of an accepted treatment regime [54].

The 2010 retrospective trial by Hachem et al. [30] determined that there was no increased risk of BOS with preemptive treatment of de novo DSA-positive patients using a single dose of rituximab and a monthly regime of IVIG (0.5 g/kg) for at least 6 months if follow-up DSA screens were negative. Monthly treatment continued if DSA screens remained positive.

It is important to recognize that these extremely potent therapies for AMR are capable of treating for all circulating antibodies that may be causing damage to the graft. However, our impression that the treatment of declining graft function in lung transplant recipients with anti-HLA DSA leads to remission of AMR may be naive. Certainly, there are other antibodies for which we do not routinely screen that may contribute to allograft dysfunction, and perhaps it is the reduction of these antibodies that actually leads to recovery of allograft function. Autoantibodies of note include Col-V and k-α1-tubulin, and multiple antibodies directed against currently unknown antigens may prove to be extremely important mediators of AMR-associated graft dysfunction but have yet to be discovered.

Future Directions

As a lung transplant community, it appears we may finally be nearing the threshold of answering the enigma of why the transplanted lung fails even in the absence of cellular rejection or infection. Allograft rejection is, perhaps not surprisingly, due to lack of tolerance to the graft and its components, as the lung allograft is variably challenged by the vicissitudes of constant exposure to the external environment but ultimately at the mercy of the immune system, which has had millennia to develop sophisticated responses to nonself-antigens, however presented to immune surveillance.

With this understanding, combined with an expanding technology platform, we can now look forward to offering our patients the hope of better survival and quality of life, although the cynics amongst us might reply that all we can hope to know is why the graft failed. That at least is a beginning to solving the problem of lung allograft rejection.

References

1. Takemoto SK, Zeevi A, Feng S, Colvin RB, Jordan S, Kobashigawa J, et al. National conference to assess antibody-mediated rejection in solid organ transplantation. Am J Transplant. 2004;4(7):1033–41.
2. Solez K, Colvin RB, Racusen LC, Sis B, Halloran PF, Birk PE, et al. Banff '05 meeting report: differential diagnosis of chronic allograft injury and elimination of chronic allograft nephropathy ('CAN'). Am J Transplant. 2007;7(3):518–26.
3. Cooper NR. The classical complement pathway: activation and regulation of the first complement component. Adv Immunol. 1985;37:151–216.
4. Lanier LL, Phillips JH. Evidence for three types of human cytotoxic lymphocyte. Immunol Today. 1986;7(5):132–4.
5. Piertney SB, Oliver MK. The evolutionary ecology of the major histocompatibility complex. Heredity. 2006;96(1):7–21.
6. Glanville AR, Tazelaar HD, Theodore J, Imoto E, Rouse RV, Baldwin JC, et al. The distribution of MHC class I and II antigens on bronchial epithelium. Am Rev Respir Dis. 1989;139(2):330–4.
7. Steimle V, Siegrist CA, Mottet A, Lisowska-Grospierre B, Mach B. Regulation of MHC class II expression by interferon-gamma mediated by the transactivator gene CIITA. Science. 1994;265(5168):106–9.
8. Montgomery RA, Cozzi E, West LJ, Warren DS. Humoral immunity and antibody-mediated rejection in solid organ transplantation. Semin Immunol. 2011;23(4):224–34.
9. Goers TA, Ramachandran S, Aloush A, Trulock E, Patterson GA, Mohanakumar T. De novo production of K-alpha1 tubulin-specific antibodies: role in chronic lung allograft rejection. J Immunol. 2008;180(7):4487–94.
10. Burlingham WJ, Love RB, Jankowska-Gan E, Haynes LD, Xu Q, Bobadilla JL, et al. IL-17-dependent cellular immunity to collagen type V predisposes to obliterative bronchiolitis in human lung transplants. J Clin Invest. 2007;117(11):3498–506.
11. Tiriveedhi V, Angaswamy N, Brand D, Weber J, Gelman AG, Hachem R, et al. A shift in the collagen V antigenic epitope leads to T helper phenotype switch and immune response to self-antigen leading to chronic lung allograft rejection. Clin Exp Immunol. 2012;167(1):158–68.
12. Williams GM, Hume DM, Hudson Jr RP, Morris PJ, Kano K, Milgrom F. "Hyperacute" renal-homograft rejection in man. N Engl J Med. 1968;279(12):611–8.
13. Sis B, Mengel M, Haas M, Colvin RB, Halloran PF, Racusen LC, et al. Banff '09 meeting report: antibody mediated graft deterioration and implementation of Banff working groups. Am J Transplant. 2010;10(3):464–71.
14. (SRTR). OPaTNOaSRoTR. OPTN/SRTR 2010 Annual Data Report. Rockville, MD: Department of Health and Human Services HRaSA, Healthcare Systems Bureau, Division of Transplantation; 2011.

15. Morris PJ, Mickey MR, Singal DP, Terasaki PI. Serotyping for homotransplantation. XXII. Specificity of cytotoxic antibodies developing after renal transplantation. BMJ. 1969; 1(5646):758–9.
16. Lee P-C, Terasaki PI, Takemoto SK, Lee PH, Hung CJ, Chen YL, et al. All chronic rejection failures of kidney transplants were preceded by the development of HLA antibodies. Transplantation. 2002;74(8):1192–4.
17. Mauiyyedi S, Pelle PD, Saidman S, Collins AB, Pascual M, Tolkoff-Rubin NE, et al. Chronic humoral rejection: identification of antibody-mediated chronic renal allograft rejection by C4d deposits in peritubular capillaries. J Am Soc Nephrol. 2001;12(3):574–82.
18. Worthington JE, Martin S, Dyer PA, Johnson RW. An association between posttransplant antibody production and renal transplant rejection. Transplant Proc. 2001;33(1–2):475–6.
19. Einecke G, Sis B, Reeve J, Mengel M, Campbell PM, Hidalgo LG, et al. Antibody-mediated microcirculation injury is the major cause of late kidney transplant failure. Am J Transplant. 2009;9(11):2520–31.
20. Tambur AR, Bray RA, Takemoto SK, Mancini M, Costanzo MR, Kobashigawa JA, et al. Flow cytometric detection of HLA-specific antibodies as a predictor of heart allograft rejection. Transplantation. 2000;70(7):1055–9.
21. Worthington JE, Martin S, Al-Husseini DM, Dyer PA, Johnson RWG. Posttransplantation production of donor HLA-specific antibodies as a predictor of renal transplant outcome. Transplantation. 2003;75(7):1034–40.
22. Mao Q, Terasaki PI, Cai J, Briley K, Catrou P, Haisch C, et al. Extremely high association between appearance of HLA antibodies and failure of kidney grafts in a five-year longitudinal study. Am J Transplant. 2007;7(4):864–71.
23. Herzenberg AM, Gill JS, Djurdjev O, Magil AB. C4d deposition in acute rejection: an independent long-term prognostic factor. J Am Soc Nephrol. 2002;13(1):234–41.
24. Nickeleit V, Zeiler M, Gudat F, Thiel G, Mihatsch MJ. Detection of the complement degradation product C4d in renal allografts: diagnostic and therapeutic implications. J Am Soc Nephrol. 2002;13(1):242–51.
25. Kieran N, Wang X, Perkins J, Davis C, Kendrick E, Bakthavatsalam R, et al. Combination of peritubular c4d and transplant glomerulopathy predicts late renal allograft failure. J Am Soc Nephrol. 2009;20(10):2260–8.
26. Rodriguez ER, Skojec DV, Tan CD, Zachary AA, Kasper EK, Conte JV, et al. Antibody-mediated rejection in human cardiac allografts: evaluation of immunoglobulins and complement activation products C4d and C3d as markers. Am J Transplant. 2005;5(11):2778–85.
27. Lefaucheur C, Suberbielle-Boissel C, Hill GS, Nochy D, Andrade J, Antoine C, et al. Clinical relevance of preformed HLA donor-specific antibodies in kidney transplantation. Am J Transplant. 2008;8(2):324–31.
28. Smith MA, Sundaresan S, Mohanakumar T, Trulock EP, Lynch JP, Phelan DL, et al. Effect of development of antibodies to HLA and cytomegalovirus mismatch on lung transplantation survival and development of bronchiolitis obliterans syndrome. J Thorac Cardiovasc Surg. 1998;116(5):812–20.
29. Sundaresan S, Mohanakumar T, Smith MA, Trulock EP, Lynch J, Phelan D, et al. HLA-A locus mismatches and development of antibodies to HLA after lung transplantation correlate with the development of bronchiolitis obliterans syndrome. Transplantation. 1998;65(5):648–53.
30. Hachem RR, Yusen RD, Meyers BF, Aloush AA, Mohanakumar T, Patterson GA, et al. Anti-human leukocyte antigen antibodies and preemptive antibody-directed therapy after lung transplantation. J Heart Lung Transplant. 2010;29(9):973–80.
31. Magro CM, Pope Harman A, Klinger D, Orosz C, Adams P, Waldman J, et al. Use of C4d as a diagnostic adjunct in lung allograft biopsies. Am J Transplant. 2003;3(9):1143–54.
32. Magro CM, Ross Jr P, Kelsey M, Waldman WJ, Pope-Harman A. Association of humoral immunity and bronchiolitis obliterans syndrome. Am J Transplant. 2003;3(9):1155–66.
33. Wallace WD, Reed EF, Ross D, Lassman CR, Fishbein MC. C4d staining of pulmonary allograft biopsies: an immunoperoxidase study. J Heart Lung Transplant. 2005;24(10): 1565–70.

34. Ionescu DN, Girnita AL, Zeevi A, Duquesnoy R, Pilewski J, Johnson B, et al. C4d deposition in lung allografts is associated with circulating anti-HLA alloantibody. Transpl Immunol. 2005;15(1):63–8.
35. Berry G, Burke M, Andersen C, Angelini A, Bruneval P, Calbrese F, et al. Pathology of pulmonary antibody-mediated rejection: 2012 update from the Pathology Council of the ISHLT. J Heart Lung Transplant. 2013;32(1):14–21.
36. Talbot D, Givan AL, Shenton BK, Stratton A, Proud G, Taylor RM. The relevance of a more sensitive crossmatch assay to renal transplantation. Transplantation. 1989;47(3):552–5.
37. Daud SA, Yusen RD, Meyers BF, Chakinala MM, Walter MJ, Aloush AA, et al. Impact of immediate primary lung allograft dysfunction on bronchiolitis obliterans syndrome. Am J Respir Crit Care Med. 2007;175(5):507–13.
38. Hagedorn PH, Burton CM, Carlsen J, Steinbrüchel D, Andersen CB, Sahar E, et al. Chronic rejection of a lung transplant is characterized by a profile of specific autoantibodies. Immunology. 2010;130(3):427–35.
39. Fukami N, Ramachandran S, Saini D, Walter M, Chapman W, Patterson GA, et al. Antibodies to MHC class I induce autoimmunity: role in the pathogenesis of chronic rejection. J Immunol. 2009;182(1):309–18.
40. Shah AS, Nwakanma L, Simpkins C, Williams J, Chang DC, Conte JV. Pretransplant panel reactive antibodies in human lung transplantation: an analysis of over 10,000 patients. Ann Thorac Surg. 2008;85(6):1919–24.
41. Patel R, Terasaki PI. Significance of the positive crossmatch test in kidney transplantation. N Engl J Med. 1969;280(14):735–9.
42. Reinsmoen NL, Nelson K, Zeevi A. Anti-HLA antibody analysis and crossmatching in heart and lung transplantation. Transpl Immunol. 2004;13(1):63–71.
43. Fuller TC, Fuller AA, Golden M, Rodey GE. HLA alloantibodies and the mechanism of the antiglobulin-augmented lymphocytotoxicity procedure. Hum Immunol. 1997;56(1–2):94–105.
44. Piatosa B, Rubik J, Grenda R. Is positive flow cytometric cross-match a risk factor for early cadaveric kidney graft dysfunction? Transplant Proc. 2006;38(1):53–5.
45. Pajaro OE, George JF. On solid-phase antibody assays. J Heart Lung Transplant. 2010;29(11):1207–9.
46. Gebel HM, Bray RA. Sensitization and sensitivity: defining the unsensitized patient. Transplantation. 2000;69(7):1370–4.
47. Gebel HM, Bray RA, Ruth JA, Zibari GB, McDonald JC, Kahan BD, et al. Flow PRA to detect clinically relevant HLA antibodies. Transplant Proc. 2001;33(1–2):477.
48. Vlad G, Ho EK, Vasilescu ER, Colovai AI, Stokes MB, Markowitz GS, et al. Relevance of different antibody detection methods for the prediction of antibody-mediated rejection and deceased-donor kidney allograft survival. Hum Immunol. 2009;70(8):589–94.
49. Ho EK, Vasilescu ER, Colovai AI, Stokes MB, Hallar M, Markowitz GS, et al. Sensitivity, specificity and clinical relevance of different cross-matching assays in deceased-donor renal transplantation. Transpl Immunol. 2008;20(1–2):61–7.
50. Berry GJ, Burke M, Anderson C, Angelini A, Bruneval P, Calbrese F, et al. The pathology of pulmonary antibody mediated rejection: 2012 update from the Pathology Council of ISHLT. J Heart Lung Transplant. 2012;32(1):14–21.
51. Mengel M, Sis B, Haas M, Colvin RB, Halloran PF, Racusen LC, et al. Banff 2011 meeting report: new concepts in antibody-mediated rejection. Am J Transplant. 2012;12(3):563–70.
52. Glanville AR. Antibody-mediated rejection in lung transplantation: myth or reality? J Heart Lung Transplant. 2010;29(4):395–400.
53. Jordan SC, Toyoda M, Vo AA. Intravenous immunoglobulin a natural regulator of immunity and inflammation. Transplantation. 2009;88(1):1–6.
54. Archdeacon P, Chan M, Neuland C, Velidedeoglu E, Meyer J, Tracy L, et al. Summary of FDA antibody-mediated rejection workshop. Am J Transplant. 2011;11(5):896–906.

Chapter 8
Innate Immune Responses and Bronchiolitis Obliterans Syndrome

Jamie L. Todd and Scott M. Palmer

Abstract The innate immune system, central to host defense, is now recognized to play a critical role in regulating adaptive immune responses, including allograft rejection. Innate immunity is of particular importance in lung transplantation, given the specialized innate defense mechanisms within the lung and the constant interaction between the allograft and the external environment. A central principle of innate immunity is the recognition of highly conserved molecular patterns present on microbial pathogens or injured tissue by host innate pattern recognition receptors (PRRs). The Toll-like receptors (TLRs) are the best described and most extensively studied PRRs of relevance to transplant rejection. For example, in animal models, genetic inhibition of TLR signaling attenuates allograft rejection, while TLR activation impedes successful transplant tolerance. These findings have been translated into clinical lung transplantation, as we have shown that functional polymorphisms in the innate receptors TLR4 and CD14 impact the risk for acute rejection and bronchiolitis obliterans syndrome (BOS). Consequently, a more complex view of BOS pathogenesis that considers the influence of previously identified clinical risk factors on activation of both innate and adaptive immunity has emerged. While additional studies are needed to define the full spectrum of innate ligands and PRRs relevant to lung transplantation, it is clear that innate mechanisms are likely to play a central role in mediating lung allograft rejection and BOS. Selective inhibition of innate pathways represents an attractive approach that could complement existing immunosuppressive strategies to reduce rejection after lung transplantation.

Keywords Bronchiolitis obliterans • Allograft tolerance • Innate immunity • Toll-like receptor • Pattern recognition receptor

---

J.L. Todd, M.D. (✉) • S.M. Palmer, M.D., M.H.S.
Division of Pulmonary, Allergy, and Critical Care Medicine, Department of Internal Medicine, Duke University Medical Center, DUMC Box 2629, Durham, NC 27710, USA
e-mail: Jamie.Todd@duke.edu; Jamie.Todd@dm.Duke.edu

K.C. Meyer and A.R. Glanville (eds.), *Bronchiolitis Obliterans Syndrome in Lung Transplantation*, Respiratory Medicine 8, DOI 10.1007/978-1-4614-7636-8_8,

Introduction

The lung represents a unique challenge as compared to other commonly transplanted solid organs in that it is in constant interaction with the external environment. As a result of this direct interface, the lung has developed a sophisticated and complex system of innate defense mechanisms in order to protect the host from invading pathogens and other injurious events. The complexity and central importance of innate immunity became apparent with the description of a novel family of innate pattern recognition receptors (PRRs), the Toll-like receptors (TLRs). Specialized cells within the lung, including resident alveolar macrophages (AMs), are equipped with TLRs and other innate PRRs that enable rapid and efficient responses to inhaled toxins or infections. Beyond PRRs, an array of important secreted and soluble proteins produced by the pulmonary epithelium and alveolar pneumocytes also contribute to the maintenance of host defense.

While most of the early work in pulmonary innate immunity focused on its actions related to pathogen defense, it is now clear that innate mechanisms are relevant to almost all aspects of pulmonary health and disease, including the response to allotransplantation. In this chapter we provide a brief overview of the basic mechanisms of pulmonary innate immunity, including the relevant PRRs and their respective ligands. We then describe important experimental and clinical evidence supporting a role for the innate immune system in allograft rejection, highlighting key studies specific to lung transplantation. This growing body of research supports a more complex view of bronchiolitis obliterans syndrome (BOS) risk factors and pathogenic mechanisms than previous primarily T cell-focused work. An enhanced understanding of innate immunity in lung transplantation is critical to the development of more effective therapeutic strategies to reduce the high burden of lung rejection and BOS and improve long-term patient outcomes.

Overview of Pulmonary Innate Immunity

The innate immune system is a highly conserved mechanism of host defense that evolutionarily long predates adaptive immunity. As shown in Table 8.1, the innate immune system differs from adaptive immunity in that it provides an immediate response, distinguishes self from nonself, and uses germline-encoded receptors to recognize patterns distinct to invading pathogens or injured tissues [1]. It also differs such that, in isolation, the innate response cannot confer longstanding immunological memory. While recent studies suggest some of these distinctions are less absolute than originally hypothesized, the diverse and complementary functions of innate and adaptive immunity provide a highly coordinated host response effective against a wide range of potential pathogens. In addition, it is now recognized that extensive cross-talk occurs between these two facets of the immune system, and this appears critical to allow for the most mature and effective host response [2].

Table 8.1 Important differences in innate and adaptive immunity

	Innate	Adaptive
Antigen specificity	Nonspecific	Exquisite specificity
	Limited number PAMPs/DAMPs	>10^{14} unique epitopes
Germline encoded	Yes	No
Response time	Rapid, active before exposure	Days, clonal proliferation
Immunologic memory	No	Yes, robust second response
Distinguish self vs. non	Yes	No, delete self-reactive

PAMP pathogen-associated molecular pattern, *DAMP* damage-associated molecular pattern

Innate pathways are of particular importance in the lung given the extensive alveolar surface area and continuous exposure to a wide array of airborne particles and invading microbes during normal respiration. The lung presents unique challenges because the degree of host response needs to be appropriate to resolve the infection or airborne challenge, but not so excessive as to damage the delicate alveolar structures necessary for gas exchange. The lung is able to achieve this balance by relying on several layers of pulmonary innate immunity that can be divided into tissue- and cell-specific structural properties, soluble or secreted proteins in the airway and alveolar space, and cells that reside within or are recruited to the lung [3].

The anatomical design of the upper and lower airways represents the initial barrier to foreign invaders. Particles larger than 5 μm are sequestered in the tortuous channels of the upper airway and in the mucociliary lining of the trachea, bronchi, and larger bronchioles [3]. The cough reflex and highly coordinated ciliary beat facilitate movement of trapped particles toward the oropharynx for expectoration [4]. Smaller particles, including most bacterial, viral, and mycobacterial components, gain access to the terminal airways and alveolar spaces where they encounter a variety of soluble proteins critical to the maintenance of a sterile intrapulmonary environment.

Numerous soluble or secreted proteins have been described to include defensins, collectins (surfactant proteins A and D), lysozyme, lactoferrin, fibronectin, complement, and immunoglobulins A and G [3–7]. These secreted or soluble components of the innate immune system are present in the fluid of the epithelial lining where they exert direct microbicidal effects, act as opsonins and agglutinins to facilitate subsequent phagocytosis, and play an important role in regulating local inflammation [3].

The cellular innate immune response becomes activated either by the action of these soluble protein mediators or in direct response to invading pathogens. Cells important to the innate response include airway and alveolar epithelial cells, AMs and recruited natural killer (NK) cells, dendritic cells (DCs), and neutrophils. AMs account for the vast majority of leukocytes in the normal, healthy lung, where they phagocytose and eradicate inhaled particles on an ongoing basis [8]. In the event of a large particulate load or exceptionally virulent pathogen, AMs produce proinflammatory cytokines and chemokines to initiate recruitment of neutrophils, DCs, and monocyte-derived macrophages from the pulmonary vasculature in order to generate a robust local inflammatory response. Additionally, AMs act as antigen-presenting cells (APCs), carrying foreign antigens to regional lymph nodes, where they are taken up by DCs and presented to naïve lymphocytes, thus invoking clonal T-cell proliferation and promoting robust adaptive immune responses [8]. Importantly, recent literature also suggests that the lung itself can act as a tertiary lymphoid organ, with local antigen presentation and cell maturation occurring even in the absence of extrapulmonary lymphoid tissue, a novel finding with contextual relevance to lung transplantation [9].

Receptors and Ligands of the Innate Immune System

Initiation of the innate immune response depends on a series of germline-encoded PRRs that recognize highly conserved molecular patterns on microorganisms (pathogen-associated molecular patterns [PAMPs]). More recently, it has been noted that in addition to recognition of foreign molecular patterns, PRRs also provide an internal mechanism by which to mount a response to injured self-tissue via recognition of damage-associated molecular patterns (DAMPs). PRRs can be secreted into the bloodstream or expressed either intracellularly or on the cell surface, where they serve a variety of functions depending on the cell type and location of expression. For example, secreted PRRs activate the complement cascade and promote microbial opsonization and phagocytosis, while ligation of cell surface PRRs stimulates maturation of APCs and inflammatory cytokine production [10–15].

The earliest identified and best described PRRs are those in the TLR family. TLRs are expressed by a wide variety of cells important in pulmonary innate immunity, including AMs, DCs, neutrophils, and epithelial cells of the alveoli and conducting airways. To date, there are 11 well-described TLRs (numbered TLR1 through TLR11), and their ligand specificity, location of expression, and functions demonstrate a high degree of specialization in pathogen recognition (Table 8.2) [11, 13, 16]. Notably, myeloid differentiation factor 88 (MyD88) is an adaptor protein shared by all TLRs with the exception of TLR3, and signaling can occur in a MyD88-dependent or independent fashion, with the MyD88-independent signaling pathway utilizing the adaptor protein TRIF [11, 12, 16]. While some TLRs do not have known co-receptor requirements, others have been shown to associate with co-receptors in a tissue-specific manner in order to detect microbial antigens. TLR4, for example, utilizes co-receptor CD14 to recruit lipopolysaccharide (LPS) for subsequent direct receptor-ligand interaction. Interestingly, in addition to tissue- and location-specific specialization of function, TLRs have also recently been reported to form heterodimers, and this cooperativity is believed to further diversify the range of recognizable molecular motifs [15]. Certainly, the complexity of TLR signaling and its integration into the full host response is only now just beginning to be understood.

Microbial PAMPs and endogenous DAMPs demonstrated to signal in a TLR-dependent fashion are outlined in Table 8.2 [11, 13, 16]. Ligation of the TLR by

Table 8.2 Toll-like receptors with known ligands and location of expression

Toll-like receptor	Ligand(s)	Location
TLR1	Triacyl lipopeptides, bacteria, and mycobacteria	Cell surface
TLR2	Hemagglutinin proteins, measles virus	Cell surface
	Lipoarabinomannan, mycobacteria	
	Phospholipomannan, yeast	
	Zymosan, yeast	
	Porins, *Neisseria*	
	Peptidoglycan, gram-positive bacteria	
	Lipoteichoic acid, *group B Streptococcus*	
TLR3	Ds RNA, viruses	Intracellular
	Polyinosine:cytosine, viruses	
TLR4	Lipopolysaccharide, gram-negative bacteria	Cell surface
	F protein, respiratory syncytial virus	
	Mannan, yeast	
	Fibrinogen, tissue injury	
	Hyaluronic acid, tissue injury	
	Heat-shock proteins, tissue injury	
TLR5	Flagellin, flagellated bacteria	Cell surface
TLR6	Zymosan, yeast	Cell surface
	Lipoteichoic acid, *group B Streptococcus*	
TLR7	Ss RNA, RNA viruses	Intracellular
TLR8	Ss RNA, RNA viruses	Intracellular
TLR9	Unmethylated CpG DNA, bacteria and mycobacteria	Intracellular
	DNA, viruses	
TLR10	Uncertain	Uncertain
TLR11	Profilin-like molecules, *Toxoplasma gondii*	Intracellular

CpG cytidyl phosphate guanosine oligodeoxynucleotides

these and other yet to be identified PAMPs and DAMPs initiates a complex intracellular kinase cascade either in a MyD88-dependent or independent fashion. While the MyD88-independent pathway results in upregulation of interferons important in host response to viral infection, the MyD88-dependent pathway ultimately activates transcription factor NFκ(kappa)B, thus promoting DC maturation and proinflammatory cytokine and costimulatory molecule production that in turn direct a Th1 immune response [11]. Hence, TLR signaling is a critical mechanism by which the immune system can distinguish healthy self from injured self and microbial nonself and instruct downstream adaptive immune reactivity.

TLR Signaling in Transplant Rejection and Tolerance

Registry data suggest that long-term outcomes after lung transplantation remain inferior when compared to most other solid organs, despite aggressive immunosuppression protocols [17]. Given that the lung is in constant interaction with the external environment, it has been hypothesized that these inferior outcomes are mediated by an amplified immune response in the setting of concomitant exposure to alloantigens and environmental PAMPs or endogenous DAMPs [18, 19]. Because of the complexity and central importance of pulmonary innate immunity in host defense, it is plausible that similar innate mechanisms also contribute to the relative frequency of lung allograft rejection. The failure of aggressive T cell-based immunosuppression to adequately prevent the onset of BOS after lung transplant substantiates this hypothesis; however, much of the early work that established a role for innate immunity in allograft rejection primarily focused on models of skin and non-lung solid organ transplantation.

One of these early studies, for example, demonstrated the development of a robust inflammatory response in murine cardiac allografts, even in the absence of functional donor and recipient lymphocytes [20]. Later, a novel hierarchical cluster analysis of gene expression at multiple time points after murine heterotopic cardiac transplantation revealed two distinct phases of rejection, with genes important in innate immunity, including the TLR co-receptor CD14, being expressed as early as 6 h post-transplant [21]. These data suggested that the full host response to solid organ transplant includes both innate and adaptive components and, furthermore, implicated a role for TLR signaling in the pathobiology of allograft rejection.

Since these initial descriptions, a series of elegant experimental and clinical studies have enhanced our understanding of the significance of TLR signaling in transplant rejection and tolerance. In a seminal study, Goldstein and colleagues demonstrated a critical role for the TLR adaptor molecule MyD88 in acute skin allograft rejection [22]. Using a minor antigen mismatched skin transplant model in mice with targeted deletions of TLR2, TLR4, or their downstream signal MyD88, Goldstein et al. showed that recipients and donors lacking MyD88 had indefinite allograft survival. Furthermore, the authors demonstrated a reduction in the number of DCs in draining lymph nodes, impaired generation of alloreactive T cells, and reduced Th1 immunity as measured by interferon-γ (gamma) (IFN-γ) in the absence of MyD88, indicating that skin graft rejection across minor mismatch was critically dependent upon innate immune MyD88 signaling [22].

Subsequent studies, however, have generated inconsistent results with respect to innate signaling in murine solid organ transplant rejection and in fully major histocompatibility complex (MHC) mismatched skin transplant models. For example, in contrast to the dramatic results in the minor antigen skin transplant model, Goldstein et al. later found that in the context of completely allogeneic transplantation, both skin and heart rejection occurred despite targeted deletion of MyD88 or TLRs, although notably the tempo of rejection was reduced [23]. In contrast, McKay et al. demonstrated that combined deletion of both MyD88 and TRIF signaling prevented skin allograft rejection across major and minor MHC mismatch barriers [24]. The disparate results of these studies suggest that there are likely to be important organ-specific differences in the innate signaling mechanisms that contribute to allograft rejection. Perhaps due to the limited model systems in which to study lung rejection or BOS, similar studies have not yet been performed in the context of experimental lung transplantation.

As an alternative approach to understanding the importance of TLRs in the context of transplantation, several investigators have demonstrated that administration of TLR agonists is sufficient to prevent the establishment and maintenance of long-term allograft acceptance [25, 26]. These studies provide strong and consistent evidence that various PAMPs are able to break allograft tolerance even in the setting of otherwise tolerizing regimens. Chen et al., for example, administered the bacterial PAMP cytidyl phosphate guanosine oligodeoxynucleotides (CpG) perioperatively in a completely MHC mismatched murine cardiac allograft model in which the mice were treated with a CD154 monoclonal antibody tolerizing regimen known to mediate long-term graft acceptance. CpG injection broke the tolerance that is normally induced by anti-CD154, invoking prompt acute allograft rejection [26].

Perhaps more relevant to lung transplantation, a similar potentiation of alloimmune lung injury was observed after intrapulmonary administration of the bacterial PAMP LPS or the viral PAMP polyinosinic:polycytidylic acid (poly I:C) in a fully mismatched murine bone marrow transplantation (BMT) model. The model is relevant in that the observed pathology of alloimmune injury in BMT-related pulmonary graft versus host disease (GVHD) overlaps considerably with that observed after lung transplantation. The results suggested these PAMPs contribute to exacerbations of pulmonary GVHD. Furthermore, the development of lymphocytic lung inflammation after LPS administration was found to be dependent on functional TLR4 on donor-derived hematopoietic cells [27, 28].

The distinct mechanisms underlying the impedance of tolerance in these models are becoming better understood and emphasize the important immunomodulatory functions of $CD4^{+}Foxp3^{+}$ T-regulatory (Treg) cells in mediating graft acceptance. Indeed the TLR ligand CpG was shown to eradicate Treg proliferation in the murine cardiac allograft model, while mice that underwent allogeneic BMT had diminished numbers of Tregs and thereby an attenuated Treg response to poly I:C exposure compared to their syngeneic counterparts [26, 28, 29]. Still other studies demonstrate that, apart from Tregs, the production of proinflammatory cytokines, specifically interleukin-6 and interleukin-17, represents a critical mechanism by which bacterial PAMP exposure abrogates allograft tolerance [30, 31].

While much remains to be learned, these influential lines of experimental research have established that defects in TLR signaling modulate allograft rejection, TLR activation by a variety of environmental PAMPs impedes successful experimental transplant tolerance, and that this reversal of tolerance is facilitated by favoring proinflammatory cytokine production and the differentiation of Th1 and Th17 type responses while inhibiting a T-regulatory response. The translation of these laboratory findings into the human transplant setting, specifically lung transplantation, has served to substantiate the clinical relevance of TLR signaling in mediating lung allograft rejection and BOS.

Given the heterogeneity in the timing and severity of BOS onset after lung transplant and the notable variation in innate immune responses in humans [32], we hypothesized that single nucleotide polymorphisms (SNPs) in innate immune genes may account for the clinically apparent differential susceptibility to BOS. Two loss-of-function SNPs in the TLR4 gene had previously been described as associated with an attenuated inflammatory response to inhaled endotoxin and protective with respect to the development of inflammatory-mediated diseases, such as vascular atherogenesis [33].

These two SNPs were subsequently genotyped in a large cohort of lung-transplant recipients and evaluated for their correlation with acute rejection, BOS, survival, and burden of post-transplant infections. Strikingly, compared with wild-type recipients, a significant reduction in the absolute rate of acute rejection was noted amongst lung-transplant recipients heterozygous for either TLR4 loss-of-function SNP [34]. A follow-up study in 170 patients confirmed the low rate of acute rejection in TLR4 heterozygotes over an extended period post-transplant, and, furthermore, it indicated a trend towards improved BOS-free survival [19].

Perhaps due to standard antimicrobial prophylaxis employed after lung transplantation, no difference in the rate or type of post-transplant infections was noted between the groups [19]. Additionally, only recipient, not donor, TLR4 polymorphisms were noted to be associated with the risk for allograft rejection, consistent with the idea that TLR signaling in recipient-derived cells, such as AMs, but not donor structural lung cells, contribute directly to the development of acute rejection [34]. Importantly, these findings parallel those in previous experimental transplant models, particularly studies of pulmonary GVHD, where TLR4 signaling in bone marrow-derived hematopoietic cells rather than structural lung tissue was necessary for LPS-induced disease exacerbation [27].

To further test our hypothesis, we later went on to characterize CD14 SNPs amongst 252 lung allograft recipients and demonstrated that recipients homozygous for the CD14 SNP TT, associated with endotoxin *hyperresponsiveness*, had an earlier onset of BOS (Fig. 8.1) and overall worse survival when compared to wild-type recipients. Consistent with a dose response effect of this SNP, heterozygous patients had intermediate rates of acute rejection and BOS. Furthermore, markers of systemic inflammation, including levels of IFN-γ (gamma) and interleukin-6, were higher in TT recipients, even in the absence of active infection or allograft rejection [35].

In summary, these important clinical studies indicate that BOS develops as a consequence of intricate interactions between environmental stimuli and host genetic susceptibilities and confirms experimental findings that TLR activation and signaling play a critical role in modulating allograft rejection. As many patients with protective TLR4 polymorphisms still went on to develop BOS, however, it is very likely that BOS susceptibility is regulated by multiple genes with overlying complex, and yet to be elucidated, gene–gene and gene–environment interactions occurring in the context of varying post-transplant PAMP/DAMP exposure and PRR activation.

Additional Innate Immune Mechanisms in Transplant Rejection and Tolerance

Although TLRs have been the most extensively described and studied elements of the innate immune system in the context of transplantation, additional basic and clinical studies suggest the importance of other innate immune components in the

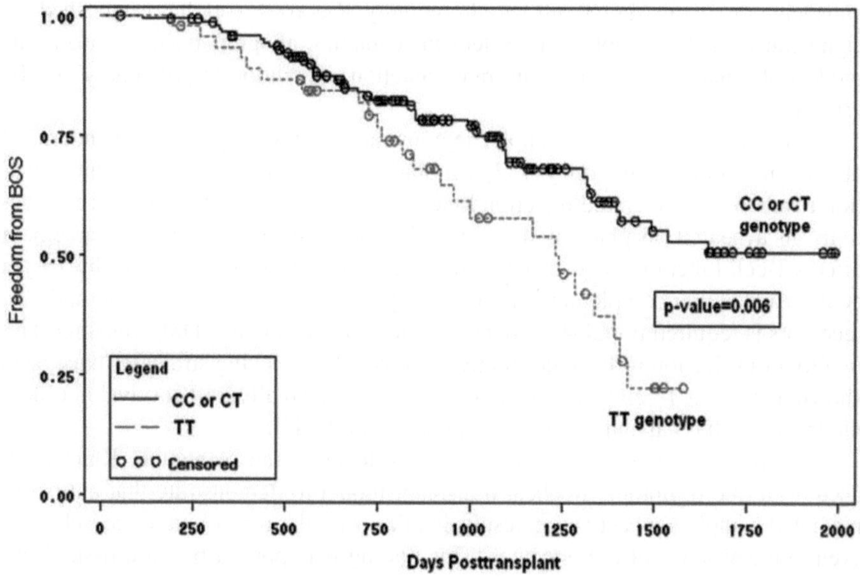

Fig. 8.1 Recipient CD14 polymorphisms impact the risk for BOS after lung transplantation. Lung-transplant recipients with the homozygous for the TT CD14 genotype have a significantly worse freedom from BOS as compared to those with CC or CT genotypes ($p=0.006$). *BOS* bronchiolitis obliterans syndrome. Reproduced with permission from Palmer SM, Klimecki W, Yu L, Reinsmoen NL, Snyder LD, Ganous TM, et al. Genetic regulation of rejection and survival following human lung transplantation by the innate immune receptor CD14. Am J Transplant. 2007 Mar;7(3):693–9

development or maintenance of allograft rejection, including complement activation, proteins secreted into the epithelial lining, and local innate immune cell-mediated responses.

Complement and Soluble Innate Proteins

The soluble and secreted protein components of the pulmonary innate immune system are essential to local pathogen control and furthermore maintain the ability to invoke and modulate local inflammatory responses. While the function of many of these secreted proteins as it relates to transplantation remains to be fully evaluated, activation of the complement cascade and alterations in the levels of mannose-binding lectin (MBL), alpha defensins, and surfactant protein A (SP-A), in particular, have been demonstrated to impact the risk for allograft rejection.

The complement system is a highly complex cascade involving three pathways—the classical, alternative, and lectin—all of which converge to generate C3 convertases that cleave C3 to C3a and C3b. While complement activation results in neutrophil and epithelial activation and cell lysis, it can also regulate the alloimmune response by enhancing or suppressing T cell-based immunity. Rigorous work has established the significance of the complement system in regulating allograft rejection in murine models of renal, cardiac, and skin transplantation in addition to pulmonary GVHD [36–41].

Pratt and colleagues, for example, demonstrated that wild-type mice do not reject allogeneic C3-deficient kidneys [37]. Similarly, enhanced local complement activation resulted in accelerated rejection kinetics and amplified anti-donor T-cell reactivity in a heart transplant model [38]. The mechanisms by which complement affects T-cell function are also becoming better understood. Experiments by Vieyra et al. revealed that complement production by DCs and expression of C3a and C5a receptors is required for $CD4^+$ lymphocytes to provide help to $CD8^+$ cells important in allograft rejection [40]. Accordingly, C5a receptor blocking strategies have been shown to prevent T-cell priming and result in prolonged allograft survival in rodent models of both renal and cardiac transplantation [39, 41].

More recently, and of increased relevance to lung transplantation, Khan et al. used a murine orthotopic tracheal transplant model to demonstrate that antibody-mediated complement activation results in microvascular injury and tissue ischemia, even in the absence of lymphocytes. This finding is important because tissue ischemia and loss of microcirculation are events thought to precede the development of obliterative airways disease [42] and furthermore is consistent with the observation that C4d deposition on pulmonary capillaries precedes vascular disruption during acute allograft rejection in models of rat orthotopic lung transplantation [43].

Clinical studies have corroborated the relevance of complement in human transplantation. Tissue from rejecting heart and kidney allografts has higher quantities of mRNA for the C5a and C3a complement receptors [36], and polymorphic variants in donor C3 have been demonstrated to impact recipient outcomes after renal transplantation [44]. Additional studies have invoked a potential role for complement activation, particularly of the lectin pathway by MBL, in modifying outcomes after lung transplantation [45–47]. MBL levels vary in the population owing to genetic variation and, importantly, deficiency has been shown to predispose to a variety of infections [4]. While current data remain inconclusive, alterations in MBL level may also impact susceptibility to lung allograft rejection and moderate post-transplant outcomes.

Beyond complement, others have noted that variations in pulmonary surfactant proteins [48], specifically surfactant protein A (SP-A), and the antimicrobial peptide alpha defensin [49–51] can be associated with the presence of BOS or even potentially predict its future onset. Nelsestuen and colleagues performed proteomic analysis on bronchoalveolar lavage (BAL) specimens from 57 lung allograft recipients and demonstrated that alpha defensin levels were 10–100 times greater in allograft recipients with BOS compared to stable post-transplant patients. Furthermore, the authors showed that alpha defensin levels begin to increase in the BAL up to 15 months prior to BOS diagnosis [50]. In contrast, a separate study demonstrated *reduced* SP-A levels in the BAL of patients with BOS. This decrease was detectable early after transplant, preceding BOS onset in most patients [48].

Interestingly, while SP-A has been demonstrated to have inhibitory effects on T-cell proliferation and DC maturation [5], alpha defensins are chemotactic for memory T cells and DCs [6] and may promote lung fibroblast proliferation and collagen synthesis [52]. It is therefore plausible that a reduction in SP-A eliminates an important immunoregulatory mechanism while increased levels of alpha defensins facilitate a robust inflammatory response. Further research into the specific role for these and other protein components in lung allograft rejection, specifically as they relate to long-term outcomes and BOS, is necessary. A focus on complement activation, in particular, is attractive because novel small molecule inhibitors of complement receptors are emerging and may offer selective therapeutic benefit.

Antigen-Presenting Cells

APCs, including DCs and macrophages, are central to innate immunity and represent a critical link between innate and adaptive responses. Consistent with this idea, in the context of transplant biology, ample evidence exists across numerous experimental systems illustrating a key role for DCs and macrophages in priming the alloimmune response.

DCs, in particular, are a heterogeneous population of innate cells that exist in a variety of functional states and may be derived from plasmacytoid cells (pDCs) or myeloid precursors such as monocytes (mDCs) [53]. While immature DCs are poor APCs and may even contribute to maintenance of tolerance, mature DCs are highly potent APCs that, upon activation, upregulate costimulatory molecules necessary for effective adaptive responses and express inflammatory cytokines that direct local immune processes [54]. Importantly, pDCs and mDCs have been described to have differential effects on T-cell activation. Whereas pDCs exert an immunoregulatory role and polarize toward a Th2 response, mDCs promote a strong Th1 type inflammatory response.

Initial work depleting and restoring these so-called graft passenger leukocytes in a kidney allograft model implicated DCs as key to alloantigen presentation, with donor organs devoid of incompatible leukocytes promoting graft acceptance and subsequent DC infusion reinstating immunogenicity [55]. More recent experiments in a murine orthotopic lung transplant model have confirmed the importance of donor-derived DCs in alloantigen-induced priming of recipient T cells [56]. Benson et al. evaluated the effect of either donor pDC or mDC depletion or concomitant depletion of both cell types in modulating experimental lung allograft rejection. While eradication of either cell type alone had minimal effect on the tempo or degree of acute rejection, elimination of both DC populations attenuated the severity of acute allograft rejection and decreased recipient T-cell proliferation [56].

Macrophages, like DCs, are important in antigen presentation and furthermore secrete growth factors that may play a role in mediating fibrotic airway responses after lung transplantation. Oyaizu et al. hypothesized that pharmacologic depletion of macrophages in a rat model of heterotopic tracheal transplantation would prevent the development of obliterative airway disease. Indeed, the authors demonstrated that macrophage-deplete recipients had a significant reduction in tracheal obliteration and profibrotic growth factors, including decreased expression of platelet-derived growth factor, a factor known to promote fibroblast proliferation [57]. This finding is consistent with later work in a murine cardiac allograft model that reported a 70 % reduction in the development of chronic cardiac allograft vasculopathy in macrophage-deplete hosts, an effect independent of T-cell or B-cell alloreactivity [58]. Interestingly, with a focus on graft obliteration, these studies also indicate that macrophages or macrophage-derived products may be important end-effector mechanisms in the profibrotic processes relevant to chronic allograft rejection [57, 58].

To date, very few studies have characterized DC and macrophage populations in the setting of clinical lung transplantation. The results of one small study evaluating peripheral blood leukocyte chimerism in lung allograft recipients suggest that while donor-derived mDCs persist and can be detected in the blood up to 1 year post-transplantation, pDCs are conspicuously and consistently absent, a finding of interest given the purported immunoregulatory function of pDCs [59]. Adjunctive work by Rizzo and colleagues demonstrated increased expression of adhesion molecules and the inflammatory cytokine interleukin-6 by AMs isolated from the BAL of lung-transplant recipients with acute rejection compared to stable controls, implicating AMs as important mediators of mononuclear cell adhesion and extravasation during allograft rejection [60].

Effector Cells of Innate Immunity

In addition to APCs, effector cells of innate immunity including neutrophils and NK cells have been implicated to play a role in the complex sequence of events culminating in airway fibrosis after lung transplantation. Kreisel et al. demonstrated that syngeneic lung transplantation stimulates granulopoiesis and accumulation of neutrophils within allograft tissues, suggesting that the transplant procedure itself or ischemic injury promotes neutrophils influx into the graft [61]. Furthermore, infiltrating neutrophils were recently shown to interact directly with graft donor-derived DCs in a murine model of orthotopic lung transplantation, and this interaction was associated with production of interleukin-12 and potentiation of Th1 alloimmunity and acute rejection [62]. As such, this neutrophil-DC interaction may represent a previously unrecognized link between innate and alloimmune responses after lung transplantation.

Neutrophil chemotaxis and angiogenesis have been shown to be promoted by ELR$^+$ CXC chemokines (such as interleukin-8) that utilize the CXCR2 receptor. Belperio et al. demonstrated that the CXCR2/CXCR2 ligand axis is critical in mediating early neutrophil recruitment and late vascular remodeling important to the development of fibro-obliterative airway disease in a heterotopic tracheal transplantation model, and, furthermore, levels of ELR$^+$ CXC chemokines in the BAL positively correlated with the presence of BOS in human lung allograft recipients

[63]. The neutrophil is by far the most predominant cell type in the BAL fluid of patients with BOS, even in the absence of concurrent infection or acute rejection, and the degree of BAL neutrophilia increases in correlation with increasing BOS stage. Going beyond a simple association, several studies have demonstrated the value of elevated BAL neutrophil counts prior to the onset of BOS as a factor useful in predicting its future development [64–66]. Neurohr et al., for example, followed 63 patients for 3 years post-transplant and showed that neutrophil proportions greater than 20 % predicted BOS onset a median of 232 days post-bronchoscopy [65].

NK cells are also important innate effector cells of increasingly recognized complexity. Recent work has validated that NK cells contribute to the development of solid organ transplant rejection in experimental models. In a mouse model of cardiac transplantation CD28 knockout mice depleted of NK cells were unable to reject heart allografts, while reconstitution of NK cells facilitated acute rejection via activation of CD28-negative cells, suggesting that NK cells provoke rejection through mechanisms that are not dependent on T-cell costimulation [67]. Interestingly, NK cells have also been demonstrated to play a role in chronic cardiac allograft rejection [68]. Although the precise function of innate immune cells as it relates to the mechanisms of allograft rejection in lung transplant recipients remains to be clarified, the results of one small study suggest that in recipients with BOS, there is both an increase in the number of NK cells present in lung tissue and increased activation of NK cells in the peripheral blood [69].

Together these studies implicate DCs, macrophages, and neutrophils, in particular, as important innate immune cells of particular relevance to lung transplant rejection. Further mechanistic studies characterizing the complex relationship between innate immune cells and T-cell reactivity in the context of transplantation may reveal novel strategies to polarize toward tolerant responses or minimize alloimmune and profibrotic processes.

Impact of Innate Immunity on Environmental Risk Factors for BOS

Evolving evidence supporting a central role for innate immune activation in regulating the host alloimmune response to lung transplantation provides an opportunity to reconsider the pathogenic mechanisms of established BOS risk factors. In fact, as outlined in Table 8.3, many of the previously established and more recently reported clinical risk factors for BOS are factors that could activate pulmonary innate immunity and include ischemia reperfusion injury (IRI), gastroesophageal reflux disease (GERD), exposure to air pollutants, and infection or colonization with viral or fungal pathogens, respectively [70–75].

Consistent with this idea, multiple studies have shown that endogenous DAMPs, such as high-mobility group box-1 and hyaluronic acid, released from ischemic or dying tissues in the setting of IRI, can activate innate pathways via TLR2, TLR4,

Table 8.3 Clinical BOS risk factors that activate pulmonary innate immunity

Ischemia reperfusion injury	Community respiratory virus infection
Cytomegalovirus pneumonitis	Gastroesophageal reflux disease
Aspergillus colonization	Air pollutants

BOS bronchiolitis obliterans syndrome

and the innate PRRs pentraxin-3 and receptor for advanced glycation end products [76–81]. This response may potentiate alloimmune reactivity and account for the increased risk for BOS in lung allograft recipients with a history of primary graft dysfunction. Interestingly, other noninfectious insults, such as GERD and chronic inhalation of environmental particulate matter, may also cause tissue injury and DAMP release or, alternatively, may directly activate TLRs to invoke downstream inflammation and adaptive processes. Aspiration of gastric refluxate, for example, has been noted to precipitate severe acute lung rejection and increases in innate cytokine levels in rat models of chronic sublethal aspiration [82, 83]. Still others have demonstrated a relationship between exposure to traffic air pollution and the development of BOS in a large, well-characterized sample of lung-transplant recipients from a region where air pollution levels are relatively high [73]. These latter findings are noteworthy given that genetic variations in TLR2 and TLR4 moderate responses to air pollutants in childhood asthma [84], and the functional and biological airway response to ozone has been shown to be TLR4-dependent [85].

Apart from tissue injury and DAMP release, lung-transplant recipients are also exposed to a myriad of microbial PAMPs that hold the potential to directly activate TLRs and initiate subsequent alloimmune reactivity. Lung allograft recipients, in particular, demonstrate increased susceptibility to infection due to both ongoing immunosuppression and underlying impairment in mechanical host defense [86]. Many clinical and basic studies support the link between infection and BOS. Retrospective studies suggest that community-acquired respiratory viral infections increase the risk for BOS [87–90], and experiments in a murine orthotopic tracheal transplant model indicate that infection with Sendai virus, a murine parainfluenza type I-like virus, increases tracheal fibro-obliteration and alloreactive T cells while invoking Treg apoptosis [91, 92]. Similarly, cytomegalovirus (CMV) pneumonitis has been demonstrated in large clinical cohorts to be a risk factor for BOS and death, even in the era of CMV post-transplant prophylaxis [70], and elevated levels of CCL2, a chemokine typically secreted by macrophages and chemotactic for DCs and memory T cells, have been noted in the BAL fluid from patients with CMV infection who later go on to develop BOS [93].

While literature evaluating a role for bacterial infection and colonization in BOS is inconsistent, the impact of fungal colonization is just beginning to be explored. An intriguing study by Weigt and colleagues recently implicated Aspergillus *colonization* in the lung allograft, even in the absence of frank infection, as a novel BOS risk factor that independently predicted BOS-related morbidity and mortality regardless of acute rejection burden [72]. As Aspergillus is recognized through TLR2 and TLR4, this suggests that the relationship between lung infection and BOS may not be limited to specific pathogens, but rather depend on activation of the innate immune system and subsequent alloimmune potentiation in response to a broad spectrum of pathogen-associated motifs [94].

Further identification and characterization of the specific PAMPs, DAMPs, and PRRs involved in the pulmonary allograft response to each of these clinical risk factors may offer the ability to selectively target and block subsequent adaptive immune responses. In the meantime, efforts to limit environmental infectious and noninfectious insults in addition to heightened surveillance and early recognition of allograft rejection provoked by these processes are warranted.

Future Directions

The innate immune system is now recognized to play a critical role in regulating adaptive immunity and the response to transplantation. This is of particular relevance to lung transplantation, given the constant interface between the lung allograft and external environment. Experimental evidence supports an essential role for TLR signaling and other innate processes, including complement and innate cell activation in modulating allograft rejection. Furthermore, clinical studies reinforce these experimental findings, particularly with respect to TLR activation, and indicate that BOS susceptibility is very likely to be regulated by multiple genes in the context of gene–gene and gene–environment interactions based on patterns of post-transplant PAMP/DAMP exposure and PRR activation. These data suggest a constant interplay between environmental stimuli, the innate immune response, and recipient genetic susceptibilities that together shape and regulate the subsequent adaptive response.

A major limitation of the current studies as they relate to lung transplantation is that much of the available evidence related to innate immune activation in allotransplantation has utilized experimental models of skin or heart rejection. Many opportunities now exist to take advantage of the range of newly established lung allograft models, including the murine orthotopic lung transplant model, in order to directly explore these innate processes in a context that is more relevant to human lung transplantation [95]. Such studies have already implicated a novel role for the lung as a tertiary lymphoid organ and established the importance of neutrophils in acute rejection [9, 62]. Rigorous work to further characterize the specific innate processes involved in lung rejection using these and other model systems is likely to identify novel targets for selective therapeutic intervention.

In fact, TLR inhibitors and antagonists of other innate immune receptors or protein effectors, such as CD14 and complement receptors, are being developed for use in humans, and clinical trials are already ongoing in certain immune or inflammatory conditions [96–98]. Although no substantial adverse effects have been reported to date, the efficacy of such approaches remains to be determined. In addition, studies of therapeutics targeting innate immunity must balance the risks of inhibiting protective first-line host defense with the potential benefit of attenuating harmful downstream inflammatory responses. The timing of such targeted therapies with respect to transplantation also remains to be explored, as innate stimuli are both immediate and persistent over the lifetime of the allograft.

The growing understanding of innate immunity in solid organ transplantation offers important mechanistic insights that are highly relevant to lung transplantation. Innate processes are likely to contribute to the high rates of lung rejection and BOS. As additional mechanistic details related to the innate-alloimmune interaction are discovered, there is great potential to develop novel therapies that could significantly enhance the effectiveness of current immunosuppressive regimens and reduce lung rejection. In summary, an evolving body of experimental and clinical evidence suggests that further research focused on innate immunity is critical to advance the field of lung transplantation, and an improved understanding of the role of innate immunity in lung allograft rejection could translate into therapies that substantially improve long-term patient outcomes in the future.

References

1. Medzhitov R, Janeway Jr C. Innate immunity. N Engl J Med. 2000;343(5):338–44.
2. Trinchieri G, Kubin M, Bellone G, Cassatella MA. Cytokine cross-talk between phagocytic cells and lymphocytes: relevance for differentiation/activation of phagocytic cells and regulation of adaptive immunity. J Cell Biochem. 1993;53(4):301–8.
3. Zhang P, Summer WR, Bagby GJ, Nelson S. Innate immunity and pulmonary host defense. Immunol Rev. 2000;173(1):39–51.
4. Zaas AK, Schwartz DA. Innate immunity and the lung: defense at the interface between host and environment. Trends Cardiovasc Med. 2005;15(6):195–202.
5. Wright JR. Immunoregulatory functions of surfactant proteins. Nat Rev Immunol. 2005;5(1):58–68. doi:10.1038/nri1528.
6. Ganz T. Defensins: antimicrobial peptides of innate immunity. Nat Rev Immunol. 2003;3(9):710–20. doi:10.1038/nri1180.
7. Dunkelberger JR, Song W-C. Complement and its role in innate and adaptive immune responses. Cell Res. 2009;20(1):34–50.
8. Martin TR, Frevert CW. Innate immunity in the lungs. Proc Am Thorac Soc. 2005;2(5):403–11.
9. Gelman AE, Li W, Richardson SB, Zinselmeyer BH, Lai J, Okazaki M, et al. Cutting edge: acute lung allograft rejection is independent of secondary lymphoid organs. J Immunol. 2009;182(7):3969–73.
10. Trinchieri G, Sher A. Cooperation of Toll-like receptor signals in innate immune defence. Nat Rev Immunol. 2007;7(3):179–90.
11. Kawai T, Akira S. TLR signaling. Semin Immunol. 2007;19(1):24–32.
12. Akira S, Takeda K, Kaisho T. Toll-like receptors: critical proteins linking innate and acquired immunity. Nat Immunol. 2001;2(8):675–80.
13. Medzhitov R. Toll-like receptors and innate immunity. Nat Rev Immunol. 2001;1(2):135–45.
14. Medzhitov R, Janeway Jr C. The Toll receptor family and microbial recognition. Trends Microbiol. 2000;8(10):452–6.
15. Imler JL, Hoffmann JA. Toll receptors in innate immunity. Trends Cell Biol. 2001;11(7):304–11.
16. Akira S, Takeda K. Toll-like receptor signalling. Nat Rev Immunol. 2004;4(7):499–511. doi:10.1038/nri1391.
17. OPTN/SRT 2010 Annual Report. [7 Apr 2012]; http://www.srtr.org/annual_reports.

18. Ahmed EB, Daniels M, Alegre ML, Chong AS. Bacterial infections, alloimmunity, and transplantation tolerance. Transplant Rev (Orlando). 2011;25(1):27–35.
19. Palmer SM, Burch LH, Trindade AJ, Davis RD, Herczyk WF, Reinsmoen NL, et al. Innate immunity influences long-term outcomes after human lung transplant. Am J Respir Crit Care Med. 2005;171(7):780–5.
20. He H, Stone JR, Perkins DL. Analysis of robust innate immune response after transplantation in the absence of adaptive immunity. Transplantation. 2002;73(6):853–61.
21. Christopher K, Mueller TF, Ma C, Liang Y, Perkins DL. Analysis of the innate and adaptive phases of allograft rejection by cluster analysis of transcriptional profiles. J Immunol. 2002;169(1):522–30.
22. Goldstein DR, Tesar BM, Akira S, Lakkis FG. Critical role of the Toll-like receptor signal adaptor protein MyD88 in acute allograft rejection. J Clin Invest. 2003;111(10):1571–8.
23. Tesar BM, Zhang J, Li Q, Goldstein DR. TH1 immune responses to fully MHC mismatched allografts are diminished in the absence of MyD88, a Toll-like receptor signal adaptor protein. Am J Transplant. 2004;4(9):1429–39.
24. McKay D, Shigeoka A, Rubinstein M, Surh C, Sprent J. Simultaneous deletion of MyD88 and Trif delays major histocompatibility and minor antigen mismatch allograft rejection. Eur J Immunol. 2006;36(8):1994–2002.
25. Thornley TB, Brehm MA, Markees TG, Shultz LD, Mordes JP, Welsh RM, et al. TLR agonists abrogate costimulation blockade-induced prolongation of skin allografts. J Immunol. 2006;176(3):1561–70.
26. Chen L, Wang T, Zhou P, Ma L, Yin D, Shen J, et al. TLR engagement prevents transplantation tolerance. Am J Transplant. 2006;6(10):2282–91.
27. Garantziotis S, Palmer SM, Snyder LD, Ganous T, Chen BJ, Wang T, et al. Alloimmune lung injury induced by local innate immune activation through inhaled lipopolysaccharide. Transplantation. 2007;84(8):1012–9.
28. Kinnier CV, Martinu T, Gowdy KM, Nugent JL, Kelly FL, Palmer SM. Innate immune activation by the viral PAMP poly I:C potentiates pulmonary graft-versus-host disease after allogeneic hematopoietic cell transplant. Transpl Immunol. 2011;24(2):83–93.
29. Porrett PM, Yuan X, LaRosa DF, Walsh PT, Yang J, Gao W, et al. Mechanisms underlying blockade of allograft acceptance by TLR ligands. J Immunol. 2008;181(3):1692–9.
30. Ahmed EB, Wang T, Daniels M, Alegre ML, Chong AS. IL-6 induced by Staphylococcus aureus infection prevents the induction of skin allograft acceptance in mice. Am J Transplant. 2011;11(5):936–46.
31. Chen L, Ahmed E, Wang T, Wang Y, Ochando J, Chong AS, et al. TLR signals promote IL-6/IL-17-dependent transplant rejection. J Immunol. 2009;182(10):6217–25.
32. Arbour NC, Lorenz E, Schutte BC, Zabner J, Kline JN, Jones M, et al. TLR4 mutations are associated with endotoxin hyporesponsiveness in humans. Nat Genet. 2000;25(2):187–91.
33. Goldstein DR, Palmer SM. Role of Toll-like receptor-driven innate immunity in thoracic organ transplantation. J Heart Lung Transplant. 2005;24(11):1721–9.
34. Palmer SM, Burch LH, Davis RD, Herczyk WF, Howell DN, Reinsmoen NL, et al. The role of innate immunity in acute allograft rejection after lung transplantation. Am J Respir Crit Care Med. 2003;168(6):628–32.
35. Palmer SM, Klimecki W, Yu L, Reinsmoen NL, Snyder LD, Ganous TM, et al. Genetic regulation of rejection and survival following human lung transplantation by the innate immune receptor CD14. Am J Transplant. 2007;7(3):693–9.
36. Kwan WH, van der Touw W, Heeger PS. Complement regulation of T cell immunity. Immunol Res. 2012;54(1–3):247–53.
37. Pratt JR, Basheer SA, Sacks SH. Local synthesis of complement component C3 regulates acute renal transplant rejection. Nat Med. 2002;8(6):582–7.
38. Pavlov V, Raedler H, Yuan S, Leisman S, Kwan WH, Lalli PN, et al. Donor deficiency of decay-accelerating factor accelerates murine T cell-mediated cardiac allograft rejection. J Immunol. 2008;181(7):4580–9.

39. Gueler F, Rong S, Gwinner W, Mengel M, Brocker V, Schon S, et al. Complement 5a receptor inhibition improves renal allograft survival. J Am Soc Nephrol. 2008;19(12):2302–12.
40. Vieyra M, Leisman S, Raedler H, Kwan WH, Yang M, Strainic MG, et al. Complement regulates CD4 T-cell help to CD8 T cells required for murine allograft rejection. Am J Pathol. 2011;179(2):766–74.
41. Raedler H, Vieyra MB, Leisman S, Lakhani P, Kwan W, Yang M, et al. Anti-complement component C5 mAb synergizes with CTLA4Ig to inhibit alloreactive T cells and prolong cardiac allograft survival in mice. Am J Transplant. 2011;11(7):1397–406.
42. Khan MA, Jiang X, Dhillon G, Beilke J, Holers VM, Atkinson C, et al. CD4+ T cells and complement independently mediate graft ischemia in the rejection of mouse orthotopic tracheal transplants. Circ Res. 2011;109(11):1290–301.
43. Murata K, Iwata T, Nakashima S, Fox-Talbot K, Qian Z, Wilkes DS, et al. C4d deposition and cellular infiltrates as markers of acute rejection in rat models of orthotopic lung transplantation. Transplantation. 2008;86(1):123–9.
44. Brown KM, Kondeatis E, Vaughan RW, Kon SP, Farmer CK, Taylor JD, et al. Influence of donor C3 allotype on late renal-transplantation outcome. N Engl J Med. 2006;354(19): 2014–23.
45. Hodge S, Dean M, Hodge G, Holmes M, Reynolds PN. Decreased efferocytosis and mannose binding lectin in the airway in bronchiolitis obliterans syndrome. J Heart Lung Transplant. 2011;30(5):589–95.
46. Carroll KE, Dean MM, Heatley SL, Meehan AC, Mifsud NA, Kotsimbos TC, et al. High levels of mannose-binding lectin are associated with poor outcomes after lung transplantation. Transplantation. 2011;91(9):1044–9.
47. Munster JM, van der Bij W, Breukink MB, van der Steege G, Zuurman MW, Hepkema BG, et al. Association between donor MBL promoter haplotype and graft survival and the development of BOS after lung transplantation. Transplantation. 2008;86(12):1857–63.
48. Meloni F, Salvini R, Bardoni AM, Passadore I, Solari N, Vitulo P, et al. Bronchoalveolar lavage fluid proteome in bronchiolitis obliterans syndrome: possible role for surfactant protein A in disease onset. J Heart Lung Transplant. 2007;26(11):1135–43.
49. Anderson RL, Hiemstra PS, Ward C, Forrest IA, Murphy D, Proud D, et al. Antimicrobial peptides in lung transplant recipients with bronchiolitis obliterans syndrome. Eur Respir J. 2008;32(3):670–7.
50. Nelsestuen GL, Martinez MB, Hertz MI, Savik K, Wendt CH. Proteomic identification of human neutrophil alpha-defensins in chronic lung allograft rejection. Proteomics. 2005;5(6):1705–13.
51. Ross DJ, Cole AM, Yoshioka D, Park AK, Belperio JA, Laks H, et al. Increased bronchoalveolar lavage human beta-defensin type 2 in bronchiolitis obliterans syndrome after lung transplantation. Transplantation. 2004;78(8):1222–4.
52. Han W, Wang W, Mohammed KA, Su Y. α-Defensins increase lung fibroblast proliferation and collagen synthesis via the β-catenin signaling pathway. FEBS J. 2009;276(22):6603–14.
53. Lechler R, Ng WF, Steinman RM. Dendritic cells in transplantation—friend or foe? Immunity. 2001;14(4):357–68.
54. Murphy SP, Porrett PM, Turka LA. Innate immunity in transplant tolerance and rejection. Immunol Rev. 2011;241(1):39–48.
55. Lechler RI, Batchelor JR. Restoration of immunogenicity to passenger cell-depleted kidney allografts by the addition of donor strain dendritic cells. J Exp Med. 1982;155(1):31–41.
56. Benson HL, Suzuki H, Lott J, Fisher AJ, Walline C, Heidler KM, et al. Donor lung derived myeloid and plasmacytoid dendritic cells differentially regulate T cell proliferation and cytokine production. Respir Res. 2012;13:25.
57. Oyaizu T, Okada Y, Shoji W, Matsumura Y, Shimada K, Sado T, et al. Reduction of recipient macrophages by gadolinium chloride prevents development of obliterative airway disease in a rat model of heterotopic tracheal transplantation. Transplantation. 2003;76(8):1214–20.

58. Kitchens WH, Chase CM, Uehara S, Cornell LD, Colvin RB, Russell PS, et al. Macrophage depletion suppresses cardiac allograft vasculopathy in mice. Am J Transplant. 2007;7(12):2675–82.
59. Paantjens AW, van de Graaf EA, Heerkens HD, Kwakkel-van Erp JM, Hoefnagel T, van Kessel DA, et al. Chimerism of dendritic cell subsets in peripheral blood after lung transplantation. J Heart Lung Transplant. 2011;30(6):691–7.
60. Rizzo M, SivaSai KS, Smith MA, Trulock EP, Lynch JP, Patterson GA, et al. Increased expression of inflammatory cytokines and adhesion molecules by alveolar macrophages of human lung allograft recipients with acute rejection: decline with resolution of rejection. J Heart Lung Transplant. 2000;19(9):858–65.
61. Kreisel D, Sugimoto S, Tietjens J, Zhu J, Yamamoto S, Krupnick AS, et al. Bcl3 prevents acute inflammatory lung injury in mice by restraining emergency granulopoiesis. J Clin Invest. 2011;121(1):265–76.
62. Kreisel D, Sugimoto S, Zhu J, Nava R, Li W, Okazaki M, et al. Emergency granulopoiesis promotes neutrophil-dendritic cell encounters that prevent mouse lung allograft acceptance. Blood. 2011;118(23):6172–82.
63. Belperio JA, Keane MP, Burdick MD, Gomperts B, Xue YY, Hong K, et al. Role of CXCR2/CXCR2 ligands in vascular remodeling during bronchiolitis obliterans syndrome. J Clin Invest. 2005;115(5):1150–62.
64. Slebos D-J, Postma DS, Koëter GH, van der Bij W, Boezen M, Kauffman HF. Bronchoalveolar lavage fluid characteristics in acute and chronic lung transplant rejection. J Heart Lung Transplant. 2004;23(5):532–40.
65. Neurohr C, Huppmann P, Samweber B, Leuschner S, Zimmermann G, Leuchte H, et al. Prognostic value of bronchoalveolar lavage neutrophilia in stable lung transplant recipients. J Heart Lung Transplant. 2009;28(5):468–74.
66. Reynaud-Gaubert M, Thomas P, Badier M, Cau P, Giudicelli R, Fuentes P. Early detection of airway involvement in obliterative bronchiolitis after lung transplantation. Am J Respir Crit Care Med. 2000;161(6):1924–9.
67. Maier S, Tertilt C, Chambron N, Gerauer K, Huser N, Heidecke C-D, et al. Inhibition of natural killer cells results in acceptance of cardiac allografts in CD28–/– mice. Nat Med. 2001;7(5):557–62. doi:10.1038/87880.
68. Uehara S, Chase CM, Kitchens WH, Rose HS, Colvin RB, Russell PS, et al. NK cells can trigger allograft vasculopathy: the role of hybrid resistance in solid organ allografts. J Immunol. 2005;175(5):3424–30.
69. Fildes JE, Yonan N, Tunstall K, Walker AH, Griffiths-Davies L, Bishop P, et al. Natural killer cells in peripheral blood and lung tissue are associated with chronic rejection after lung transplantation. J Heart Lung Transplant. 2008;27(2):203–7.
70. Snyder LD, Finlen-Copeland CA, Turbyfill WJ, Howell D, Willner DA, Palmer SM. Cytomegalovirus pneumonitis is a risk for bronchiolitis obliterans syndrome in lung transplantation. Am J Respir Crit Care Med. 2010;181(12):1391–6.
71. Kumar D, Erdman D, Keshavjee S, Peret T, Tellier R, Hadjiliadis D, et al. Clinical impact of community-acquired respiratory viruses on bronchiolitis obliterans after lung transplant. Am J Transplant. 2005;5(8):2031–6.
72. Weigt SS, Elashoff RM, Huang C, Ardehali A, Gregson AL, Kubak B, et al. Aspergillus colonization of the lung allograft is a risk factor for bronchiolitis obliterans syndrome. Am J Transplant. 2009;9(8):1903–11.
73. Nawrot TS, Vos R, Jacobs L, Verleden SE, Wauters S, Mertens V, et al. The impact of traffic air pollution on bronchiolitis obliterans syndrome and mortality after lung transplantation. Thorax. 2011;66(9):748–54.
74. Lee JC, Christie JD. Primary graft dysfunction. Proc Am Thorac Soc. 2009;6(1):39–46.
75. Davis Jr RD, Lau CL, Eubanks S, Messier RH, Hadjiliadis D, Steele MP, et al. Improved lung allograft function after fundoplication in patients with gastroesophageal reflux disease undergoing lung transplantation. J Thorac Cardiovasc Surg. 2003;125(3):533–42.

76. Diamond JM, Lederer DJ, Kawut SM, Lee J, Ahya VN, Bellamy S, et al. Elevated plasma long pentraxin-3 levels and primary graft dysfunction after lung transplantation for idiopathic pulmonary fibrosis. Am J Transplant. 2011;11(11):2517–22.
77. Pelaez A, Force SD, Gal AA, Neujahr DC, Ramirez AM, Naik PM, et al. Receptor for advanced glycation end products in donor lungs is associated with primary graft dysfunction after lung transplantation. Am J Transplant. 2010;10(4):900–7.
78. Christie JD, Shah CV, Kawut SM, Mangalmurti N, Lederer DJ, Sonett JR, et al. Plasma levels of receptor for advanced glycation end products, blood transfusion, and risk of primary graft dysfunction. Am J Respir Crit Care Med. 2009;180(10):1010–5.
79. Wu H, Ma J, Wang P, Corpuz TM, Panchapakesan U, Wyburn KR, et al. HMGB1 contributes to kidney ischemia reperfusion injury. J Am Soc Nephrol. 2010;21(11):1878–90.
80. Wu H, Chen G, Wyburn KR, Yin J, Bertolino P, Eris JM, et al. TLR4 activation mediates kidney ischemia/reperfusion injury. J Clin Invest. 2007;117(10):2847–59.
81. Shigeoka AA, Holscher TD, King AJ, Hall FW, Kiosses WB, Tobias PS, et al. TLR2 is constitutively expressed within the kidney and participates in ischemic renal injury through both MyD88-dependent and -independent pathways. J Immunol. 2007;178(10):6252–8.
82. Appel III JZ, Lee SM, Hartwig MG, Li B, Hsieh CC, Cantu III E, et al. Characterization of the innate immune response to chronic aspiration in a novel rodent model. Respir Res. 2007;8:87.
83. Hartwig MG, Appel JZ, Li B, Hsieh CC, Yoon YH, Lin SS, et al. Chronic aspiration of gastric fluid accelerates pulmonary allograft dysfunction in a rat model of lung transplantation. J Thorac Cardiovasc Surg. 2006;131(1):209–17.
84. Kerkhof M, Postma DS, Brunekreef B, Reijmerink NE, Wijga AH, de Jongste JC, et al. Toll-like receptor 2 and 4 genes influence susceptibility to adverse effects of traffic-related air pollution on childhood asthma. Thorax. 2010;65(8):690–7.
85. Li Z, Potts-Kant EN, Garantziotis S, Foster WM, Hollingsworth JW. Hyaluronan signaling during ozone-induced lung injury requires TLR4, MyD88, and TIRAP. PLoS One. 2011;6(11):e27137.
86. Fishman JA. Infection in solid-organ transplant recipients. N Engl J Med. 2007;357(25): 2601–14.
87. Billings JL, Hertz MI, Savik K, Wendt CH. Respiratory viruses and chronic rejection in lung transplant recipients. J Heart Lung Transplant. 2002;21(5):559–66.
88. Holt ND, Gould FK, Taylor CE, Harwood JF, Freeman R, Healy MD, et al. Incidence and significance of noncytomegalovirus viral respiratory infection after adult lung transplantation. J Heart Lung Transplant. 1997;16(4):416–9.
89. Palmer Jr SM, Henshaw NG, Howell DN, Miller SE, Davis RD, Tapson VF. Community respiratory viral infection in adult lung transplant recipients. Chest. 1998;113(4):944–50.
90. Vilchez RA, Dauber J, Kusne S. Infectious etiology of bronchiolitis obliterans: the respiratory viruses connection—myth or reality? Am J Transplant. 2003;3(3):245–9.
91. Kuo E, Bharat A, Goers T, Chapman W, Yan L, Street T, et al. Respiratory viral infection in obliterative airway disease after orthotopic tracheal transplantation. Ann Thorac Surg. 2006;82(3):1043–50.
92. Bharat A, Kuo E, Saini D, Steward N, Hachem R, Trulock EP, et al. Respiratory virus-induced dysregulation of T-regulatory cells leads to chronic rejection. Ann Thorac Surg. 2010;90(5):1637–44; discussion 44.
93. Weigt SS, Elashoff RM, Keane MP, Strieter RM, Gomperts BN, Xue YY, et al. Altered levels of CC chemokines during pulmonary CMV predict BOS and mortality post-lung transplantation. Am J Transplant. 2008;8(7):1512–22.
94. Garantziotis S, Palmer SM. An unwelcome guest: Aspergillus colonization in lung transplantation and its association with bronchiolitis obliterans syndrome. Am J Transplant. 2009;9(8):1705–6.
95. Kreisel D, Gelman AE, Palmer SM. In pursuit of new experimental models of obliterative bronchiolitis. Am J Transplant. 2011;11(5):882–3.

96. Hennessy EJ, Parker AE, O'Neill LA. Targeting Toll-like receptors: emerging therapeutics? Nat Rev Drug Discov. 2010;9(4):293–307.
97. Axtelle T, Pribble J. An overview of clinical studies in healthy subjects and patients with severe sepsis with IC14, a CD14-specific chimeric monoclonal antibody. J Endotoxin Res. 2003;9(6):385–9.
98. Testa L, Van Gaal WJ, Bhindi R, Biondi-Zoccai GGL, Abbate A, Agostoni P, et al. Pexelizumab in ischemic heart disease: a systematic review and meta-analysis on 15,196 patients. J Thorac Cardiovasc Surg. 2008;136(4):884–93.

Chapter 9
Mechanisms of Fibrogenesis in Post-transplant Bronchiolitis Obliterans

Anish Wadhwa and Vibha N. Lama

Abstract Bronchiolitis obliterans (BO) post-lung transplant is a fibroproliferative disease of the small airways. Among all fibrotic diseases, BO is unique in that we have the opportunity to follow the evolution of airway remodeling and fibrosis via serial lung samplings. Although there is a definite role of immune and nonimmune injury in the pathogenesis of this disease, the physiological impairment in BO is related to fibrogenesis. Hence, understanding the pathogenesis of fibroproliferation in BO is critical for identifying targets for future therapeutic interventions and the timing of such therapy. This review updates the understanding of the cellular and molecular participants in fibrotic remodeling of the lung allograft.

Keywords Bronchiolitis obliterans • Fibrosis • Mesenchymal cell • Collagen • Remodeling • Lung transplant • Fibroproliferation • Myofibroblast • Fibrogenesis • Mesenchymal stem cell

A. Wadhwa, M.D.
Pulmonary and Critical Care Medicine, University of Michigan Health System, 6301 MSRB III/5642, 1150 West Medical Center Drive, Ann Arbor, MI 48109-5642, USA
e-mail: anishw@med.umich.edu

V.N. Lama, M.D., M.S. (✉)
Department of Internal Medicine, University of Michigan, 6340, MSRB III, 1150 West Medical Center Drive, Ann Arbor, MI 48103, USA
e-mail: vlama@umich.edu

K.C. Meyer and A.R. Glanville (eds.), *Bronchiolitis Obliterans Syndrome in Lung Transplantation*, Respiratory Medicine 8, DOI 10.1007/978-1-4614-7636-8_9,

Fibrosis as a Prominent Histological Feature of Chronic Allograft Rejection

Architectural remodeling with fibrosis and scarring of airways and blood vessels is the most prominent histological feature noted in lung allografts undergoing chronic allograft dysfunction [1, 2]. Basement membrane fragmentation, intra-luminal, or subepithelial infiltration of mesenchymal cells, and dense collagen deposition are noted in the membranous and respiratory bronchioles. This fibroproliferative process results in partial or complete obliteration of the lumen [3] and in late stages the small airways can be completely replaced by a fibrous scar (Fig. 9.1).

Role of Allo- and Autoimmune Injury in Pathogenesis of Fibrosis Accompanying BO in Lung Transplant Recipients

While the pathological diagnosis of bronchiolitis obliterans (BO) is not limited to lung transplant recipients, its predominance in patients with either bone marrow transplantation or lung transplantation—scenarios marked by allogeneic mismatch of the lung with the hematopoietic cells—suggests an important role for alloimmune insults in perpetuating this process. Further evidence is provided by an association of acute rejection episodes with the development of BOS in lung transplant recipients [4–8]. Specifically, lymphocytic infiltration of small airways is thought to precede fibrotic obliteration [9–11]. Both T and B lymphocytes have been implicated in development of airway obliteration in murine models, suggesting a role for cell-mediated and humoral immunity in the resultant fibrotic responses [12–15]. Alloimmune injury can also potentially initiate development of an autoimmune response. Work in this field demonstrates development of collagen(V)-specific cellular immunity prior to development of BOS [16]. Thus, BO can be characterized as an aberrant repair response of the donor lung to chronic/recurrent allo- or autoimmune insults and can be compared to wound healing.

Myofibroblasts: The Central Effector Cell in BO

Recruitment and proliferation of mesenchymal cells and their differentiation to myofibroblasts represent the hallmark of fibroproliferative disorders [17]. Myofibroblasts demonstrate phenotypic and behavioral features of fibroblasts and smooth muscle cells and are characterized by expression of the contractile protein, α(alpha)-smooth muscle actin (α-SMA). BO lesions in human lungs demonstrate luminal or subintimal infiltration by myofibroblasts [18] (Fig. 9.1). Due to their increased collagen synthetic function and contractile phenotype, these cells play a crucial role in the resulting fibrotic pathology and associated obstructive physiology.

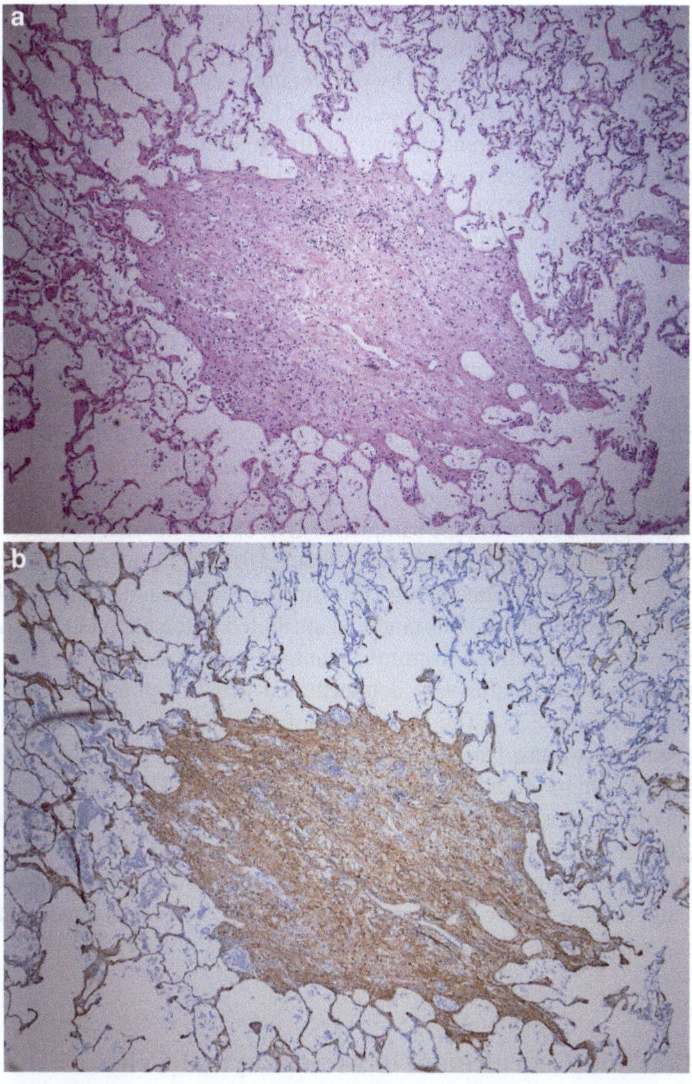

Fig. 9.1 Myofibroblasts in a bronchiolitis obliterans lesion. Bronchiolitis obliterans is noted as demonstrated by complete fibrotic obliteration of a terminal bronchus. (**a**) H&E staining, ×40 magnification. (**b**) Alpha-smooth muscle actin-positive mesenchymal cells (myofibroblasts) can be identified in the lesion by immunohistochemical staining

Origin of Mesenchymal Cells in Graft Fibrogenesis

Understanding the origin of myofibroblasts is crucial to targeting molecular mechanisms that underlie the recruitment and differentiation of mesenchymal cells in fibrotic lung diseases. In the context of lung transplantation, the potential sources of mesenchymal cells can be divided into those of donor vs. recipient origin. Resident mesenchymal or epithelial somatic cells in the lung graft can contribute to augmentation of the mesenchymal cell pool by proliferation or trans-differentiation, respectively. Donor lungs also contain a population of long-lived mesenchymal progenitor cells with an ability to differentiate into multiple mesenchymal lineages, including myofibroblasts. The presence of mesenchymal stem cells in the bone marrow and an increased expression of CD45-positive collagen-expressing cells termed fibrocytes in the blood of patients with BOS also suggests that the recipient has the ability to contribute to the mesenchymal pool in the transplanted lung [19, 20]. These multiple potential sources, combined with the lack of unique markers of origin, make it difficult to determine the relative contribution of a specific compartment to lung fibrogenesis. However, recent studies of sex-mismatched patients and comparison of lung-derived to bone marrow-derived mesenchymal progenitor cells have shed more light on this issue. Newer methodology that combines staining for mesenchymal markers with fluorescent in situ hybridization (FISH) for detection of sex chromosomes can be utilized to identify the origin of cells in lung grafts. This technique, when applied to histologic samples of BO, carries the risk of overestimating recipient contribution, because hematopoietic cells can lie in close proximity to mesenchymal cells [21]. Nonetheless, in a study of BO lesions utilizing this technique, only a minority of the cells could be attributed to the recipient [22]. Analysis of mesenchymal cells derived from transplanted lungs of sex-mismatched patients at a single cell level conclusively demonstrated that this population is predominantly donor in origin [23]. The persistence of mesenchymal cells of donor origin up to 11 years post-transplant emphasizes the ability of the graft to self-perpetuate and self-replenish its cellular populations (Fig. 9.2) [23]. Furthermore, unique expression of embryonic lung mesenchyme-associated transcription factors such as forkhead/winged helix transcription factor forkhead box (FOXF1) in graft-derived mesenchymal progenitor cells as well as in the myofibroblasts in biopsy samples strongly suggest that the mesenchymal component of the transplanted adult lung is the major contributor to fibrogenesis occurring in the graft [24].

Migration and Recruitment of Mesenchymal Cells Within an Allograft

Mobilization of mesenchymal cell populations within an allograft has been demonstrated by quantification of fibroblast colony-forming units in bronchoalveolar lavage fluid (BAL) [23]. An increase in mesenchymal cells in the airspaces is noted early post-transplant, suggesting a role for these cells in lung repair [25]. An increase in mesenchymal cell numbers in the BAL fluid also accompanies and predates development of BOS [25]. These finding are in contrast to normal lungs or quiescent allografts, which do not demonstrate a significant mesenchymal cell population in the BAL [23].

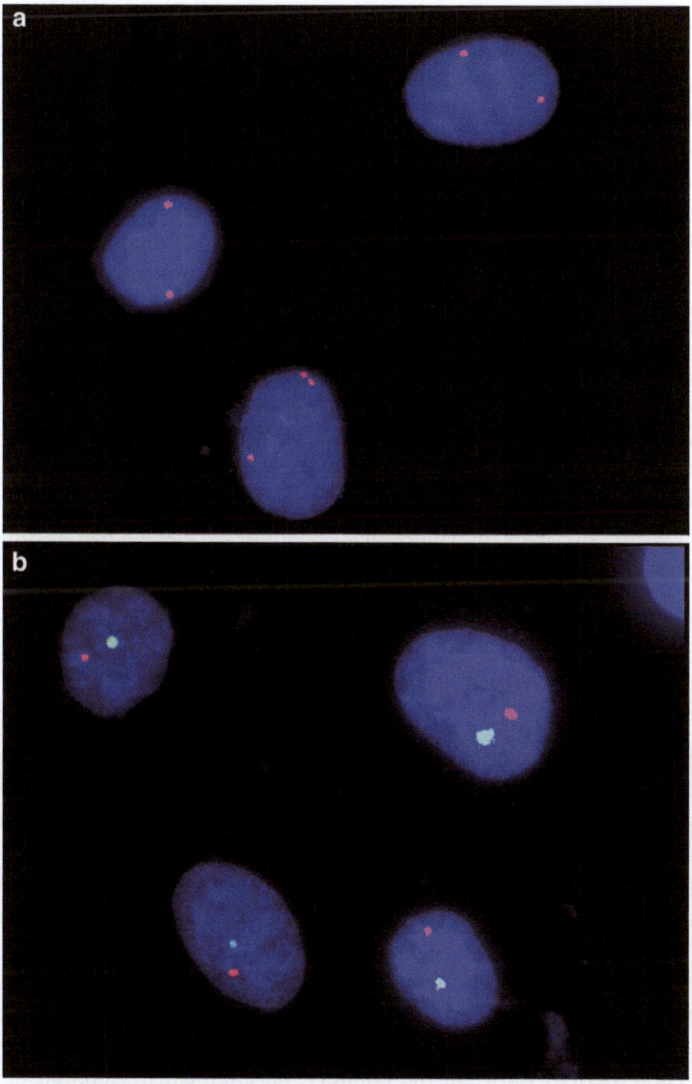

Fig. 9.2 Mesenchymal cells in an allograft are donor derived. XY chromosome analysis in sex-mismatched recipients demonstrates donor origin of mesenchymal progenitor cells population derived from bronchoalveolar lavage of human lung allografts. Red signal indicates X chromosome, and green signal indicates Y chromosome. Cells shown in (**a**) demonstrate female sex chromosome pattern and were obtained from a male patient who received a female donor lung. (**b**) demonstrates the male sex chromosome status of mesenchymal cells obtained from BAL of a male donor lung transplanted into a female recipient. Republished with permission of American Society for Clinical Investigation, from Lama VN, Smith L, Badri L, Flint A, Andrei AC, Murray S, et al. Evidence for tissue-resident mesenchymal stem cells in human adult lung from studies of transplanted allografts. J Clin Invest 2007;117:989–96; permission conveyed through Copyright Clearance Center, Inc.

Mesenchymal cell recruitment and migration during wound healing can be mediated by a wide array of chemokines, growth factors, and lipid mediators. Several of these mesenchymal chemotactic factors have been demonstrated to be present in a human lung allograft milieu and could potentially be relevant in migration of mesenchymal cells within an allograft. Endothelin-1 (ET-1), a potent mitogenic and pro-fibrotic peptide produced by pulmonary vascular endothelial cells, is increased in BAL [26] and also stimulates migration of mesenchymal progenitor cells isolated from allograft airspaces [27]. BAL derived from human lung allografts can induce migration of mesenchymal cells in vitro [28]. The predominant factor responsible for this capacity was found to be a bioactive lipid mediator, lysophosphatidic acid (LPA) [28]. LPA levels in BAL correlate with number of mesenchymal cells, and antagonism of LPA receptor can counteract the majority of the mesenchymal chemoattractant ability of BAL. LPA-induced migration of lung allograft–derived mesenchymal cells is mediated via activation of β(beta)-catenin, an integral cell–cell adhesion adaptor protein and a transcriptional co-regulator. LPA-induced ligation of the G protein coupled receptor, LPA1, induces PKC-mediated GSK3β (beta) phosphorylation, which results in cytoplasmic accumulation and nuclear translocation of β(beta)-catenin [28].

Altered Mesenchymal Cell Phenotype in BOS

Investigation of mesenchymal cells post-transplant suggests a stable phenotypic alteration in patients with BOS [24, 29]. Increased extracellular matrix synthetic capacity as well as higher α(alpha)-SMA expression is seen in mesenchymal cells isolated from allografts of patients with BOS [24], and these functional alterations appear to predate development of BOS. Failure of anti-fibrotic mechanisms and an augmentation of pro-fibrotic mediators likely contribute to skewing of the mesenchymal progenitor cells in the lung allograft towards fibrotic differentiation. Prostaglandin (PG) E_2, a well-recognized anti-fibrotic lipid mediator, can inhibit proliferation and myofibroblast differentiation of mesenchymal cells of normal lung allografts. However, a decreased synthesis and response to PGE_2 is noted in mesenchymal cells in BOS [30]. On the contrary, an augmented secretion of the pro-fibrotic mediator, endothelin-1, is described in mesenchymal cells in BOS [27].

Mesenchymal Cell and Myeloid Cell Interactions in the Allograft

The allograft milieu, which is marked by infiltration with recipient immune cells and mobilization of donor lung-resident progenitor cells, provides a fertile ground for interaction of these cell types. Macrophages are the foremost adaptive immune cell that can regulate mesenchymal cell recruitment and differentiation directly by secreting pro-fibrotic growth factors such as TGF-β(transforming growth factor-beta) and PDGF (platelet derived growth factor). Alveolar macrophage secretion and BALF levels of TGF-β1 are both increased in BOS [31, 32]. Similarly, increased concentrations of PDGF and IGF-1 (insulin like growth factor-1) are seen in BALF from patients with BO [33, 34]. Neutrophils, recruited to the graft by variety of chemoattractants such as interleukin(IL)-8, IL-17, and proline-glycine-proline (PGP), are also of great significance in BOS [35, 36]. A large body of literature supports a strong association of an increase in neutrophil numbers in the BAL and development of BOS [35, 37–41]. Furthermore, their persistence during the course of the disease supports their role in ensuing fibroproliferation in BOS.

Critical to regulation of mesenchymal cell function by the innate immune response is the balance of pro-inflammatory cytokines such as IL-1β, TNF-α (tumor necrosis factor-alpha), and IFN-α (interferon-gamma) to pro-fibrotic cytokines such as IL-13. IFN-α inhibits mesenchymal cell proliferation and myofibroblast differentiation. Both IFN-α and IL-1β are potent inducers of cyclooxygenase 2 and, hence, upregulate secretion of PGE_2, and the augmented production of PGE_2, which is a potent anti-fibrotic mediator, can ameliorate TGF-β-induced myofibroblast differentiation of lung allograft-derived mesenchymal cells. While preponderance of these pro-inflammatory cytokines is noted in ischemia reperfusion and acute rejection [42–46], the allograft milieu in BOS is characterized by predominance of IL-13, a pro-fibrotic Th2 cytokine, and growth factors such as TGF-β. IL-13 released by graft-infiltrating host cells acts as a critical effector cytokine that drives fibroproliferation in BO [18]. Myofibroblasts in the human lung allograft express IL-13 Rα(alpha)1 [18], and IL-13 promotes collagen secretion and α-SMA expression in graft-resident mesenchymal progenitor cells [24]. IL-13 is also a well-characterized inhibitor of PGE_2 synthesis by mesenchymal cells. Thus, a switch from pro-inflammatory to pro-fibrotic cytokines can promote maladaptive repair responses leading to remodeling. However, the interaction of various myeloid cells among themselves and with the resident mesenchymal cells is likely much more complex and involves both soluble mediators and cell–cell contact. An interesting example is the ability of donor lung mesenchymal cells to inhibit T-cell proliferation and modulate cytokine secretion [47]. Soluble mediators, among them PGE_2 that is secreted by mesenchymal cells when cocultured with allogeneic T cells, play an important role in mediating this effect [47]. But in BOS, a stable phenotypic change in mesenchymal cells characterized by a loss of PGE_2 synthetic function combined with preponderance of TH1 rather than TH2 cytokines can explain a "switch" of the function of these cells from immunoregulatory to pro-fibrotic.

Mesenchymal Epithelial Interaction in the Allograft

Epithelial cell injury and dysregulation of homeostatic epithelial-mesenchymal interaction is key to the development of fibrosis. Compelling evidence about the importance of epithelium in the pathogenesis of the fibrotic lesion in BO is provided by animal studies where re-epithelization of donor trachea by recipient cells prevents fibrotic obliteration [48–50]. Epithelium has been shown to be an important target of immune responses following human lung transplantation. Bronchial epithelial cells are capable of inducing T-cell proliferation, and upregulation of major histocompatibility class I and class II antigen expression is seen in bronchial epithelial cells in BOS [51, 52], making them prone to binding by anti-HLA antibodies [53, 54]. Non-HLA antibodies directed against alveolar epithelial cells are also present in BOS patients [55], and ligation of antibodies leads to upregulation of pro-fibrotic growth factors in epithelial cells [55, 56]. Epithelial cell injury can also be induced by infections such as cytomegalovirus, which are associated with development of BOS [8, 57–59]. Furthermore, microvascular loss and resulting airway ischemia have been shown to lead to epithelial cell injury. While epithelial cells can also potentially contribute directly to fibrosis via acquisition of a mesenchymal phenotype [60], epithelial cell injury by immune and nonimmune mechanisms likely plays a major pathogenic role by inducing of mesenchymal cell migration, proliferation, and differentiation.

Studying Fibrogenesis in the Allograft

As the physiologic abnormalities seen in BOS are a direct consequence of progressive matrix deposition and airway obliteration, there has been an increasing emphasis on understanding cellular types and signaling pathways involved in fibroproliferation. The de novo development of fibrosis during the allograft life can be studied longitudinally, thus providing an ideal opportunity to investigate fibroproliferative responses over time. Furthermore, human lung is unique among transplanted solid organs because of the easy accessibility to lung tissue and the allograft milieu via bronchoscopy. This ability to repeatedly specimens from the lung has been utilized to identify biomarkers and biomodulaters of BO onset via translational studies. However, factors leading to a disorganized remodeling response in the allograft remain to be completely determined. An important question is whether, once initiated, fibrosis can self-perpetuate itself independent of allo- or autoimmune stimulation. This is indeed suggested by the failure of augmented immunosuppressive medications to alter the progressive course of BOS and further underscores the need to develop anti-fibroproliferative therapies.

Animal Models of BO

Attempts have been made to model fibrotic airway obliteration that occurs in alloimmune transplantation in small animals. Allogeneic rodent tracheal transplant into subcutaneous sites, while anatomically incorrect, provides a simple and reproducible model of fibroproliferation and luminal obliteration [61]. The histologic lesions progress from immune cell infiltration and epithelial injury to complete fibrotic obliteration, thus allowing for studies of alloimmune mechanisms as well as fibrogenesis. An orthotopic transplant model where donor trachea is re-anastomosed to the recipient trachea is technically more challenging, but it offers the advantage of allowing airflow through the lumen and revascularization of the graft. In this model, while acute alloimmune injury leads to immune cell infiltration, epithelial regeneration from migration of recipient-derived epithelial cells limits development of overt fibrotic airway intra-luminal obstruction [50]. This model has highlighted the role of epithelial injury in fibroproliferation and continues to be utilized for studying mechanisms of alloimmune injury [18, 62–64]. However, both heterotopic and orthotopic tracheal transplant models share the drawback of having a histologically incorrect graft placed in an extra-pulmonary environment. Refinements have been made to the latter in a recently described intrapulmonary tracheal transplant model [64–66].

Whole lung transplant offers a significant advantage for investigating the cellular interactions and mechanistic pathways in an allograft milieu. However, the use of large-animal models of orthotopic lung transplantation is limited by the expense of animal care and cost of housing. Initial work using a rat model of orthotopic aerated, vascularized lung transplantation provided a realistic model to approximate lung transplantation in humans [67], and modifications of the protocol have made the model more reproducible for study [68]. Fully mismatched allografts are acutely rejected without immunosuppression, and attempts to mimic BO have been made by using moderately histocompatible strains without immunosuppression [69]. However, fibrotic remodeling has not been validated or extensively applied in this model. The limited availability of specific antibodies and transgenic or knockout strains has shifted the focus to the development of an orthotopic lung transplant model in mice [70, 71]. An obliterative bronchiolitis model using minor histo-incompatible antigen murine orthotopic single-left lung transplants has been recently described [72]. While still requiring further validation, this model opens exciting new avenues for investigating the pathogenesis of fibroproliferation in a lung allograft.

Conclusion

Bronchiolitis obliterans is a fibrotic remodeling response of the donor lung. Epithelial injury from persistent or recurrent immune-mediated or infectious insults leads to mesenchymal cell migration and infiltration (Fig. 9.3). However, the development of a persistently altered phenotype of mesenchymal cells in this disease suggests its independence from continuing immune injury and the need to directly target mesenchymal cells to arrest its progression. As the fibroproliferation of BO develops de novo in a transplanted graft during the period of active surveillance, this disease process provides an ideal scenario in which one can study novel anti-fibrotic therapies.

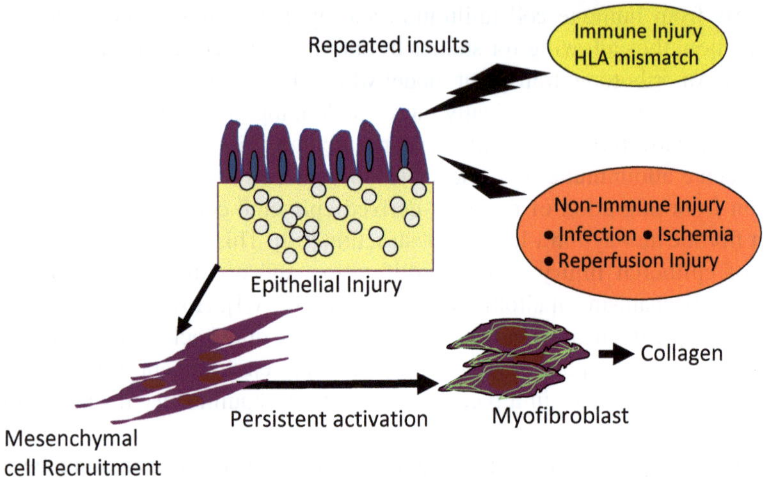

Fig. 9.3 Proposed paradigm of pathogenesis of bronchiolites obliterans post-lung transplantation. Immune and nonimmune mechanisms participate in epithelial injury, initiating mobilization of local progenitors including mesenchymal cell population. Repeated or persistent injurious insults likely play a role in the disorganized repair response marked by a stable phenotypic change in the mesenchymal cell population. Persistent activation of mesenchymal cells results in continuing matrix deposition and loss of tissue function

References

1. Yousem SA, Suncan SR, Ohori NP, Sonmez-Alpan E. Architectural remodeling of lung allografts in acute and chronic rejection. Arch Pathol Lab Med. 1992;116:1175–80.
2. Burke CM, Theodore J, Dawkins KD, Yousem SA, Blank N, Billingham ME, et al. Post-transplant obliterative bronchiolitis and other late lung sequelae in human heart-lung transplantation. Chest. 1984;86:824–9.
3. Stewart S, Fishbein MC, Snell GI, Berry GJ, Boehler A, Burke MM, et al. Revision of the 1996 working formulation for the standardization of nomenclature in the diagnosis of lung rejection. J Heart Lung Transplant. 2007;26:1229–42.
4. Davis WA, Finlen Copeland CA, Todd JL, Snyder LD, Martissa JA, Palmer SM. Spirometrically significant acute rejection increases the risk for BOS and death after lung transplantation. Am J Transplant. 2012;12:745–52.
5. Burton CM, Iversen M, Carlsen J, Mortensen J, Andersen CB, Steinbruchel D, et al. Acute cellular rejection is a risk factor for bronchiolitis obliterans syndrome independent of post-transplant baseline FEV1. J Heart Lung Transplant. 2009;28:888–93.
6. Hachem RR, Khalifah AP, Chakinala MM, Yusen RD, Aloush AA, Mohanakumar T, et al. The significance of a single episode of minimal acute rejection after lung transplantation. Transplantation. 2005;80:1406–13.
7. Khalifah AP, Hachem RR, Chakinala MM, Yusen RD, Aloush A, Patterson GA, et al. Minimal acute rejection after lung transplantation: a risk for bronchiolitis obliterans syndrome. Am J Transplant. 2005;5:2022–30.
8. Heng D, Sharples LD, McNeil K, Stewart S, Wreghitt T, Wallwork J. Bronchiolitis obliterans syndrome: incidence, natural history, prognosis, and risk factors. J Heart Lung Transplant. 1998;17:1255–63.

9. Scott AI, Sharples LD, Stewart S. Bronchiolitis obliterans syndrome: risk factors and therapeutic strategies. Drugs. 2005;65:761–71.
10. Sharples LD, McNeil K, Stewart S, Wallwork J. Risk factors for bronchiolitis obliterans: a systematic review of recent publications. J Heart Lung Transplant. 2002;21:271–81.
11. Husain AN, Siddiqui MT, Holmes EW, Chandrasekhar AJ, McCabe M, Radvany R, et al. Analysis of risk factors for the development of bronchiolitis obliterans syndrome. Am J Respir Crit Care Med. 1999;159:829–33.
12. Fukami N, Ramachandran S, Takenaka M, Weber J, Subramanian V, Mohanakumar T. An obligatory role for lung infiltrating B cells in the immunopathogenesis of obliterative airway disease induced by antibodies to MHC class I molecules. Am J Transplant. 2012;12:867–76.
13. Jaramillo A, Fernandez FG, Kuo EY, Trulock EP, Patterson GA, Mohanakumar T. Immune mechanisms in the pathogenesis of bronchiolitis obliterans syndrome after lung transplantation. Pediatr Transplant. 2005;9:84–93.
14. Srinivasan M, Flynn R, Price A, Ranger A, Browning JL, Taylor PA, et al. Donor B-cell alloantibody deposition and germinal center formation are required for the development of murine chronic GVHD and bronchiolitis obliterans. Blood. 2012;119:1570–80.
15. Xue J, Zhu X, George MP, Myerburg MM, Stoner MW, Pilewski JW, et al. A human-mouse chimeric model of obliterative bronchiolitis after lung transplantation. Am J Pathol. 2011;179:745–53.
16. Burlingham WJ, Love RB, Jankowska-Gan E, Haynes LD, Xu Q, Bobadilla JL, et al. IL-17-dependent cellular immunity to collagen type V predisposes to obliterative bronchiolitis in human lung transplants. J Clin Invest. 2007;117:3498–506.
17. Serini G, Gabbiani G. Mechanisms of myofibroblast activity and phenotypic modulation. Exp Cell Res. 1999;250:273–83.
18. Lama VN, Harada H, Badri LN, Flint A, Hogaboam CM, McKenzie A, et al. Obligatory role for interleukin-13 in obstructive lesion development in airway allografts. Am J Pathol. 2006;169:47–60.
19. Gilpin SE, Lung KC, Sato M, Singer LG, Keshavjee S, Waddell TK. Altered progenitor cell and cytokine profiles in bronchiolitis obliterans syndrome. J Heart Lung Transplant. 2012;31:222–8.
20. LaPar DJ, Burdick MD, Emaminia A, Harris DA, Strieter BA, Liu L, et al. Circulating fibrocytes correlate with bronchiolitis obliterans syndrome development after lung transplantation: a novel clinical biomarker. Ann Thorac Surg. 2011;92:470–7; discussion 477.
21. Lama VN, Phan SH. The extrapulmonary origin of fibroblasts: stem/progenitor cells and beyond. Proc Am Thorac Soc. 2006;3:373–6.
22. Brocker V, Langer F, Fellous TG, Mengel M, Brittan M, Bredt M, et al. Fibroblasts of recipient origin contribute to bronchiolitis obliterans in human lung transplants. Am J Respir Crit Care Med. 2006;173:1276–82.
23. Lama VN, Smith L, Badri L, Flint A, Andrei AC, Murray S, et al. Evidence for tissue-resident mesenchymal stem cells in human adult lung from studies of transplanted allografts. J Clin Invest. 2007;117:989–96.
24. Walker N, Badri L, Wettlaufer S, Flint A, Sajjan U, Krebsbach PH, et al. Resident tissue-specific mesenchymal progenitor cells contribute to fibrogenesis in human lung allografts. Am J Pathol. 2011;178:2461–9.
25. Badri L, Murray S, Liu LX, Walker NM, Flint A, Wadhwa A, et al. Mesenchymal stromal cells in bronchoalveolar lavage as predictors of bronchiolitis obliterans syndrome. Am J Respir Crit Care Med. 2011;183:1062–70.
26. Salama M, Jaksch P, Andrukhova O, Taghavi S, Klepetko W, Aharinejad S. Endothelin-1 is a useful biomarker for early detection of bronchiolitis obliterans in lung transplant recipients. J Thorac Cardiovasc Surg. 2010;140:1422–7.
27. Salama M, Andrukhova O, Jaksch P, Taghavi S, Kelpetko W, Dekan G, et al. Endothelin-1 governs proliferation and migration of bronchoalveolar lavage-derived lung mesenchymal stem cells in bronchiolitis obliterans syndrome. Transplantation. 2011;92:155–62.

28. Badri L, Lama VN. Lysophosphatidic acid induces migration of human lung-resident mesenchymal stem cells through the beta-catenin pathway. Stem Cells. 2012;30(9):2010–9.
29. Andersson-Sjoland A, Thiman L, Nihlberg K, Hallgren O, Rolandsson S, Skog I, et al. Fibroblast phenotypes and their activity are changed in the wound healing process after lung transplantation. J Heart Lung Transplant. 2011;30:945–54.
30. Walker NM, Badri LN, Wadhwa A, Wettlaufer S, Peters-Golden M, Lama VN. Prostaglandin E2 as an inhibitory modulator of fibrogenesis in human lung allografts. Am J Respir Crit Care Med. 2012;185:77–84.
31. Elssner A, Jaumann F, Dobmann S, Behr J, Schwaiblmair M, Reichenspurner H, et al. Elevated levels of interleukin-8 and transforming growth factor-beta in bronchoalveolar lavage fluid from patients with bronchiolitis obliterans syndrome: proinflammatory role of bronchial epithelial cells. Munich Lung Transplant Group. Transplantation. 2000;70:362–7.
32. Magnan A, Mege JL, Escallier JC, Brisse J, Capo C, Reynaud M, et al. Balance between alveolar macrophage IL-6 and TGF-beta in lung-transplant recipients. Marseille and Montreal Lung Transplantation Group. Am J Respir Crit Care Med. 1996;153:1431–6.
33. Hertz MI, Henke CA, Nakhleh RE, Harmon KR, Marinelli WA, Fox JM, et al. Obliterative bronchiolitis after lung transplantation: a fibroproliferative disorder associated with platelet-derived growth factor. Proc Natl Acad Sci U S A. 1992;89:10385–9.
34. Charpin JM, Stern M, Grenet D, Israel-Biet D. Insulinlike growth factor-1 in lung transplants with obliterative bronchiolitis. Am J Respir Crit Care Med. 2000;161:1991–8.
35. DiGiovine B, Lynch III JP, Martinez FJ, Flint A, Whyte RI, Iannettoni MD, et al. Bronchoalveolar lavage neutrophilia is associated with obliterative bronchiolitis after lung transplantation: role of IL-8. J Immunol. 1996;157:4194–202.
36. Hardison MT, Galin FS, Calderon CE, Djekic UV, Parker SB, Wille KM, et al. The presence of a matrix-derived neutrophil chemoattractant in bronchiolitis obliterans syndrome after lung transplantation. J Immunol. 2009;182:4423–31.
37. Devouassoux G, Drouet C, Pin I, Brambilla C, Brambilla E, Colle PE, et al. Alveolar neutrophilia is a predictor for the bronchiolitis obliterans syndrome, and increases with degree of severity. Transpl Immunol. 2002;10:303–10.
38. Neurohr C, Huppmann P, Samweber B, Leuschner S, Zimmermann G, Leuchte H, et al. Prognostic value of bronchoalveolar lavage neutrophilia in stable lung transplant recipients. J Heart Lung Transplant. 2009;28:468–74.
39. Riise GC, Williams A, Kjellstrom C, Schersten H, Andersson BA, Kelly FJ. Bronchiolitis obliterans syndrome in lung transplant recipients is associated with increased neutrophil activity and decreased antioxidant status in the lung. Eur Respir J. 1998;12:82–8.
40. Zheng L, Walters EH, Ward C, Wang N, Orsida B, Whitford H, et al. Airway neutrophilia in stable and bronchiolitis obliterans syndrome patients following lung transplantation. Thorax. 2000;55:53–9.
41. Zheng L, Whitford HM, Orsida B, Levvey BJ, Bailey M, Walters EH, et al. The dynamics and associations of airway neutrophilia post lung transplantation. Am J Transplant. 2006;6:599–608.
42. Bharat A, Kuo E, Steward N, Aloush A, Hachem R, Trulock EP, et al. Immunological link between primary graft dysfunction and chronic lung allograft rejection. Ann Thorac Surg. 2008;86:189–95; discussion 196–7.
43. Blocher S, Wilker S, Sucke J, Pfeil U, Dietrich H, Weimer R, et al. Acute rejection of experimental lung allografts: characterization of intravascular mononuclear leukocytes. Clin Immunol. 2007;124:98–108.
44. Geudens N, Vanaudenaerde BM, Neyrinck AP, Van De Wauwer C, Vos R, Verleden GM, et al. The importance of lymphocytes in lung ischemia-reperfusion injury. Transplant Proc. 2007;39:2659–62.
45. Hodge G, Hodge S, Chambers D, Reynolds PN, Holmes M. Acute lung transplant rejection is associated with localized increase in T-cell IFNgamma and TNFalpha proinflammatory cytokines in the airways. Transplantation. 2007;84:1452–8.

46. Rizzo M, SivaSai KS, Smith MA, Trulock EP, Lynch JP, Patterson GA, et al. Increased expression of inflammatory cytokines and adhesion molecules by alveolar macrophages of human lung allograft recipients with acute rejection: decline with resolution of rejection. J Heart Lung Transplant. 2000;19:858–65.
47. Jarvinen L, Badri L, Wettlaufer S, Ohtsuka T, Standiford TJ, Toews GB, et al. Lung resident mesenchymal stem cells isolated from human lung allografts inhibit T cell proliferation via a soluble mediator. J Immunol. 2008;181:4389–96.
48. Adams BF, Berry GJ, Huang X, Shorthouse R, Brazelton T, Morris RE. Immunosuppressive therapies for the prevention and treatment of obliterative airway disease in heterotopic rat trachea allografts. Transplantation. 2000;69:2260–6.
49. Adams BF, Brazelton T, Berry GJ, Morris RE. The role of respiratory epithelium in a rat model of obliterative airway disease. Transplantation. 2000;69:661–4.
50. Ikonen TS, Brazelton TR, Berry GJ, Shorthouse RS, Morris RE. Epithelial re-growth is associated with inhibition of obliterative airway disease in orthotopic tracheal allografts in non-immunosuppressed rats. Transplantation. 2000;70:857–63.
51. Glanville AR, Tazelaar HD, Theodore J, Imoto E, Rouse RV, Baldwin JC, et al. The distribution of MHC class I and II antigens on bronchial epithelium. Am Rev Respir Dis. 1989;139:330–4.
52. Taylor PM, Rose ML, Yacoub MH. Expression of MHC antigens in normal human lungs and transplanted lungs with obliterative bronchiolitis. Transplantation. 1989;48:506–10.
53. Reznik SI, Jaramillo A, Zhang L, Patterson GA, Cooper JD, Mohanakumar T. Anti-HLA antibody binding to HLA class I molecules induces proliferation of airway epithelial cells: a potential mechanism for bronchiolitis obliterans syndrome. J Thorac Cardiovasc Surg. 2000; 119:39–45.
54. Mauck KA, Hosenpud JD. The bronchial epithelium: a potential allogeneic target for chronic rejection after lung transplantation. J Heart Lung Transplant. 1996;15:709–14.
55. Jaramillo A, Naziruddin B, Zhang L, Reznik SI, Smith MA, Aloush AA, et al. Activation of human airway epithelial cells by non-HLA antibodies developed after lung transplantation: a potential etiological factor for bronchiolitis obliterans syndrome. Transplantation. 2001;71:966–76.
56. Goers TA, Ramachandran S, Aloush A, Trulock E, Patterson GA, Mohanakumar T. De novo production of k-alpha1 tubulin-specific antibodies: role in chronic lung allograft rejection. J Immunol. 2008;180:4487–94.
57. Keenan RJ, Lega ME, Dummer JS, Paradis IL, Dauber JH, Rabinowich H, et al. Cytomegalovirus serologic status and postoperative infection correlated with risk of developing chronic rejection after pulmonary transplantation. Transplantation. 1991;51:433–8.
58. Reichenspurner H, Girgis RE, Robbins RC, Conte JV, Nair RV, Valentine V, et al. Obliterative bronchiolitis after lung and heart-lung transplantation. Ann Thorac Surg. 1995;60:1845–53.
59. Sharples LD, Tamm M, McNeil K, Higenbottam TW, Stewart S, Wallwork J. Development of bronchiolitis obliterans syndrome in recipients of heart-lung transplantation—early risk factors. Transplantation. 1996;61:560–6.
60. Hodge S, Holmes M, Banerjee B, Musk M, Kicic A, Waterer G, et al. Posttransplant bronchiolitis obliterans syndrome is associated with bronchial epithelial to mesenchymal transition. Am J Transplant. 2009;9:727–33.
61. Hertz MI, Jessurun J, King MB, Savik SK, Murray JJ. Reproduction of the obliterative bronchiolitis lesion after heterotopic transplantation of mouse airways. Am J Pathol. 1993;142:1945–51.
62. Cao H, Lan Q, Shi Q, Zhou X, Liu G, Liu J, et al. Anti-IL-23 antibody blockade of IL-23/IL-17 pathway attenuates airway obliteration in rat orthotopic tracheal transplantation. Int Immunopharmacol. 2011;11:569–75.
63. Deuse T, Schrepfer S, Reichenspurner H, Hoyt G, Fischbein MP, Robbins RC, et al. Techniques for experimental heterotopic and orthotopic tracheal transplantations—when to use which model? Transpl Immunol. 2007;17:255–61.

64. Sato M, Hirayama S, Hwang DM, Lara-Guerra H, Wagnetz D, Waddell TK, et al. The role of intrapulmonary de novo lymphoid tissue in obliterative bronchiolitis after lung transplantation. J Immunol. 2009;182:7307–16.
65. Sato M, Hirayama S, Lara-Guerra H, Anraku M, Waddell TK, Liu M, et al. MMP-dependent migration of extrapulmonary myofibroblast progenitors contributing to posttransplant airway fibrosis in the lung. Am J Transplant. 2009;9:1027–36.
66. Sato M, Liu M, Anraku M, Ogura T, D'Cruz G, Alman BA, et al. Allograft airway fibrosis in the pulmonary milieu: a disorder of tissue remodeling. Am J Transplant. 2008;8:517–28.
67. Asimacopoulos PJ, Molokhia FA, Pegg CA, Norman JC. Lung transplantation in the rat. Transplant Proc. 1971;3:583–5.
68. Zhai W, Ge J, Inci I, Hillinger S, Markus C, Korom S, et al. Simplified rat lung transplantation by using a modified cuff technique. J Invest Surg. 2008;21:33–7.
69. Matsumura Y, Marchevsky A, Zuo XJ, Kass RM, Matloff JM, Jordan SC. Assessment of pathological changes associated with chronic allograft rejection and tolerance in two experimental models of rat lung transplantation. Transplantation. 1995;59:1509–17.
70. Jungraithmayr WM, Korom S, Hillinger S, Weder W. A mouse model of orthotopic, single-lung transplantation. J Thorac Cardiovasc Surg. 2009;137:486–91.
71. Okazaki M, Krupnick AS, Kornfeld CG, Lai JM, Ritter JH, Richardson SB, et al. A mouse model of orthotopic vascularized aerated lung transplantation. Am J Transplant. 2007;7:1672–9.
72. Suzuki H, Fan L, Wilkes DS. Development of obliterative bronchiolitis in a murine model of orthotopic lung transplantation. J Vis Exp. 2012;(65). pii: 3947.

Chapter 10
The Role of Autoimmunity in the Pathogenesis of Obliterative Bronchiolitis

Rudolf K. Braun, Keith C. Meyer, and William J. Burlingham

Abstract Many risk factors and post-transplant events have been linked to the development of bronchiolitis obliterans syndrome. Evolving research suggests that the development of cell-mediated and humoral reactivity to self-antigens (collagen V, K-α1 tubulin) in the lung allograft may play a very significant role in the bronchiolar inflammation and fibrosis that lead to obliterative bronchiolitis and progressive graft dysfunction and loss. Alloimmune and autoimmune mechanisms likely work together to mediate chronic lung allograft rejection. This chapter examines the role of autoimmunity in bronchiolitis obliterans syndrome with a focus on the role of Th17 lymphocytes, IL-17, and immune regulatory mechanisms in the development and progression of obliterative bronchiolitis.

Keywords Autoimmunity • Alloimmunity • Lung transplant • Bronchiolitis obliterans syndrome • Obliterative bronchiolitis • Chronic rejection

R.K. Braun, Ph.D.
Department of Pediatrics, University of Wisconsin Madison, 600 Highland Avenue, Clinical Science Center, H6/551, Madison, WI 53792, USA
e-mail: rkbraun@wisc.edu

K.C. Meyer, M.D., M.S.
Department of Internal Medicine, Section of Allergy, Pulmonary and Critical Care Medicine, University of Wisconsin School of Medicine and Public Health, K4/910 Clinical Science Center, 600 Highland Avenue, Madison, WI 53792-9988, USA
e-mail: Kcm@medicine.wisc.edu

W.J. Burlingham, Ph.D. (✉)
Department of Surgery, University of Wisconsin, 600 Highland Avenue, G4/702, Madison, WI 53792, USA
e-mail: burlingham@surgery.wisc.edu

K.C. Meyer and A.R. Glanville (eds.), *Bronchiolitis Obliterans Syndrome in Lung Transplantation*, Respiratory Medicine 8, DOI 10.1007/978-1-4614-7636-8_10,

Introduction

Bronchiolitis obliterans syndrome (BOS) is a major cause of allograft dysfunction and loss following lung transplantation. The histopathologic correlate of lung allograft dysfunction due to BOS is obliterative bronchiolitis (OB), which is generally considered to be caused by chronic lung allograft rejection. BOS is recognized as a major cause of graft dysfunction following lung transplantation and is the major cause of graft loss and patient death for patients who survive beyond 1 year post-transplant [1–3]. Lung histopathology in patients with BOS can show striking similarities to the OB that can lead to progressive pulmonary function decline in allogeneic bone marrow or stem cell transplant recipients as well as the constrictive bronchiolitis that can occur in patients with connective tissue diseases (CTD). These airway changes are perceived as alloimmune or autoimmune disorders, respectively.

Numerous risk factors have been associated with the development of BOS. Alloimmunity is still the most widely accepted and "logical" cause of delayed allograft dysfunction in all types of organ transplantation, including that due to BOS after lung transplantation. Mismatching of tissue antigens, particularly HLA-A, HLA-B, and DR/DQ, tends to cause recipient alloimmune rejection responses to foreign tissue that are not adequately suppressed by currently available post-transplant immunosuppressive therapies [4–6]. Risk factors for BOS that have been linked to alloimmune rejection responses include acute cellular rejection, lymphocytic bronchiolitis, greater degrees of human leukocyte antigen (HLA) mismatch, and generation of de novo anti-HLA antibodies. Additional risk factors associated with BOS include pathologic gastroesophageal reflux (GER) with microaspiration, primary graft dysfunction (PGD), infection (viral, bacterial, and fungal), and exposure to high levels of ambient air pollution.

The idea of HLA mismatch as the *proximal* cause of BOS has been brought into question by studies of HLA-mismatching in the European Collaborative Transplant Study data base. Opelz and colleagues [7] found relatively few HLA-0MM (mismatched) transplants [$n=28/8{,}020$], but these had a very high graft failure rate despite having no mismatches, suggesting that factors other than HLA may be driving lung allograft rejection. Recent investigations have linked autoimmunity to solid organ allograft dysfunction. Evolving research has shown that de novo immune responses to self-antigens (e.g., myosin or vimentin in heart transplantation, collagen IV or VI in renal transplantation, and collagen V or K-α(alpha)1 tubulin in lung transplantation) can develop post-transplantation, and such autoimmune responses may be triggered or induced by alloimmune responses in the setting of orthotopic organ transplantation [8, 9]. Hagedorn et al. [10] have reported that sera from patients with higher grades of BOS contain autoantibodies that react to a number of self-antigens. This chapter will review findings from investigations into the role of autoimmunity in lung allograft rejection and focus especially on collagen V autoimmunity, which has been identified as a key risk factor for developing BOS [11–13] and which may be present in some individuals with advanced lung disease prior to lung transplant [14].

Autoimmunity and Chronic Lung Diseases

As in other forms of end-stage organ failure, autoimmunity underlies many of the diseases typical of patients presenting for lung transplantation. Indeed, autoimmunity appears to play a role in an expanding number of lung diseases. Many patients with CTD, such as rheumatoid arthritis (RA), systemic sclerosis (SS), inflammatory myopathies, systemic lupus erythematosus (SLE), Sjogren's syndrome, and mixed CTD, develop CTD-associated lung disease [15, 16]. The CTD disorders are recognized as systemic autoimmune diseases, and diagnosis is made via a combination of clinical presentation and patterns of autoantibodies that are present in the circulation [17]. Multiple patterns of involvement (airway-predominant, parenchymal inflammation, pulmonary fibrosis, pleural inflammation) and different idiopathic interstitial pneumonia (IIP) pathologies (e.g., nonspecific interstitial pneumonia [NSIP], usual interstitial pneumonia [UIP]) may develop in patients diagnosed with CTD [15, 16]. Interestingly, a UIP pattern is the typical and defining histopathologic pattern in patients with idiopathic pulmonary fibrosis (IPF), and areas of NSIP are also frequently present in the lungs of patients with IPF [18], but CTD-associated autoantibodies are usually not detected in patients diagnosed as having IPF.

Recent studies suggest that autoantibodies and T cells associated with autoreactivity can be found in IPF [14, 19–21]. Bobadilla et al. [14] found that T-cell autoimmunity to collagen type V was specifically elevated in many patients with end-stage IPF prior to lung transplantation. Feghali-Bostwick et al. [19] found abnormal proliferation of CD4+ T-cell clones and IgG autoantibodies directed against a number of cellular antigens in the majority of a cohort of 48 IPF patients, and extracts of IPF lung could stimulate autologous CD4 T-cell proliferation (but not preparations from normal lung or non-IPF lung disease), suggesting that these responses were driven by autoantigens in the IPF lung. Additionally, Kurosu et al. [20] reported that CD4+ T-lymphocyte proliferation to the N-terminal region of annexin-1 was associated with acute exacerbation of IPF, and Taille et al. [21] identified anti-periplakin antibodies in both serum and bronchoalveolar lavage (BAL) fluid from patients with IPF; 16 of 40 patients with IPF had anti-periplakin antibodies in sera versus none of the 40 healthy control subjects or patients with COPD. Additionally, although periplakin was expressed in both normal and IPF lung specimens, expression of periplakin in alveolar epithelium of IPF lungs was significantly altered from the pattern observed for normal lungs. In addition to evidence of both T-cell and humoral autoreactivity in IPF, the appearance of unusual T-cell subsets such as CD4+CD28 null lymphocytes (suggesting antigen-driven proliferation) by Gilani et al. [22] correlated with more aggressive disease. Kotsianidis et al. [23] found that suppressor function by regulatory T cells (Treg) was impaired in both BAL and peripheral blood in patients with IPF as well as patients with CTD-ILD.

Evidence for sensitization to self-antigens has also been reported for obstructive lung disease. Rinaldi et al. [24] examined plasma and peripheral blood mononuclear cell (PBMC) from 320 patients with chronic obstructive pulmonary disease (COPD). They report a significant increase in T-cell sensitization to collagen V in both smokers and patients with COPD vs. those who had never smoked. Similarly, Liu et al. [25] found that patients with asthma had higher concentrations of anti-collagen V antibodies vs. controls, and higher antibody levels correlated with more severe asthma and with use of corticosteroids. Antibodies to other self-antigens were also detected; these included epidermal growth factor receptor, activin A type 1 receptors, and α(alpha)-catenin. Additionally, Nunez et al. [26] detected circulating anti-tissue antibodies in 26 % of 328 patients with COPD.

Animal Research

Because therapies for BOS are generally ineffective, several different animal models have been developed to study the mechanisms of chronic rejection and OB and to investigate treatment options. Small- and large-animal models have been developed that allow the study of acute rejection (AR) and therapies for its treatment and prevention, and a number of models have also been developed to study chronic rejection and OB.

Tracheal transplantation has been used for tracheobronchial restorative surgery [27, 28], and Hertz et al. [29] subsequently used the mouse model of heterotopic tracheal transplantation to study development of OB lesions. This model has since been widely used to study OB in mice and rats and also dogs [30, 31]. Common observations include evidence of epithelial damage, lymphocytic inflammation, and luminal obliteration. However, some major differences as compared to OB in the human lung allograft remained and limited the use of this model for mechanistic studies of OB. OB is a disease of small airways, and the heterotopic tracheal graft is not vascularized and aerated. Similarly, the use of a heterotopic model of lung transplantation showed little success because of the complete loss of lung structure, making it impossible to differentiate AR and OB [29, 32]. A more successful model of heterotopic airway transplantation was developed in swine by Ikonen et al. [33, 34]. In contrast to the rodent model, the use of terminal bronchi leads to lesions that resemble OB much more closely, although some remaining disadvantages include the lack of vascularization and aeration. Additionally, orthotopic tracheal transplants have also been used to study tracheal repair and to reduce the shortcomings of heterotopic transplantations [35–37]. However, the pathology is significantly different in these models; the lack of fibrosis and the replacement of the airway epithelium by host cells are the main differences as compared to the heterotopic models.

A much better model to investigate lung transplant rejection is provided by orthotopic lung transplantation in the mouse or rat. This procedure is significantly more technically demanding compared to orthotopic or heterotopic tracheal transplantation, but the results provide a much closer approximation of clinical AR and OB. The original method for lung transplantation in rats used sutures to anastomose the vessels, but this was shown to be difficult and time consuming [38–40]. A considerably improved technique was introduced by Mizuta et al. and later improved by Zhai et al. in 2008 using a cuff technique for rat lung transplantation [41–43], and the same technique was applied by Okazaki et al. to achieve lung transplantation in the mouse [44]. This method was further developed by Jungraithmayr et al. [45, 46] and has become the major model used to study AR and OB in animals. Acute rejection can be observed in any transplant with differences in MHC or non-MHC molecules between donor and recipient.

The extent of the antigenic difference (e.g., MHC plus non-MHC vs. non-MHC only mismatch) influences the speed of rejection but does not guarantee a switch from AR to OB. When it occurs, the development of OB lesions is not apparent in all animals, and only a few approaches will lead to the occlusion of small airways typical of clinical OB. In Lewis rats that are sensitized with skin from brown Norway (BN) rats 7 days before receiving left lung transplants from donors that were Lew×BN F(1) hybrids, fibroproliferative lesions with partial obliteration of airways develop in the presence of CsA and rapamycin treatment [47]. A breakthrough was reported in 2011 by Fan et al. [48] when lungs from C57BL/10 mice were transplanted into C57BL/6 mice. These mouse strains are MHC compatible, but minor histocompatibility antigen incompatible, which leads to the development of OB in about 55 % of the animals within 21 days. A different mouse model was introduced by a Swiss group using completely MHC-mismatched mice with additional treatment with CsA and steroids [49]. This leads to the development of OB lesions in approximately 30 % of the animals. The difference in MHC antigens drives the alloimmune response after transplantation, and the allo-response induced by the instillation of allogeneic (C57BL/6) BAL cells into the lungs of recipient BALB/c mice generated the histology and immunology associated with acute lung allograft rejection. This was thought to result from the presentation of donor lung alloantigens to recipient lymphocytes [50], and the deposition of IgG2a in the perivascular and peribronchiolar tissues seemed to confirm this conclusion. However, the antigen recognized by these antibodies was not the donor MHC molecule but was identified as collagen type V (colV), a minor fibrillar collagen required for collagen fiber production in lung tissue [51, 52]. Moreover, only the α(alpha)1 chain of colV is recognized, although several different collagens are found in the lung. The response to colV may be induced through the extensive remodeling during rejection and inflammation associated with up-regulated activity of MMP-2 and MMP-9, which are capable of cleaving collagen molecules [53, 54]. Subsequent studies revealed a new and previously unknown role for this antigen. Tolerance to colV induced by instillation of colV or colV-pulsed autologous macrophages before the instillation of allogeneic macrophages inhibited development of rejection pathology in the lung induced by the transfer of allogeneic BAL cells [55]. Similarly, induction of oral tolerance to colV prior to lung transplantation in rats abrogated graft rejection [56]. More detailed analysis revealed that rejection pathology was mediated by colV-specific CD4+ effector T cells [12] and protection from rejection was associated with regulatory CD4+ T cells [57]. Adoptive transfer of CD4+ T cells from colV-tolerant rats induced similar protection in allograft recipients [58]. The colV-specific T-cell-mediated reactivity is sufficient to induce rejection-like pathology in lung isografts, and transfer of colV-specific CD4+ T cells or lymph node cells from colV-immunized rats into well-healed lung isografts induced rejection-like pathology, whereas other specificities did not show an effect [11, 12].

Although most animal models show acute rejection pathology, development of OB has so far only been observed in a small proportion of experimental lung transplant recipients. In contrast, development of OB or BOS is a major concern in human lung transplantation. OB was first observed after bone marrow and lung transplantation [59–61]. As mentioned in the introduction to this chapter, the driving mechanism leading to OB was originally thought to be an alloimmune response resulting in the production of antibodies and activated T cells to mismatched HLA antigens [6, 62]. However, in many cases of OB, no antibodies to HLA antigens were detected, an observation that is similar to the finding in mice [55]. Inspired by the animal data, analysis of cellular reactivity in human lung transplant recipients revealed a strong correlation between the risk of developing BOS and the presence of colV immune reactivity [13]. Observation of human lung transplantation recipients over a 7-year period using a trans-vivo delayed-type hypersensitivity (TV-DTH) assay to monitor colV reactivity showed a tenfold increased risk of developing severe BOS (level 2 or 3) in patients with elevated colV-specific cell-mediated immunity [13]. Interestingly, in the same group of lung transplant patients, the relative risk for severe BOS imparted by an HLA-DR mismatch was only twofold [13]. Collagen V sensitization has also been associated with PGD [14, 63] and the induction of alloimmune injury to the lung allograft potentiates the production of anti-colV antibodies [9, 65].

Autoimmunity after lung transplantation is not restricted to colV, nor is the phenomenon of allo-induced autoimmunity restricted to lung transplants. After lung transplantation, antibodies and T-cell reactivity to K-α(alpha)1 tubulin and collagen type V (colV) have been identified and characterized [11, 65, 66]. Experimental evidence for autoimmunity was also shown in a mouse heart transplant model where vasculopathy persisted when the allograft was retransplanted into a syngeneic host, suggesting that the recognition of an autoantigen contributes to the rejection [67].

Anti-colV responses in lung transplant recipients have been identified as IL23-, IL17-, and Th17 cell-dependent [12, 13, 58], which is similar to what has been observed in non-transplant-related autoimmune disorders. IL-10-producing regulatory T cells that are dependent on the presence of regulatory CD4+CD25+ cells may suppress collagen V autoimmune sensitization, and these IL-10-secreting cells decline in peripheral blood of human lung transplant recipients when BOS appears [68, 69].

IL8 (CXCL8), a key chemoattractant and activating factor for neutrophils, was identified as one of the major mediators of airway inflammation in human BOS [70]. The concentration of CXCL8 in BAL fluid of BOS patients correlates with airway neutrophilia [70] and is produced by epithelial cells, endothelial cells, macrophages, and smooth muscle cells in response to IL-17 [71, 72]. In addition, IL-17 increases E-selectin-dependent leukocyte rolling on microvascular endothelium and enhances endothelial expression of the chemokines, CXCL1, CXCL2, and CXCL5, which leads to CXCR2-dependent neutrophil but not T-cell transmigration [73]. IL-17 was discovered by subtracted cDNA library cloning from mouse T cells [74] and by sequence homology from human T cells [75]. Six cytokines are part of the interleukin-17 family of cytokines, IL-17A, IL-17B, IL-17C, IL-17D, IL-17E (also called IL-25), and IL-17F. IL-17A and IL-17F can be secreted as both disulfide-linked homodimeric and heterodimeric glycoproteins with the IL-17A homodimer being the most potent [76]. Of particular interest is the rather restricted set of T cells that produced IL-17 with a group of CD4+ T helper cells being the predominant producer [76]. These T cells were shown to be different from Th1 and Th2 cells and are called Th17 [77, 78]. However, IL-17A and IL-17F homodimers and heterodimers are also produced by CD8+ T cells (Tc17), γδ(gamma, delta) T cells, natural killer T (NKT) cells, activated monocytes, and neutrophils [79]. IL-17 and, therefore, Th17 cells are critical to the adaptive immune response against bacterial and fungal infections [80].

The production of IL-17 is associated with the development of autoimmunity in animal disease models and human diseases, and it was also found to be associated with the occurrence of BOS after lung transplantation before Th17 cells were identified [81–88]. Bettelli et al. discovered the association of increased Th17 cell number and disease severity in the development of experimental autoimmune encephalitis (EAE) [89], and earlier work associated the cytokine IL-23 with the development of EAE and collagen-induced arthritis, distinguishing the effect of IL-12 from IL-23 [90]. Because IL-23 is a key cytokine for the development of pathogenic Th17 cells, these findings had already suggested that IL-17 mediates autoimmunity. The relationship of IL23 to endogenous production of TGF β(beta)3, which is critical for conversion of the harmless Th17 precursor (induced by TGF β1 plus IL-6 into a fully pathogenic Th17 effector cell), has recently been elucidated by Lee et al. [91]. Several autoimmune diseases are now associated with the presence and activity of pathogenic Th17 effector cells. The evidence has accumulated on several levels including the production of IL-17, IL-23, or CCL20, the ligand for CCR6, that mediate recruitment of Th17 cells [92]. Human diseases include psoriasis, rheumatoid arthritis, multiple sclerosis, and inflammatory bowel disease, and corresponding animal disease models show a strong correlation between disease severity and Th17 cell number in the tissue.

As mentioned above, autoreactivity to colV is associated with BOS after lung transplantation. The production of IL-17 is up-regulated in bronchoalveolar fluid of transplant patients during acute rejection [93]. In animal models transfer of colV reactivity or tolerance was strictly associated to lung graft destruction or survival [48, 56, 58]. Furthermore, in the mouse model of BOS recently published by Fan et al. [48, 56, 58], IL17 blockade using a recombinant IL17R/Fc approach completely prevented formation of the OB lesion. However, the relative contribution of autoimmune vs. alloimmune and innate immune T cells to the critical event of IL-17A production remains to be established.

Autoimmunity and Allograft Dysfunction in Humans

A prospective study that monitored PBMC responses in 54 lung transplant recipients over a 7-year period showed a strong correlation of collagen V-specific cell-mediated immune responses with the incidence (HR 5.4 for BOS-1, HR 9.8 for

BOS-2) and severity of BOS [13]. The colV-specific response was detected using the trans-vivo DTH assay [94, 95]. This is a relatively simple assay that measures the swelling of a SCID mouse footpad 24 h after injection of human PBMC plus antigen. Because the study was begun in 2000 when the Th17 cell was completely unknown and IFNγ-producing Th1 cells were the standard target for in vitro monitoring of transplant recipients, this remarkably strong correlation of colV autoimmunity with severe BOS development would undoubtedly have been missed if we had chosen a IFNγ(gamma)-based monitoring assay. However, fortuitously, IL-17–producing CD4 T cells are efficient inducers of foot pad swelling in SCID mice, even though the mechanism involved is quite different from that used by Th1 cells [13] (see also below). ColV-specific autoimmunity was detected with the same assay in PBMC obtained prior to lung transplant in a subset of patients with end-stage lung disease, particularly those with a diagnosis of IPF, and pre-transplant reactivity to colV was found to be associated with PGD immediately after lung transplant [64]. Because IPF had been previously associated with GER disease, induction of collagen V reactivity was studied in relation to abnormal GER and the development of BOS, and it was found to be associated with both [14]. Also of interest is the recent report by Saini et al. [96] that found a strong correlation of the appearance of donor-specific anti-HLA antibodies with the detection of antibodies directed against self-antigens (collagen V and K-α(alpha)1 tubulin) in a retrospective analysis of 42 lung transplant recipients with BOS.

One of the mysteries regarding autoimmune etiologies of late allograft failures is the role of the passenger leukocyte and microchimerism. Particularly in the lung, which may contain upwards of 10^{10} donor leukocytes at the time of transplant, the activities of T cells, B cells, and myeloid components in the generation of allo- and autoimmunity cannot be underestimated. Just as the presence of bronchus-associated lymphoid tissue (BALT) and lymphoid neogenesis can be associated with lung transplant tolerance [97], so the presence of so many donor tissue-resident memory T cells may exert a powerful influence on subsequent development of autoimmunity. Microchimerism resulting from a donor with immune response genes (including HLA-DR/DQ) different from that of the recipient, might conceivably impart susceptibility or resistance to development of an autoimmune response directed against collagen V or other potential targets of an autoimmune response in the lung. Such a pathway has recently been invoked to explain the observed protection from rheumatoid arthritis in HLA-DR "susceptible" women after pregnancy with a fetus bearing a DR "resistance" allele [98].

Treg Suppression of Th17 Autoimmunity

Certain unusual features of Th17 cell biology deserve mention in the context of understanding which regulatory T cells are best equipped to control Th17 autoimmunity. One feature that appears to distinguish these cells from Th1 cells is their unique dependence on monocytes [99]. This dependence also appears to be linked to a requirement for IL-1β(beta) and for extracellular ATP (Sullivan, Hegde, Jankowska-Gan, and Burlingham, manuscript in preparation), which is needed for the P2X7-dependent processing of pro-IL1β(beta) to its mature bioactive form. Recent studies have shown that a subset of CD4+CD25+ Treg cells expressing the ectonuclease CD39, which cleaves extracellular ATP, is essential for control of TH17 cell function. Removal of these Tregs does not compromise regulation of Th1 proliferation or IFN-γ(gamma)-mediated immunity, but it completely abolishes the regulation of Th17 cells [100, 101].

In light of these new insights, the observation that Th17 responses to collagen V can be suppressed by CD4+CD45RC^{high} regulatory T cells [57, 58] is of interest. It has been postulated that such regulatory T cells likely account for the suppression of rejection responses and the consequent airway pathologic changes via the collagen V-induced oral tolerance that has been observed in animal models of lung transplantation [56, 102, 103]. Both TGFβ(beta)- and IL-10-producing regulatory T cells (suppressor IL-10 T cells) that are dependent on the presence of natural T regulatory CD4+25^{high} cells have been reported to suppress collagen V autoimmune sensitization [56]. The suppressive cytokine-producing regulatory T cells, most likely iTregs (induced type) appear to decline along with loss of nTregs in peripheral blood of human lung transplant recipients when BOS appears [68, 69]. However, the loss of CD39 ectonuclease activity in Tregs may be even more critical than the loss of nTregs as a whole; recent studies in our lab indicate a negative correlation between colV-specific Th17 activity in PBMC and the percent of CD39+ Tregs (manuscript in preparation). Similarly, the role of the novel suppressive cytokine IL-35, which is produced by a subset of Treg cells, is relatively unexplored [104, 105].

Conclusion

Sensitization to self-antigens such as colV may play a key role in the development of autoimmune responses directed against airways of the lung allograft following lung transplantation along with cell-mediated and humoral alloimmune responses (Fig. 10.1). Patients with lung disease (especially those with IPF) may already have sensitization to colV prior to transplantation, and T17 responses directed against the allograft as well as compromised regulatory mechanisms to suppress such responses likely play a key role in the initiation and progression of chronic lung allograft dysfunction due to the development of OB. An improved understanding of how autoimmune responses are induced and regulated may lead to the development of novel therapies to prevent and treat BOS, which remains the major cause of graft loss and patient death beyond the first post-transplant year.

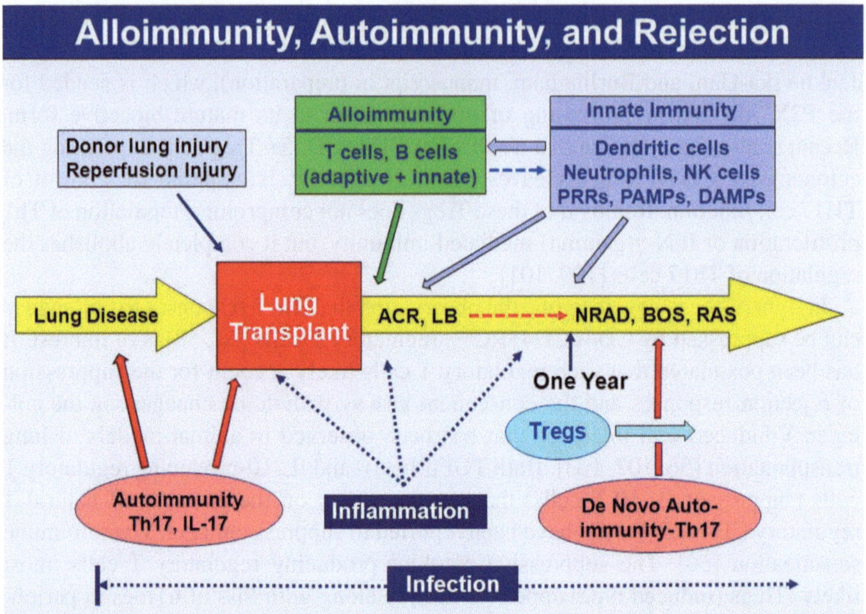

Fig. 10.1 Autoimmunity in lung allograft dysfunction. Autoimmune sensitization to self-antigens (e.g., collagen V) may be present prior to transplant and may play a role in early allograft dysfunction. Additionally, such sensitization may develop post-transplant (especially if not adequately suppressed by regulatory T cells) and contribute to chronic lung allograft dysfunction due to the development of neutrophilic reversible allograft dysfunction (NRAD), bronchiolitis obliterans syndrome (BOS), or restrictive allograft syndrome (RAS). *PRR* pattern recognition receptor, *PAMP* pathogen-associated molecular pattern, *DAMP* damage-associated molecular pattern, *ACR* acute cellular rejection, *LB* lymphocytic bronchiolitis

Future Directions

We are currently investigating the immunogenetics of colV-specific autoimmunity, the role of CD39 Tregs in control of BOS, and the interplay of TGFβ(beta)1, TGFβ3, IL1β, and IL23 in the generation of pathogenesis vs. “reg-like” TH17 cells. We speculate that if we could keep Treg cells fully functional in our patients following lung transplantation (as in healthy controls), they might be protected from the development and expansion of pathogenic anti-colV, anti-Kat, anti-vimentin Th17 cells that have been linked to the pathogenesis of BOS.

References

1. Christie JD, Edwards LB, Aurora P, Dobbels F, Kirk R, Rahmel AO, et al. The registry of the International Society for Heart and Lung Transplantation: twenty-sixth official adult lung and heart-lung transplantation report-2009. J Heart Lung Transplant. 2009;28(10):1031–49.

2. Cooper JD, Billingham M, Egan T, Hertz MI, Higenbottam T, Lynch J, et al. A working formulation for the standardization of nomenclature and for clinical staging of chronic dysfunction in lung allografts. International Society for Heart and Lung Transplantation. J Heart Lung Transplant. 1993;12(5):713–6.
3. Estenne M, Maurer JR, Boehler A, Egan JJ, Frost A, Hertz M, et al. Bronchiolitis obliterans syndrome 2001: an update of the diagnostic criteria. J Heart Lung Transplant. 2002;21(3):297–310.
4. Verleden GM, Vos R, De Vleeschauwer SI, Willems-Widyastuti A, Verleden SE, Dupont LJ, et al. Obliterative bronchiolitis following lung transplantation: from old to new concepts? Transpl Int. 2009;22(8):771–9.
5. Kinnier CV, Martinu T, Gowdy KM, Nugent JL, Kelly FL, Palmer SM. Innate immune activation by the viral PAMP poly I:C potentiates pulmonary graft-versus-host disease after allogeneic hematopoietic cell transplant. Transpl Immunol. 2011;24(2):83–93.
6. Todd JL, Palmer SM. Bronchiolitis obliterans syndrome: the final frontier for lung transplantation. Chest. 2011;140(2):502–8.
7. Opelz G, Susal C, Ruhenstroth A, Dohler B. Impact of HLA compatibility on lung transplant survival and evidence for an HLA restriction phenomenon: a collaborative transplant study report. Transplantation. 2010;90(8):912–7.
8. Nath DS, Basha HI, Mohanakumar T. Antihuman leukocyte antigen antibody-induced autoimmunity: role in chronic rejection. Curr Opin Organ Transplant. 2010;15(1):16–20.
9. Fukami N, Ramachandran S, Saini D, Walter M, Chapman W, Patterson GA, et al. Antibodies to MHC class I induce autoimmunity: role in the pathogenesis of chronic rejection. J Immunol. 2009;182(1):309–18.
10. Hagedorn PH, Burton CM, Carlsen J, Steinbruchel D, Andersen CB, Sahar E, et al. Chronic rejection of a lung transplant is characterized by a profile of specific autoantibodies. Immunology. 2010;130(3):427–35.
11. Haque MA, Mizobuchi T, Yasufuku K, Fujisawa T, Brutkiewicz RR, Zheng Y, et al. Evidence for immune responses to a self-antigen in lung transplantation: role of type V collagen-specific T cells in the pathogenesis of lung allograft rejection. J Immunol. 2002;169(3):1542–9.
12. Yoshida S, Haque A, Mizobuchi T, Iwata T, Chiyo M, Webb TJ, et al. Anti-type V collagen lymphocytes that express IL-17 and IL-23 induce rejection pathology in fresh and well-healed lung transplants. Am J Transplant. 2006;6(4):724–35.
13. Burlingham WJ, Love RB, Jankowska-Gan E, Haynes LD, Xu Q, Bobadilla JL, et al. IL-17-dependent cellular immunity to collagen type V predisposes to obliterative bronchiolitis in human lung transplants. J Clin Invest. 2007;117(11):3498–506.
14. Bobadilla JL, Love RB, Jankowska-Gan E, Xu Q, Haynes LD, Braun RK, et al. TH-17, monokines, collagen type V, and primary graft dysfunction in lung transplantation. Am J Respir Crit Care Med. 2008;177:660–8.
15. Fischer A, du Bois R. Interstitial lung disease in connective tissue disorders. Lancet. 2012;380(9842):689–98.
16. Swigris JJ, Brown KK, Flaherty KR. The idiopathic interstitial pneumonias and connective tissue disease-associated interstitial lung disease. Curr Rheumatol Rev. 2010;6:91–8.
17. Self SE. Autoantibody testing for autoimmune disease. Clin Chest Med. 2010;31(3):415–22.
18. Flaherty KR, Travis WD, Colby TV, Toews GB, Kazerooni EA, Gross BH, et al. Histopathologic variability in usual and nonspecific interstitial pneumonias. Am J Respir Crit Care Med. 2001;164(9):1722–7.
19. Feghali-Bostwick CA, Tsai CG, Valentine VG, Kantrow S, Stoner MW, Pilewski JM, et al. Cellular and humoral autoreactivity in idiopathic pulmonary fibrosis. J Immunol. 2007;179(4):2592–9.

20. Kurosu K, Takiguchi Y, Okada O, Yumoto N, Sakao S, Tada Y, et al. Identification of annexin 1 as a novel autoantigen in acute exacerbation of idiopathic pulmonary fibrosis. J Immunol. 2008;181(1):756–67.
21. Taille C, Grootenboer-Mignot S, Boursier C, Michel L, Debray MP, Fagart J, et al. Identification of periplakin as a new target for autoreactivity in idiopathic pulmonary fibrosis. Am J Respir Crit Care Med. 2011;183(6):759–66.
22. Gilani SR, Vuga LJ, Lindell KO, Gibson KF, Xue J, Kaminski N, et al. CD28 down-regulation on circulating CD4 T-cells is associated with poor prognoses of patients with idiopathic pulmonary fibrosis. PLoS One. 2010;5(1):e8959.
23. Kotsianidis I, Nakou E, Bouchliou I, Tzouvelekis A, Spanoudakis E, Steiropoulos P, et al. Global impairment of CD4+CD25+FOXP3+ regulatory T cells in idiopathic pulmonary fibrosis. Am J Respir Crit Care Med. 2009;179(12):1121–30.
24. Rinaldi M, Lehouck A, Heulens N, Lavend'homme R, Carlier V, Saint-Remy JM, et al. Antielastin B-cell and T-cell immunity in patients with chronic obstructive pulmonary disease. Thorax. 2012;67(8):694–700.
25. Liu M, Subramanian V, Christie C, Castro M, Mohanakumar T. Immune responses to self-antigens in asthma patients: clinical and immunopathological implications. Hum Immunol. 2012;73(5):511–6.
26. Nunez B, Sauleda J, Anto JM, Julia MR, Orozco M, Monso E, et al. Anti-tissue antibodies are related to lung function in chronic obstructive pulmonary disease. Am J Respir Crit Care Med. 2011;183(8):1025–31.
27. Goffrini P. Sulla possibilita di conservazione e di utilizzazione del tessuto tracheale nella chirurgia riparatrice della trachea e dei grossi bronchi. [Possibility of serving and using tracheal tissue in surgical repair of the trachea and bronchi]. Minerva Chir. 1952;7(15):583–6.
28. Depaulis J. Les plasties tracheobronchiques. [Tracheobronchial restorative surgery]. J Med Bord. 1952;129(4):291–5.
29. Hertz MI, Jessurun J, King MB, Savik SK, Murray JJ. Reproduction of the obliterative bronchiolitis lesion after heterotopic transplantation of mouse airways. Am J Pathol. 1993;142(6):1945–51.
30. Nakanishi R, Shirakusa T, Hanagiri T. Early histopathologic features of tracheal allotransplant rejection: a study in nonimmunosuppressed dogs. Transplant Proc. 1994;26(6):3715–8.
31. Nakanishi R, Shirakusa T, Mitsudomi T. Maximum length of tracheal autografts in dogs. J Thorac Cardiovasc Surg. 1993;106(6):1081–7.
32. Xavier-Elsas P, Santos-Maximiano E, Queto T, Mendonca-Sales S, Joseph D, Gaspar-Elsas MI, et al. Ectopic lung transplantation induces the accumulation of eosinophil progenitors in the recipients' lungs through an allergen- and interleukin-5-dependent mechanism. Clin Exp Allergy. 2007;37(1):29–38.
33. Ikonen T, Uusitalo M, Taskinen E, Korpela A, Salminen US, Morris RE, et al. Small airway obliteration in a new swine heterotopic lung and bronchial allograft model. J Heart Lung Transplant. 1998;17(10):945–53.
34. Salminen US, Ikonen T, Uusitalo M, Taskinen E, Korpela A, Maasilta P, et al. Obliterative lesions in small airways in an immunosuppressed porcine heterotopic bronchial allograft model. Transpl Int. 1998;11 Suppl 1:S515–8.
35. Ikonen TS, Brazelton TR, Berry GJ, Shorthouse RS, Morris RE. Epithelial re-growth is associated with inhibition of obliterative airway disease in orthotopic tracheal allografts in non-immunosuppressed rats. Transplantation. 2000;70(6):857–63.
36. Nakanishi R. Revascularization of trachea in lung and tracheal transplantation. Clin Transplant. 2007;21(5):668–74.
37. Nakanishi R. Cryopreservation of the tracheal grafts: review and perspective. Organogenesis. 2009;5(3):113–8.
38. Asimacopoulos PJ, Molokhia FA, Pegg CA, Norman JC. Lung transplantation in the rat. Transplant Proc. 1971;3(1):583–5.
39. Marck KW, Prop J, Wildevuur CR, Nieuwenhuis P. Lung transplantation in the rat: histopathology of left lung iso- and allografts. J Heart Transplant. 1985;4(2):263–6.

40. Marck KW, Wildevuur CR. Lung transplantation in the rat: I. Technique and survival. Ann Thorac Surg. 1982;34(1):74–80.
41. Mizuta T, Kawaguchi A, Nakahara K, Kawashima Y. Simplified rat lung transplantation using a cuff technique. J Thorac Cardiovasc Surg. 1989;97(4):578–81.
42. Mizuta T, Nakahara K, Shirakura R, Fujii Y, Kawaguchi A, Minami M, et al. Total nonmicrosuture technique for rat lung transplantation. J Thorac Cardiovasc Surg. 1991;102(1):159–60.
43. Zhai W, Ge J, Inci I, Hillinger S, Markus C, Korom S, et al. Simplified rat lung transplantation by using a modified cuff technique. J Invest Surg. 2008;21(1):33–7.
44. Okazaki M, Krupnick AS, Kornfeld CG, Lai JM, Ritter JH, Richardson SB, et al. A mouse model of orthotopic vascularized aerated lung transplantation. Am J Transplant. 2007;7(6):1672–9.
45. Jungraithmayr WM, Korom S, Hillinger S, Weder W. A mouse model of orthotopic, single-lung transplantation. J Thorac Cardiovasc Surg. 2009;137(2):486–91.
46. Jungraithmayr W, Weder W. The technique of orthotopic mouse lung transplantation as a movie-improved learning by visualization. Am J Transplant. 2012;12(6):1624–6.
47. Jungraithmayr W, Vogt P, Inci I, Hillinger S, Arni S, Korom S, et al. A model of chronic lung allograft rejection in the rat. Eur Respir J. 2010;35(6):1354–63.
48. Fan L, Benson HL, Vittal R, Mickler EA, Presson R, Fisher AJ, et al. Neutralizing IL-17 prevents obliterative bronchiolitis in murine orthotopic lung transplantation. Am J Transplant. 2011;11(5):911–22.
49. De Vleeschauwer S, Jungraithmayr W, Wauters S, Willems S, Rinaldi M, Vaneylen A, et al. Chronic rejection pathology after orthotopic lung transplantation in mice: the development of a murine BOS model and its drawbacks. PLoS One. 2012;7(1):e29802.
50. Wilkes DS, Heidler KM, Bowen LK, Quinlan WM, Doyle NA, Cummings OW, et al. Allogeneic bronchoalveolar lavage cells induce the histology of acute lung allograft rejection, and deposition of IgG2a in recipient murine lungs. J Immunol. 1995;155(5):2775–83.
51. Linsenmayer TF, Gibney E, Igoe F, Gordon MK, Fitch JM, Fessler LI, et al. Type V collagen: molecular structure and fibrillar organization of the chicken alpha 1(V) NH2-terminal domain, a putative regulator of corneal fibrillogenesis. J Cell Biol. 1993;121(5):1181–9.
52. Wenstrup RJ, Florer JB, Brunskill EW, Bell SM, Chervoneva I, Birk DE. Type V collagen controls the initiation of collagen fibril assembly. J Biol Chem. 2004;279(51):53331–7.
53. Wilkes DS, Heidler KM, Yasufuku K, Devito-Haynes L, Jankowska-Gan E, Meyer KC, et al. Cell-mediated immunity to collagen V in lung transplant recipients: correlation with collagen V release into BAL fluid. J Heart Lung Transplant. 2001;20(2):167.
54. Trello CA, Williams DA, Keller CA, Crim C, Webster RO, Ohar JA. Increased gelatinolytic activity in bronchoalveolar lavage fluid in stable lung transplant recipients. Am J Respir Crit Care Med. 1997;156(6):1978–86.
55. Mares DC, Heidler KM, Smith GN, Cummings OW, Harris ER, Foresman B, et al. Type V collagen modulates alloantigen-induced pathology and immunology in the lung. Am J Respir Cell Mol Biol. 2000;23(1):62–70.
56. Yasufuku K, Heidler KM, O'Donnell PW, Smith Jr GN, Cummings OW, Foresman BH, et al. Oral tolerance induction by type V collagen downregulates lung allograft rejection. Am J Respir Cell Mol Biol. 2001;25(1):26–34.
57. Mizobuchi T, Yasufuku K, Zheng Y, Haque MA, Heidler KM, Woods K, et al. Differential expression of Smad7 transcripts identifies the CD4(+)CD45RC(high) regulatory T cells that mediate type V collagen-induced tolerance to lung allografts. J Immunol. 2003;171(3):1140–7.
58. Braun RK, Molitor-Dart M, Wigfield C, Xiang Z, Fain SB, Jankowska-Gan E, et al. Transfer of tolerance to collagen type V suppresses Th-17 lymphocyte mediated acute lung transplant rejection. Transplantation. 2009;88(12):1341–8.
59. McGregor CG, Jamieson SW, Baldwin JC, Burke CM, Dawkins KD, Stinson EB, et al. Combined heart-lung transplantation for end-stage Eisenmenger's syndrome. J Thorac Cardiovasc Surg. 1986;91(3):443–50.

60. Tazelaar HD, Yousem SA. The pathology of combined heart-lung transplantation: an autopsy study. Hum Pathol. 1988;19(12):1403–16.
61. Ostrow D, Buskard N, Hill RS, Vickars L, Churg A. Bronchiolitis obliterans complicating bone marrow transplantation. Chest. 1985;87(6):828–30.
62. Tiriveedhi V, Sarma N, Mohanakumar T. An important role for autoimmunity in the immunopathogenesis of chronic allograft rejection. Int J Immunogenet. 2012;39(5):373–80.
63. Iwata T, Chiyo M, Yoshida S, Smith Jr GN, Mickler EA, Presson Jr R, et al. Lung transplant ischemia reperfusion injury: metalloprotease inhibition down-regulates exposure of type V collagen, growth-related oncogene-induced neutrophil chemotaxis, and tumor necrosis factor-alpha expression. Transplantation. 2008;85(3):417–26.
64. Iwata T, Philipovskiy A, Fisher AJ, Presson Jr RG, Chiyo M, Lee J, et al. Anti-type V collagen humoral immunity in lung transplant primary graft dysfunction. J Immunol. 2008;181(8):5738–47.
65. Benichou G, Alessandrini A, Charrad RS, Wilkes DS. Induction of autoimmunity after allotransplantation. Front Biosci. 2007;12:4362–9.
66. Goers TA, Ramachandran S, Aloush A, Trulock E, Patterson GA, Mohanakumar T. De novo production of K-alpha1 tubulin-specific antibodies: role in chronic lung allograft rejection. J Immunol. 2008;180(7):4487–94.
67. Izutani H, Miyagawa S, Shirakura R, Matsumiya G, Nakata S, Shimazaki Y, et al. Evidence that graft coronary arteriosclerosis begins in the early phase after transplantation and progresses without chronic immunoreaction. Histopathological analysis using a retransplantation model. Transplantation. 1995;60(10):1073–9.
68. Bharat A, Fields RC, Steward N, Trulock EP, Patterson GA, Mohanakumar T. CD4+25+ regulatory T cells limit Th1-autoimmunity by inducing IL-10 producing T cells following human lung transplantation. Am J Transplant. 2006;6(8):1799–808.
69. Bharat A, Fields RC, Trulock EP, Patterson GA, Mohanakumar T. Induction of IL-10 suppressors in lung transplant patients by CD4+25+ regulatory T cells through CTLA-4 signaling. J Immunol. 2006;177(8):5631–8.
70. Boehler A, Estenne M. Post-transplant bronchiolitis obliterans. Eur Respir J. 2003;22(6):1007–18.
71. Fossiez F, Banchereau J, Murray R, Van Kooten C, Garrone P, Lebecque S. Interleukin-17. Int Rev Immunol. 1998;16(5–6):541–51.
72. Linden A. Role of interleukin-17 and the neutrophil in asthma. Int Arch Allergy Immunol. 2001;126(3):179–84.
73. Griffin GK, Newton G, Tarrio ML, Bu DX, Maganto-Garcia E, Azcutia V, et al. IL-17 and TNF-alpha sustain neutrophil recruitment during inflammation through synergistic effects on endothelial activation. J Immunol. 2012;188(12):6287–99.
74. Rouvier E, Luciani MF, Mattei MG, Denizot F, Golstein P. CTLA-8, cloned from an activated T cell, bearing AU-rich messenger RNA instability sequences, and homologous to a herpesvirus saimiri gene. J Immunol. 1993;150(12):5445–56.
75. Fossiez F, Djossou O, Chomarat P, Flores-Romo L, Ait-Yahia S, Maat C, et al. T cell interleukin-17 induces stromal cells to produce proinflammatory and hematopoietic cytokines. J Exp Med. 1996;183(6):2593–603.
76. Pappu R, Ramirez-Carrozzi V, Ota N, Ouyang W, Hu Y. The IL-17 family cytokines in immunity and disease. J Clin Immunol. 2010;30(2):185–95.
77. Harrington LE, Hatton RD, Mangan PR, Turner H, Murphy TL, Murphy KM, et al. Interleukin 17-producing CD4+ effector T cells develop via a lineage distinct from the T helper type 1 and 2 lineages. Nat Immunol. 2005;6(11):1123–32.
78. Park H, Li Z, Yang XO, Chang SH, Nurieva R, Wang YH, et al. A distinct lineage of CD4 T cells regulates tissue inflammation by producing interleukin 17. Nat Immunol. 2005;6(11):1133–41.
79. Pappu R, Ramirez-Carrozzi V, Sambandam A. The interleukin-17 cytokine family: critical players in host defence and inflammatory diseases. Immunology. 2011;134(1):8–16.

80. Santamaria R, Rizzetto L, Bromley M, Zelante T, Lee W, Cavalieri D, et al. Systems biology of infectious diseases: a focus on fungal infections. Immunobiology. 2011;216(11):1212–27.
81. Chabaud M, Garnero P, Dayer JM, Guerne PA, Fossiez F, Miossec P. Contribution of interleukin 17 to synovium matrix destruction in rheumatoid arthritis. Cytokine. 2000;12(7):1092–9.
82. Wong CK, Ho CY, Li EK, Lam CW. Elevation of proinflammatory cytokine (IL-18, IL-17, IL-12) and Th2 cytokine (IL-4) concentrations in patients with systemic lupus erythematosus. Lupus. 2000;9(8):589–93.
83. Lubberts E, Joosten LA, Oppers B, van den Bersselaar L, Coenen-de Roo CJ, Kolls JK, et al. IL-1-independent role of IL-17 in synovial inflammation and joint destruction during collagen-induced arthritis. J Immunol. 2001;167(2):1004–13.
84. Dong G, Ye R, Shi W, Liu S, Wang T, Yang X, et al. IL-17 induces autoantibody overproduction and peripheral blood mononuclear cell overexpression of IL-6 in lupus nephritis patients. Chin Med J (Engl). 2003;116(4):543–8.
85. Lubberts E. The role of IL-17 and family members in the pathogenesis of arthritis. Curr Opin Investig Drugs. 2003;4(5):572–7.
86. Zhang GX, Gran B, Yu S, Li J, Siglienti I, Chen X, et al. Induction of experimental autoimmune encephalomyelitis in IL-12 receptor-beta 2-deficient mice: IL-12 responsiveness is not required in the pathogenesis of inflammatory demyelination in the central nervous system. J Immunol. 2003;170(4):2153–60.
87. McGeachy MJ, Anderton SM. Cytokines in the induction and resolution of experimental autoimmune encephalomyelitis. Cytokine. 2005;32(2):81–4.
88. Vanaudenaerde BM, Wuyts WA, Dupont LJ, Van Raemdonck DE, Demedts MM, Verleden GM. Interleukin-17 stimulates release of interleukin-8 by human airway smooth muscle cells in vitro: a potential role for interleukin-17 and airway smooth muscle cells in bronchiolitis obliterans syndrome. J Heart Lung Transplant. 2003;22(11):1280–3.
89. Bettelli E, Carrier Y, Gao W, Korn T, Strom TB, Oukka M, et al. Reciprocal developmental pathways for the generation of pathogenic effector TH17 and regulatory T cells. Nature. 2006;441(7090):235–8.
90. Cua DJ, Sherlock J, Chen Y, Murphy CA, Joyce B, Seymour B, et al. Interleukin-23 rather than interleukin-12 is the critical cytokine for autoimmune inflammation of the brain. Nature. 2003;421(6924):744–8.
91. Lee Y, Awasthi A, Yosef N, Quintana FJ, Xiao S, Peters A, et al. Induction and molecular signature of pathogenic T(H)17 cells. Nat Immunol. 2012;13(10):991–9.
92. Wilke CM, Bishop K, Fox D, Zou W. Deciphering the role of Th17 cells in human disease. Trends Immunol. 2011;32(12):603–11.
93. Vanaudenaerde BM, Dupont LJ, Wuyts WA, Verbeken EK, Meyts I, Bullens DM, et al. The role of interleukin-17 during acute rejection after lung transplantation. Eur Respir J. 2006; 27(4):779–87.
94. Carrodeguas L, Orosz CG, Waldman WJ, Sedmak DD, Adams PW, VanBuskirk AM. Trans vivo analysis of human delayed-type hypersensitivity reactivity. Hum Immunol. 1999;60(8):640–51.
95. VanBuskirk AM, Burlingham WJ, Jankowska-Gan E, Chin T, Kusaka S, Geissler F, et al. Human allograft acceptance is associated with immune regulation. J Clin Invest. 2000;106(1):145–55.
96. Saini D, Weber J, Ramachandran S, Phelan D, Tiriveedhi V, Liu M, et al. Alloimmunity-induced autoimmunity as a potential mechanism in the pathogenesis of chronic rejection of human lung allografts. J Heart Lung Transplant. 2011;30(6):624–31.
97. Li W, Bribriesco AC, Nava RG, Brescia AA, Ibricevic A, Spahn JH, et al. Lung transplant acceptance is facilitated by early events in the graft and is associated with lymphoid neogenesis. Mucosal Immunol. 2012;5(5):544–54.
98. Guthrie KA, Gammill HS, Madeleine MM, Dugowson CE, Nelson JL. Parity and HLA alleles in risk of rheumatoid arthritis. Chimerism. 2011;2(1):11–5.

99. Acosta-Rodriguez EV, Napolitani G, Lanzavecchia A, Sallusto F. Interleukins 1beta and 6 but not transforming growth factor-beta are essential for the differentiation of interleukin 17-producing human T helper cells. Nat Immunol. 2007;8(9):942–9.
100. Ye ZJ, Zhou Q, Zhang JC, Li X, Wu C, Qin SM, et al. CD39+ regulatory T cells suppress generation and differentiation of Th17 cells in human malignant pleural effusion via a LAP-dependent mechanism. Respir Res. 2011;12:77.
101. Fletcher JM, Lonergan R, Costelloe L, Kinsella K, Moran B, O'Farrelly C, et al. CD39+Foxp3+ regulatory T cells suppress pathogenic Th17 cells and are impaired in multiple sclerosis. J Immunol. 2009;183(11):7602–10.
102. Yasufuku K, Heidler KM, Woods KA, Smith Jr GN, Cummings OW, Fujisawa T, et al. Prevention of bronchiolitis obliterans in rat lung allografts by type V collagen-induced oral tolerance. Transplantation. 2002;73(4):500–5.
103. Yamada Y, Sekine Y, Yoshida S, Yasufuku K, Petrache I, Benson HL, et al. Type V collagen-induced oral tolerance plus low-dose cyclosporine prevents rejection of MHC class I and II incompatible lung allografts. J Immunol. 2009;183(1):237–45.
104. Collison LW, Delgoffe GM, Guy CS, Vignali KM, Chaturvedi V, Fairweather D, et al. The composition and signaling of the IL-35 receptor are unconventional. Nat Immunol. 2012;13(3):290–9.
105. Collison LW, Workman CJ, Kuo TT, Boyd K, Wang Y, Vignali KM, et al. The inhibitory cytokine IL-35 contributes to regulatory T-cell function. Nature. 2007;450(7169):566–9.

Chapter 11
The Role of Infections in BOS

Robin K. Avery

Abstract Background: Infectious agents, particularly cytomegalovirus (CMV), have long been considered to be potential triggers for BOS, although the exact magnitude of the role of infections and the mechanisms thereof remain an area of active research. Methods: This chapter will review previous literature and newer results concerning the possible roles of CMV, other herpesviruses, community-acquired respiratory viruses, bacteria (including *Pseudomonas*, other gram-negative, gram-positive, and atypical organisms), and fungi, including colonization as well as invasive infection. Results: The text reviews and evaluates the body of literature supporting a role for these infectious agents as risk factors for BOS and time to BOS. Changing patterns of infection over time are taken into account, and studies that have shown an association between BOS (or lack thereof) and CMV are reviewed. Strategies for prevention or early treatment of infections are discussed as potential means of preserving allograft function long term. Immunizations, stringent infection-control practices, and antimicrobial treatment including newer therapies will be discussed. Conclusion: In addition to the classic literature that has focused on CMV, an expanding spectrum of infectious organisms has been implicated as possible risk factors for BOS. Increasing knowledge of the impact of long-term antiviral suppression, prophylaxis, and outcomes of early therapy will help guide future recipient management.

Keywords Infection • Cytomegalovirus • Bacterial • *Pseudomonas* • Gram-positive • Gram-negative • Fungal • Prophylaxis

R.K. Avery, M.D. (✉)
Division of Infectious Disease (Transplant/Oncology), Johns Hopkins Hospital, 1830 East Monument Street, No. 434, Baltimore, MD 21205, USA
e-mail: ravery4@jhmi.edu

K.C. Meyer and A.R. Glanville (eds.), *Bronchiolitis Obliterans Syndrome in Lung Transplantation*, Respiratory Medicine 8, DOI 10.1007/978-1-4614-7636-8_11,

The CMV Controversy

Cytomegalovirus (CMV) has always been one of the most frequently identified pathogens in solid organ transplantation, despite multiple prevention strategies that have been developed over time. Lung transplant recipients, among all other solid organ transplant recipients, appear to be particularly susceptible to CMV disease, recurrences, and antiviral resistance. In the early era of lung transplantation, prior to widespread use of ganciclovir-based prophylaxis, symptomatic CMV disease including CMV pneumonitis was very common, occurring in up to 60–80 % of patients [1]. The highest-risk group was identified as the donor-seropositive, recipient-seronegative (D+/R–) group, which corresponds to the introduction of CMV from the donor organ into a recipient without antecedent CMV immunity and, thus, limited ability (at least initially) to limit viral replication. In studies by Zeevi and others, the development of CMV-specific immunity was shown to be delayed in some D+/R– lung recipients, although most did develop such immunity eventually [2]. In most early studies, both CMV disease and donor CMV-seropositive serology were associated with worse outcomes, including increased risk of BOS, shorter time to BOS, and/or mortality [3–7]. In some studies, use of CMV prophylaxis was associated with decreased mortality [3] or delayed onset of BOS [1].

Mechanisms of CMV effects on the allograft are an area of active research. Studies in animal models (rat tracheal allografts) have supported the hypothesis of a causative role for CMV, in that obliterative bronchiolitis was accentuated by CMV and prevented by ganciclovir prophylaxis or hyperimmune serum [8]. In this model, CMV effects were accompanied by increases in interleukin-2 and tumor necrosis factor-alpha expression and a decrease in interleukin-10 expression [8]. Wiebe et al. found that both rat CMV and bacterial infection increased chronic airway rejection in a rat model, and this process was associated with increased expression of intercellular adhesion molecule (ICAM)-1 on endothelium, as well as increased numbers of infiltrating leukocytes and ED-1 positive macrophages [9].

More recently, CMV has been associated with increased activity of proinflammatory chemokines such as CXCL 10 [10, 11]. Increases in CXCL 10 (IP 10) in CMV-positive BAL samples were associated with a decrease in FEV1 in a study by Weseslindtner et al. [10]. Weigt et al. found that pulmonary CMV was associated with increased levels of the chemokines CCL 2 and CCL 5, with CCL 2 being predictive of BOS development and CCL 5 predictive of mortality [12]. In addition, the role of recipient genetic polymorphisms in determining CMV risk has generated increasing interest [11], including a polymorphism affecting interferon-gamma levels [13]. Recent work has suggested that CMV levels in epithelial lining fluid are more relevant that those in plasma [14].

Studies that have assessed the putative association of CMV with BOS or allograft dysfunction are summarized in Table 11.1. Recently, the impact of treated CMV pneumonitis in the prophylaxis era has been reassessed, with studies showing disparate results: both a decreased impact [15] and a continued adverse impact [16, 17] of CMV pneumonitis on allograft function have been reported. Tamm et al.

Table 11.1 Studies of the association between CMV infection, disease, or serostatus and the risk of developing bronchiolitis obliterans syndrome and allograft dysfunction

Year	Author	References	No. of patients	Main findings
1991	Keenan et al.	[7]	27	CMV serology and CMV infection: increased risk for BOS
1992	Cerrina et al.	[5]	36	CMV D+/R–, CMV pneumonitis, and CMV recurrence: increased risk for BOS
1995	Bando et al.	[3]	239	CMV D+/R–: risk for BOS and death; survival improved with prophylaxis
1996	Girgis et al.	[49]	74	CMV added additional risk to the acute rejection score for BOS risk
1996	Soghikian et al.	[1]	89	CMV prophylaxis with ganciclovir delays BOS onset
1996	Sharples et al.	[88]	157	CMV infection and CMV disease: increased risk for BOS
1997	Kroshus et al.	[4]	132	CMV pneumonitis: increased risk for BOS and time to BOS
1998	Gutierrez et al.	[89]	61	On prophylaxis, donor serology but not CMV infection or CMV disease predicts BOS
1998	Heng et al.	[6]	230	CMV serology and CMV disease: increased risk for BOS
1998	Smith et al.	[90]	301	CMV D+/R–: increased risk for BOS within 3 years
1999	Speich et al.	[91]	22	Oral ganciclovir prophylaxis, decreased risk for BOS
2001	Schulman et al.	[92]	152	CMV pneumonitis: increased risk for BOS
2002	Fiser et al.	[93]	134	CMV infection: increased risk for BOS progression
2002	Jackson et al.	[94]	204	CMV not associated with acute-onset BOS
2003	Luckraz et al.	[95]	297	BOS in CMV D–/R– not significantly different from D+ and/or R+
2003	Westall et al.	[96]	26	Early CMV DNAemia associated with BOS risk despite prophylaxis
2004	Tamm et al.	[15]	341	Treated CMV pneumonitis and CMV serology: not risk factors for BOS
2005	Hachem et al.	[97]	157	ATG decreases BOS risk vs. basiliximab, but no difference in CMV
2005	Perreas et al.	[98]	146	CMV prophylaxis (3 months.) decreased CMV but not BOS risk
2006	Moffatt-Bruce et al.	[99]	128	Heart-lung recipients had more CMV than lung patients but BOS same
2006	Ruttmann et al.	[100]	68	CMV Ig addition to ganciclovir decreased CMV disease and BOS at 3 years
2008	Chmiel et al.	[101]	96	CMV prophylaxis decreased BOS and increased survival at 5 years
2008	Kwakkel-van Erp et al.	[102]	48	Lack of activating KIR correlates with BOS but not CMV
2008	Solidoro et al.	[103]	46	No difference in OB with combined prophylaxis

(continued)

Table 11.1 (continued)

Year	Author	References	No. of patients	Main findings
2008	Valentine et al.	[18]	151	CMV pneumonitis in 38 % of patients who stopped prophylaxis; 50 % of these developed BOS in 1 year
2008	Weigt et al.	[12]	72	CCL 2 and CCL 5 in CMV pneumonitis; CCL 2 predicted BOS risk and CCL 5 predicted mortality
2009	Manuel et al.	[35]	93	CMV detection in BAL is not associated with increased BOS risk
2009	Ranganathan et al.	[104]	599	CMVIg prophylaxis not related to BOS risk in pediatric lung recipients
2009	Valentine et al.	[17]	161	CMV pneumonitis in first 100 days increased BOS risk
2010	Snyder et al.	[16]	231	Treated CMV pneumonitis remains a risk for BOS and death
2011	Paraskeva et al.	[105]	192	CMV detection in BAL is associated with increased BOS risk
2011	Kwakkel-van Erp et al.	[106]	85	Mannose-binding-lectin deficiency increased CMV reactivation but no effect on BOS

ATG antithymocyte globulin, *CMV* cytomegalovirus, *CMV Ig* CMV hyperimmune globulin, *CMV D+/R−* CMV donor seropositive, recipient seronegative, *CMV R+* recipient seropositive, *CMV D−/R−* CMV donor seronegative, recipient seronegative, *KIR* killer immunoglobulin-like receptor, *OB* obliterative bronchiolitis

studied 341 lung recipients, including 151 with CMV pneumonia who were treated with ganciclovir, and 190 without CMV pneumonia. There were no significant differences in BOS or in patient survival at 1, 3, and 5 years [15]. There was also no association between CMV donor/recipient serostatus and BOS or survival [15]. Snyder et al., however, reported that there was an association between treated CMV pneumonitis and BOS. [16]. In 231 patients transplanted between 2000 and 2004, 1,887 biopsies were performed including CMV immunostaining. CMV pneumonitis developed in 49 (21 %). Treated CMV pneumonitis within the first 6 months increased the risk of BOS (hazard ratio 2.19) and death (hazard ratio 1.89). This remained significant in multivariable analysis [16]. Similarly, Valentine et al. assessed the impact of respiratory infections due to a variety of pathogens and found that CMV pneumonitis in the first 100 days increased BOS risk with a hazard ratio of 3.1 [17]. In another study, Valentine et al. reported that indefinite ganciclovir prophylaxis was associated with long-term freedom from CMV pneumonitis, but that in the group of patients who stopped prophylaxis, 38 % developed CMV pneumonitis, and 50 % of these developed BOS within 1 year [18].

Thus, some controversy still exists, but most evidence suggests at least some role for CMV. In the current era, several important differences have emerged as compared with the earlier era. CMV pneumonitis has notably declined, comprising, for example, only 4.3 % of a set of 559 respiratory infections in lung recipients in a

Table 11.2 Organisms that have been associated with risk of developing bronchiolitis obliterans syndrome and allograft dysfunction

Viral
Cytomegalovirus
Other herpesviruses: human herpesvirus-6, human herpesvirus-7, Epstein-Barr virus
Community respiratory viruses: influenza, parainfluenza, respiratory syncytial virus, adenovirus, metapneumovirus, rhinovirus, coronavirus, others
Bacterial
Pseudomonas aeruginosa
Other gram-negative bacteria (*Burkholderia* spp., *Klebsiella* spp., others)
Gram-positive bacteria (*Staphylococcus* spp., *Streptococcus* spp., others)
Chlamydophila (Chlamydia) *pneumoniae*
Mycobacteria
Simkania negevensis
Fungal
Aspergillus spp.
Pneumocystis jiroveci (formerly *P. carinii*)

study by Valentine et al. [19]. Longer-term viral suppression has become an option because of the availability of oral valganciclovir. In a randomized, multicenter study, CMV events and severity were significantly decreased in the group receiving 12 months as compared with 3 months of valganciclovir prophylaxis [20]. This benefit was maintained out to >4 years in a single-center subgroup [21]. Whether this enhanced freedom from CMV events improves the lifespan of the allograft is still a question. As mentioned above, the study by Valentine et al. of increased CMV pneumonitis and BOS in the group that stopped prophylaxis has led this group to call for indefinite long-term prophylaxis [18].

In addition, methods of CMV detection have become increasingly sophisticated, especially with the development of quantitative measures of blood and BAL viral loads, allowing for detection of early and/or subclinical infection [14, 22–25], with particular recent attention to the lung compartment over blood or plasma [14, 25]. There has also been increasing recognition in other solid organ transplant recipients of the importance of subclinical CMV infection on allograft function (e.g., cardiac allograft vasculopathy in heart recipients) [26, 27]. Whether such early detection, particularly of late CMV after cessation of prophylaxis, improves allograft function for lung recipients also remains to be shown. Given the results of Bauer et al. regarding CMV detection in epithelial lining fluid, it has been questioned whether monitoring of viremia is adequate for early detection [14]. Disparities in results between groups in the current era may also reflect more subtle differences. For example, the role of mixed infection with more than one CMV genotype is an area of active research [28].

Although CMV has received the most attention, multiple other organisms have been described as possible triggers for BOS. These include viral, bacterial, and fungal organisms (Table 11.2).

Other Herpesviruses

The herpesvirus family includes herpes simplex virus 1 and 2, varicella-zoster virus, CMV, Epstein-Barr virus (EBV), human herpesvirus 6 and 7 (HHV-6 and HHV-7), and human herpesvirus-8 (Kaposi's sarcoma herpesvirus). Of these, HHV-6 and 7, along with CMV, are termed the beta-herpesviruses. HHV-6 and 7 are the viruses that cause roseola in infants and can reactivate post-transplant, often in an earlier timeframe than CMV. HHV-6 reactivation, in particular, has been described to cause clinical syndromes that have some similarity to CMV, including pneumonitis, hepatitis, meningoencephalitis, and pancytopenia. [29] HHV-6 pneumonitis was identified as one of the causes of apparent culture-negative interstitial pneumonitis in bone marrow transplant recipients [30].

Of the herpesviruses listed above, HHV-6, HHV-7, and EBV have been reported in association with BOS or similar syndromes. Neurohr et al. performed a panel of viral PCR tests on BAL fluid from 87 lung recipients and found that HHV-6, which was detected in 20 patients, was an independent risk factor for BOS and death [31]. On the other hand, Ross et al. found a possible association between HHV-7 detection and bronchiolitis obliterans with organizing pneumonia after lung transplantation [32]. The possible role of EBV was studied by Engelmann et al., who monitored 385 lung transplant recipients for CMV (by pp65 antigenemia assay), EBV DNA, and adenovirus DNA in blood [33]. Over half of the patients had EBV DNA detected on at least one occasion, and repeated EBV DNA detection was associated with BOS risk [33]. Diagnosis of BOS prior to study entry, retransplantation, and the use of sirolimus or everolimus were associated with detection of EBV [33]. This latter finding was somewhat surprising, as the sirolimus group of immunosuppressive agents has been thought to have a protective effect with respect to viral infections as compared with other immunosuppressive agents [34].

In contrast to the above studies, a recent study by Manuel et al. of viral PCR detection in BAL did not show an association between CMV, HHV-6, or HHV-7, on the one hand, and BOS or acute rejection, on the other, although half of the patients had CMV detected and one-fifth each had HHV-6 and HHV-7 detected [35]. Differences in baseline patient populations, immunosuppression, prophylaxis, and detection methods might account for some of the differences in findings, but these remain largely unexplained. Manuel et al. hypothesized that prolonged antiviral prophylaxis, while not preventing viral reactivation within the allograft, might mitigate some of its damaging effects [35]. Although reports of associations of BOS with detection of these other herpesviruses are intriguing, the disparate results from different centers must introduce a note of caution when assessing the impact of these viruses overall.

Community Respiratory Viruses

Lung transplant recipients are highly susceptible to infection by community-acquired respiratory viruses (CARVs), particularly at times of intensified immunosuppression. Such infection may be asymptomatic or may involve the upper or lower respiratory tract. Occasionally infectious syndromes can be severe enough to warrant ICU admission and mechanical ventilation. In addition to such dramatically symptomatic episodes, however, less symptomatic but truly chronic infections have also been documented, even with the comparatively underrated and ubiquitous rhinovirus [36]. The major question with regard to CARVs (in addition to the direct infectious syndromes they produce) is the indirect and longer-lasting effect on the allograft. Mechanisms are being investigated, and recent attention has focused on the increase in the chemokine receptor CXCR 3 and its chemokine ligands. Weigt et al. compared BAL fluid in CARV and non-CARV-infected lung recipients and found that elevated levels of CXCL 10 and CXCL 11 correlated with greater decreases in FEV1 when measured 6 months after the initial infection episode [37].

Multiple studies have demonstrated an impact of community respiratory viral infection on allograft function, not only during the acute infectious process but also 3 and 6 months after resolution, although results have varied. Kumar et al. studied 100 patients from 2001 to 2003, comparing 50 patients with clinically diagnosed viral respiratory infections and 50 who were asymptomatic [38]. Nasopharyngeal and throat swabs revealed viral pathogens in two-thirds of the group with clinical respiratory infection [including rhinovirus, coronavirus, respiratory syncytial virus (RSV), influenza, parainfluenza, and human metapneumovirus]. The incidence of acute rejection and of decline in FEV1 over 3 months was significantly higher in the viral respiratory infections group, and for some patients, the decline in FEV1 was sustained out to 1 year [38]. A more recent prospective study by this group utilized a multiplex panel of molecular detection assays for 19 viruses on BAL samples of 93 lung recipients. Eighty-one BAL samples were positive for viruses; rhinovirus was detected in 46, and smaller numbers of recipients had parainfluenza, coronavirus, influenza, metapneumovirus, or RSV. Acute rejection or ≥20 % decline in FEV1 over 3 months occurred in 33.3 % of virus-positive vs. 6.7 % of virus-negative patients ($p=0.001$). This was true regardless of whether the viral infection was symptomatic or not [39]. In another study, Gottlieb et al. followed 388 lung recipients with nasopharyngeal and oropharyngeal viral swabs for 12 community respiratory viruses and found that 7.7 % of patients manifested a CARV infection. BOS occurred at 1 year in 25 % of CARV-positive patients vs. 9 % of CARV-negative patients ($p=0.002$) [40]. RSV and parainfluenza virus appeared to have more of an effect than rhinovirus and coronavirus. Symptomatic CARV remained a risk factor for BOS in multivariable analyses but did not appear to influence progression of preexisting BOS [40]. Khalifah et al. followed 259 adult lung recipients and found that CARV infection was associated with BOS, death, and death from BOS [41]. In this study, these effects were particularly strong for lower-tract CARV infection [41]. In a study by Vilchez et al., parainfluenza virus was especially strongly associated with subsequent BOS (32 %) [42].

A few studies have not shown the same impact of CARVs. A study of pediatric lung recipients by Liu et al. found that over half developed CARV infections, but these infections were not associated with chronic allograft dysfunction or death in this particular cohort [43]. In another report of 576 pediatric lung recipients in a multicenter study by Liu et al., CARV infection was associated with decreased 12-month survival but not with acute rejection [44]. A study of 50 adult lung recipients by Milstone et al. found that one-third developed CARV infection, but this was not associated with subsequent graft dysfunction [45]. Soccal et al. performed both BAL and nasopharyngeal swabs and found that 29.3 % of the upper respiratory and 17.2 % of the BAL samples were virus-positive. Acute rejection was not associated with viral infection but recovery of lung function was significantly slower when both infection and rejection were present [46]. Finally, Vu et al. performed an analysis of 34 pooled studies and confirmed an association between respiratory viral infections and symptoms, but not BOS [47].

Thus, there are some studies that provide evidence in favor of an association of CARV infection with BOS, but this was not confirmed in an analysis of pooled studies. Further multicenter studies would be of interest, involving uniform monitoring assays and protocols. The potential effects of antiviral therapy on preservation of allograft function are discussed in the section on treatment below.

Bacterial Infections

Whereas CMV infections have decreased in frequency, bacterial infections remain a common post-transplant complication [48]. In a study by Valentine et al., over 80 % of lung pathogens in the current era were bacterial, and more than half of these were *Pseudomonas aeruginosa* [19]. While bacterial infections in general have been identified as a risk factor for BOS [6, 49], *Pseudomonas* has been of particular interest [50]. It has been noted since the early days of lung transplantation that infection and colonization with *Pseudomonas* spp., including multidrug-resistant strains, is extremely common in lung recipients [51, 52]. Whereas many CF and bronchiectasis patients are colonized with *Pseudomonas* pre-transplant, Pseudomonas may also be acquired de novo post-transplant in any recipient, and is associated with an intense inflammatory response [52]. In one study by Botha et al., de novo acquisition of *Pseudomonas* was associated with increased risk of BOS within 2 years (23.4 % vs. 7.7 %, $p=0.006$) [53]. *Pseudomonas* colonization preceded BOS by a median of 204 days [53]. Gottlieb et al. reported that *Pseudomonas* colonization post-transplant in CF patients was a risk for BOS, whereas eradication of previous *Pseudomonas* colonization was associated with less frequent BOS ($p=0.006$) [54]. In addition, a variety of both enteric (*E. coli, Klebsiella, Enterobacter, Proteus*, etc.) and non-enteric gram-negative organisms (*Stenotrophomonas, Alcaligenes, Acinetobacter*, etc.) may be isolated from post-transplant BAL cultures, particularly in those patients with airway complications and/or protracted post-transplant recovery and ventilator courses. *Burkholderia cepacia* complex has been associated with high mortality post-transplant (particularly *B. cenocepacia* or genomovar III), although much of that mortality is due to direct infectious syndromes rather than long-term effects of colonization.

Gram-positive organisms, including methicillin-resistant *Staphylococcus aureus* (MRSA), have been increasingly identified as significant causes of post-transplant morbidity [55]. Gupta et al. reported that gram-positive infections occurred in 40 % of lung recipients, mostly *S. aureus* (of which 42 % was MRSA) [55]. MRSA can be acquired from the donor, can be related to pre-transplant colonization in the recipient, or can be acquired de novo post-transplant from sources other than the donor. In the study by Gupta et al., gram-positive lung infections were associated with risk of development of BOS and also with surgical airway complications [55]. Valentine et al. identified both gram-positive and gram-negative infections as associated with increased risk for BOS [17].

Mycobacterial infections, although less common than conventional bacterial infections, are also associated with morbidity and, in some settings, decreased survival after lung transplantation [56]. In the case of *Mycobacterium tuberculosis*, this morbidity is largely related to direct infectious syndromes, [57] whereas colonization with non-tuberculous mycobacteria can be associated with a spectrum of clinical manifestations, including asymptomatic colonization. Whether non-tuberculous mycobacterial infection predisposes to BOS is as yet uncertain, but in a study by Huang et al., non-tuberculous mycobacterial infection was associated with increased mortality independent of BOS [56].

Possible mechanisms of the allograft effects of bacterial colonization might include increased neutrophilic and other inflammatory responses [52] that lead to release of cytokines and chemokines; up-regulation of endothelin-1 [58]; or predisposition to other infections, including viral and fungal infections that might additionally increase risk for BOS. Borthwick et al. reported that *Pseudomonas* can serve as a cofactor in TGF-beta-1-driven epithelial-to-mesenchymal transition, which has been implicated in the pathogenesis of BOS [59]. The intriguing possible relationship of *Pseudomonas* colonization to gastroesophageal reflux has been explored by Vos et al. [60].

More subtle and difficult-to-culture organisms such as *Chlamydophila pneumoniae* (Chlamydia) have recently attracted interest [61], particularly as such organisms may be responsive to azithromycin. *Chlamydophila pneumoniae* is best detected by PCR from BAL fluid rather than culture. Such organisms have been studied in a variety of non-transplant settings because of their affinity for endothelium. Glanville et al. reported that *C. pneumoniae* was detected in BAL samples in 25 % of lung recipients and was associated with higher risk for early mortality, acute rejection, and BOS [61]. In another study by Kotsimbos et al. [62], Chlamydia D+/R− status was associated with a BOS incidence of 75 %; whereas low anti-*C. pneumoniae* titers in the donor and high anti-*C. pneumoniae* titers in the recipient were found to be predictive of freedom from BOS, suggesting that stronger antecedent recipient immunity to *C. pneumoniae* might be helpful in ameliorating effects of donor-derived *C. pneumoniae* in the allograft [62].

Husain et al. investigated the novel chlamydia-like organism, *Simkania negevensis*, in lung recipients [63]. This study found that detection of *S. negevensis* was frequent (40/41 recipients) and was associated with concomitant acute rejection [63]. The effects of *S. negevensis* on chronic allograft dysfunction are not yet known; however, because acute rejection is a risk factor for BOS, an association with acute rejection (if confirmed) might also mean an association with longer-term BOS risk.

Interestingly, *Clostridium difficile* colitis, although not an infection that affects the lung directly, was associated with increased risk of BOS in a study by Gunderson et al., particularly when *C. difficile* occurred in the early post-transplant period [64]. Whether early *C. difficile* is a marker for other complications that predispose to BOS or whether the inflammatory milieu induced by *C. difficile* infection itself is responsible needs further study.

Fungal Infections

Fungal infections, particularly aspergillosis, have long been identified as a source of morbidity and mortality in the lung transplant recipient [19, 49, 65]. Risk factors are described in the section on prevention below. Traditionally, fungal processes have been defined as invasive fungal infection or as colonization. The effects of fungal infection on the allograft have been less frequently studied than those of viral or bacterial infections. Valentine et al. identified fungal pneumonia as a significant risk factor for subsequent BOS [17]. Recent intriguing evidence from Weigt et al. has demonstrated that aspergillus colonization, even in the absence of invasive infection, is a risk factor for BOS and BOS-related mortality, independent of acute rejection [66]. Aspergillus colonization preceded BOS by a median of 261 days in this study [66]. However, neither fungal colonization nor pulmonary fungal infection was identified as a risk factor for chronic allograft dysfunction in a study of 55 pediatric lung recipients by Liu et al. [67], although pulmonary fungal infection was associated with greater 12-month mortality in a large multicenter pediatric cohort [68]. It would be of interest to determine whether there are differential effects of different antifungal prophylaxis strategies. The changing landscape of antifungal prophylaxis, particularly the shift towards voriconazole and away from itraconazole, is of interest [69, 70]. Although antifungal prophylaxis has traditionally been undertaken with a goal of preventing invasive fungal infection, perhaps the results of Weigt et al. (described above) will prompt reassessment of current antifungal prophylaxis strategies with an eye to decreasing colonization as well. In particular, it could be asked if the addition or substitution of inhaled amphotericin or liposomal amphotericin preparations [71, 72] might lead to decreased airway fungal colonization compared with systemic-only antifungal strategies, and long-term benefits to the allograft should be further explored.

Prevention of Infection-Associated BOS and Allograft Dysfunction

The following section assumes that infections do predispose to BOS, although in the case of each group of organisms, the evidence, including dissenting evidence, is reviewed above. If CMV does pose a significant risk for BOS development, an important question is whether the key risk factor is symptomatic CMV disease, subclinical viremia, or subclinical replication in the lung compartment [14]. As discussed above and summarized in Table 11.1, some but not all studies have suggested a beneficial effect of CMV prophylaxis on decreasing BOS risk. A variety of prevention strategies are effective in preventing symptomatic CMV disease, but prevention of subclinical viremia likely requires longer prophylaxis or preemptive therapy (or both), since asymptomatic viremia might otherwise occur without detection. As mentioned above, Valentine et al. called for indefinite prophylaxis, related to the finding that the group that stopped prophylaxis had high rates of CMV pneumonitis and progression to BOS within 1 year [18]. From the randomized, controlled trial by Palmer et al., it is known that CMV outcomes are significantly decreased with a 12-month course of valganciclovir prophylaxis compared with a 3-month course, but whether that benefit translates into improved long-term results for the allograft needs to be investigated further.

CMV prophylaxis might also work by decreasing replication of other herpesviruses such as EBV and HHV-6, but since the impact of those viruses on the allograft is controversial (see above), it cannot yet be concluded that this mechanism is contributory.

Other methods of CMV prevention include avoidance of CMV exposures for D–/R– patients (including use of CMV-free blood if any blood transfusions are needed), and the development of CMV vaccines in the future. If the highest-risk group (D+/R–) can be transformed into D+/R+ by pre-transplant vaccination, the risk of CMV might be ameliorated significantly in this group. Recent studies of a glycoprotein B CMV vaccine are promising in pre-transplant patients [73].

Regarding community respiratory viruses, the most important methods of prevention are immunization (for influenza) and rigorous infection control. Influenza immunization has been shown to be safe in transplant recipients, as larger studies have not corroborated any clinically significant increase in rejection or allograft dysfunction in solid organ transplant recipients [74]. The efficacy of influenza vaccine may be suboptimal, particularly in those recipients with recent transplants or intensified immunosuppression, but per current guidelines [74], partial protection is preferable to no immunization. It is also extremely important that family members and health care workers be immunized, to decrease risk of transmission of influenza to the patient. If the transplant recipient does acquire influenza despite these measures, early detection and antiviral treatment can reduce morbidity, including the need for ICU admission [75]. It is important to get this message out to primary care providers, urgent care, and emergency room clinicians, who may (rather than the transplant team) be the first to assess a transplant recipient with a viral illness.

Each year the types of circulating influenza strains and the patterns of antiviral resistance are different; clinicians should follow yearly updates from their national health organizations with each year's recommendations for antiviral therapy.

For any respiratory virus, stringent hospital infection control is essential. Outbreaks of respiratory infection, including RSV and parainfluenza, can be devastating to transplant wards. Early viral detection with nasopharyngeal swabs (even in minimally symptomatic patients) is important in limiting in-hospital transmission. Adherence to recommended precautions and to hand hygiene is essential, and programs that increase compliance with these measures will have a beneficial effect for all patients, including vulnerable transplant recipients. Health care workers with respiratory viral illnesses should ideally not have contact with transplant recipients at all, but if such contact is unavoidable, all possible measures should be taken to prevent transmission (including mask, gloves, limiting time in room, etc.). Transplant centers should develop policies that do not penalize employees for absenteeism due to illness. Educational efforts should emphasize that mild viral symptoms in a health care worker (that a worker might tend to ignore or to "work through") can translate into acute respiratory failure and/or long-term loss of allograft function in a lung recipient. Educating patients and family members regarding avoidance of out-of-hospital exposures, as well as the importance of early reporting of symptoms, are also important measures.

The role of antiviral therapy for non-influenza respiratory viruses is still evolving. Many centers use ribavirin preparations for treatment of symptomatic RSV infection [76] and sometimes parainfluenza virus [77] and metapneumovirus infection as well [78], although further data would be welcome. Most literature to date has reported on aerosolized ribavirin, but inconvenience and potential toxicity to health care workers has led to the study of other ribavirin preparations. Glanville et al. described the use of intravenous ribavirin plus oral corticosteroids in 18 lung recipients, in whom an initial fall in FEV1 was followed by recovery at 3 months, and only one patient developed subsequent BOS [79]. Intravenous ribavirin is not currently available in the United States. Similarly, promising preliminary results from a study by Pelaez et al. demonstrated preservation of allograft function in a group of lung recipients with RSV who received a regimen of 10 days of oral ribavirin in combination with high-dose steroids for the first 3 days [80]. In addition, Fuehner et al. reported on a nonrandomized study of 38 patients who received oral ribavirin compared with 29 who did not, during paramyxovirus infection. Whereas both groups had declines in FEV1, a greater percentage of ribavirin-treated patients recovered lung function within 1 month (84 % vs. 59 %, $p=0.02$). New-onset BOS within 6 months occurred in 5 % of the ribavirin vs. 24 % of the non-ribavirin-treated patients [77]. Novel therapies are also under development. A recent study of a small interfering RNA (siRNA) treatment for RSV infection demonstrated a decrease in new-onset BOS and progression to BOS by day 90 in the treatment group ($n=16$), as compared with others ($n=8$) who received standard care for RSV infection (6.3 % vs. 50 %, $p=0.027$) [81]. The likely availability of other antiviral therapies in the future would make larger, multicenter comparative effectiveness trials that include long enough follow up to detect effects on time to BOS desirable.

Prevention of bacterial infections is also a matter of infection control and hand hygiene. Immunizations for *Pneumococcus* and for pertussis (in the form of Tdap vaccine for adults) should be kept up to date and ideally should be updated during the pre-transplant evaluation phase [82]. Given the results of Gottlieb et al. regarding decreased risk in patients in whom prior *Pseudomonas* colonization was eradicated, strategies that enhance eradication are likely to produce long-term benefit for the allograft [54]. Such strategies might include individualized peri-transplant combinations of systemic and inhaled antibiotics, as well as pre-transplant attention to potential reservoirs such as the sinuses. If effective vaccines for prevention of *Pseudomonas* infection and colonization become available in the future, that would be an important intervention. The effects of airway interventions such as stents should also be considered, as foreign bodies in the airway can serve as a nidus for bacterial colonization, albeit an important intervention in prevention of post-obstructive pneumonia and allograft dysfunction.

The demonstrated effects of azithromycin in protecting the allograft from BOS [83, 84] do bring up the question as to whether prevention of infection, including subclinical infection with organisms that lack a cell wall (e.g., *Chlamydophila, Mycoplasma, Simkania*) might be one of the mechanisms that contribute to such protection. More work in this area would be of interest. The risk of emergence of azithromycin resistance in these organisms is also worthy of future study.

Prevention of fungal infections is informed by an understanding of risk factors. Exposures related to the external environment should be minimized, including protection from the effects of hospital construction. Transplant recipients should be educated about the risks of marijuana smoking, gardening, farming, construction work, composting, cave exploration, and other activities that they consider undertaking as they recover from the initial post-transplant phase and begin to resume a more normal life [85]. Antifungal prophylaxis is now utilized by many lung transplant programs, most frequently using azole antifungal agents, inhaled amphotericin preparations, combinations of the above, and sometimes other agents [69, 70]. Regarding the type of azole used, there has been a shift from itraconazole towards voriconazole over time [70]. However, even in the presence of antifungal prophylaxis, breakthrough fungal infections may occur. In fact, antifungal prophylaxis may select out for certain types of fungal organisms (e.g., zygomycetes in the setting of voriconazole prophylaxis.) Protocol BALs can help with detection of fungal colonization in the asymptomatic patient and might prompt either a change of prophylaxis or increased clinical and radiographic monitoring or both. The occurrence of fungal infections late in the post-transplant course (after discontinuation of prophylaxis) might be related to late rejection, environmental exposures, or a reservoir in the native lung for single-lung transplant recipients. An enhanced clinical awareness in patients falling into any of the above groups is helpful.

For prevention of *Pneumocystis jiroveci* pneumonia (PJP, formerly *P. carinii*), center-specific practices have varied, but some clinicians (e.g., Gordon et al.) have recommended to continue PJP prophylaxis long-term (lifelong) in lung recipients, as they, uniquely among solid organ recipients, continue to have significant PJP risk beyond the first year [86]. Trimethoprim-sulfamethoxazole is the most commonly used agent and has the added benefit of preventing several other infections (toxoplasmosis, listeriosis). For sulfa-allergic or intolerant patients, monthly aerosolized pentamidine, oral dapsone, or oral atovaquone are alternative prophylaxis options.

Whereas many previous studies have focused on individual infectious agents, the overall microbial ecology (the microbiome) of the allograft may be a more fruitful area of study [87]. Immune responses to different infectious agents may be intertwined, and ideally in the future, interventions should be assessed in terms of alteration of the microbiome rather than just impact on one particular organism.

Conclusion

A growing body of literature has linked the risk for new-onset or progressive BOS to a variety of infections, including CMV, other herpesviruses, CARVs, and bacterial and fungal infections. Although results from different centers have varied, it appears that infections play a role in BOS development in at least some settings, and mechanistic considerations (e.g., chemokines) and animal models support this hypothesis. Recent studies support longer durations of CMV prophylaxis. The role of colonization as opposed to active infection (in the case of bacteria or fungi) and the role of subclinical viral infection in the allograft are areas of considerable interest. To the extent that infections trigger BOS, development of newer strategies (including vaccines and immunotherapies) that enable early detection and intervention will be important in providing long-term preservation of allograft function.

References

1. Soghikian MV, Valentine VG, Berry GJ, Patel HR, Robbins RC, Theodore J. Impact of ganciclovir prophylaxis on heart-lung and lung transplant recipients. J Heart Lung Transplant. 1996;15(9):881–7.
2. Zeevi A, Morel P, Spichty K, Dauber J, Yousem S, Williams P, et al. Clinical significance of CMV-specific T helper responses in lung transplant recipients. Hum Immunol. 1998;59(12):768–75.
3. Bando K, Paradis IL, Komatsu K, Konishi H, Matsushima M, Keena RJ, et al. Analysis of time-dependent risks for infection, rejection, and death after pulmonary transplantation. J Thorac Cardiovasc Surg. 1995;109(1):49–57; discussion 57–9.
4. Kroshus TJ, Kshettry VR, Savik K, John R, Hertz MI, Bolman 3rd RM. Risk factors for the development of bronchiolitis obliterans syndrome after lung transplantation. J Thorac Cardiovasc Surg. 1997;114(2):195–202.
5. Cerrina J, Le Roy LF, Herve PH, Parquin F, Harari S, Chapelier A, et al. Role of CMV pneumonia in the development of obliterative bronchiolitis in heart-lung and double-lung transplant recipients. Transpl Int. 1992;5 Suppl 1:S242–5.
6. Heng D, Sharples LD, McNeil K, Stewart S, Wreghitt T, Wallwork J. Bronchiolitis obliterans syndrome: incidence, natural history, prognosis, and risk factors. J Heart Lung Transplant. 1998;17(12):1255–63.

7. Keenan RJ, Lega ME, Dummer JS, Paradis IL, Dauber JH, Rabinowich H, et al. Cytomegalovirus serologic status and postoperative infection correlated with risk of developing chronic rejection after pulmonary transplantation. Transplantation. 1991;51(2):433–8.
8. Tikkanen JM, Kallio EA, Bruggeman CA, Koskinen PK, Lemstrom KB. Prevention of cytomegalovirus infection-enhanced experimental obliterative bronchiolitis by antiviral prophylaxis or immunosuppression in rat tracheal allografts. Am J Respir Crit Care Med. 2001;164(4):672–9.
9. Wiebe K, Fraund S, Steinmuller C, Steinhoff G. Rat cytomegalovirus and Listeria monocytogenes infection enhance chronic rejection after allogenic rat lung transplantation. Transpl Int. 2005;18(10):1166–74.
10. Weseslindtner L, Nachbagauer R, Kundi M, Jaksch P, Kerschner H, Simon B, et al. Human cytomegalovirus infection in lung transplant recipients triggers a CXCL-10 response. Am J Transplant. 2011;11(3):542–52.
11. Uhlin M, Mattsson J, Maeurer M. Update on viral infections in lung transplantation. Curr Opin Pulm Med. 2012;18(3):264–70.
12. Weigt SS, Elashoff RM, Keane MP, Strieter RM, Gomperts BN, Xue YY, et al. Altered levels of CC chemokines during pulmonary CMV predict BOS and mortality post-lung transplantation. Am J Transplant. 2008;8(7):1512–22.
13. Mitsani D, Nguyen MH, Girnita DM, Spichty K, Kwak EJ, Silveira FP, et al. A polymorphism linked to elevated levels of interferon-gamma is associated with an increased risk of cytomegalovirus disease among Caucasian lung transplant recipients at a single center. J Heart Lung Transplant. 2011;30(5):523–9.
14. Bauer CC, Jaksch P, Aberle SW, Haber H, Lang G, Klepetko W, et al. Relationship between cytomegalovirus DNA load in epithelial lining fluid and plasma of lung transplant recipients and analysis of coinfection with Epstein-Barr virus and human herpesvirus 6 in the lung compartment. J Clin Microbiol. 2007;45(2):324–8.
15. Tamm M, Aboyoun CL, Chhajed PN, Rainer S, Malouf MA, Glanville AR. Treated cytomegalovirus pneumonia is not associated with bronchiolitis obliterans syndrome. Am J Respir Crit Care Med. 2004;170(10):1120–3.
16. Snyder LD, Finlen-Copeland CA, Turbyfill WJ, Howell D, Willner DA, Palmer SM. Cytomegalovirus pneumonitis is a risk for bronchiolitis obliterans syndrome in lung transplantation. Am J Respir Crit Care Med. 2010;181(12):1391–6.
17. Valentine VG, Gupta MR, Walker Jr JE, Seoane L, Bonvillain RW, Lombard GA, et al. Effect of etiology and timing of respiratory tract infections on development of bronchiolitis obliterans syndrome. J Heart Lung Transplant. 2009;28(2):163–9.
18. Valentine VG, Weill D, Gupta MR, Raper B, Laplace SG, Lombard GA, et al. Ganciclovir for cytomegalovirus: a call for indefinite prophylaxis in lung transplantation. J Heart Lung Transplant. 2008;27(8):875–81.
19. Valentine VG, Bonvillain RW, Gupta MR, Lombard GA, LaPlace SG, Dhillon GS, et al. Infections in lung allograft recipients: ganciclovir era. J Heart Lung Transplant. 2008;27(5):528–35.
20. Palmer SM, Limaye AP, Banks M, Gallup D, Chapman J, Lawrence EC, et al. Extended valganciclovir prophylaxis to prevent cytomegalovirus after lung transplantation: a randomized, controlled trial. Ann Intern Med. 2010;152(12):761–9.
21. Finlen Copeland CA, Davis WA, Snyder LD, Banks M, Avery R, Davis RD, et al. Long-term efficacy and safety of 12 months of valganciclovir prophylaxis compared with 3 months after lung transplantation: a single-center, long-term follow-up analysis from a randomized, controlled cytomegalovirus prevention trial. J Heart Lung Transplant. 2011;30(9):990–6.
22. Humar A, Michaels M. American Society of Transplantation recommendations for screening, monitoring and reporting of infectious complications in immunosuppression trials in recipients of organ transplantation. Am J Transplant. 2006;6(2):262–74.
23. Humar A, Snydman D. Cytomegalovirus in solid organ transplant recipients. Am J Transplant. 2009;9 Suppl 4:S78–86.

24. Kotton CN, Kumar D, Caliendo AM, Asberg A, Chou S, Snydman DR, et al. International consensus guidelines on the management of cytomegalovirus in solid organ transplantation. Transplantation. 2010;89(7):779–95.
25. Westall GP, Michaelides A, Williams TJ, Snell GI, Kotsimbos TC. Human cytomegalovirus load in plasma and bronchoalveolar lavage fluid: a longitudinal study of lung transplant recipients. J Infect Dis. 2004;190(6):1076–83.
26. Tu W, Potena L, Stepick-Biek P, Liu L, Dionis KY, Luikart H, et al. T-cell immunity to subclinical cytomegalovirus infection reduces cardiac allograft disease. Circulation. 2006;114(15):1608–15.
27. Potena L, Holweg CT, Vana ML, Bashyam L, Rajamani J, McCormick AL, et al. Frequent occult infection with cytomegalovirus in cardiac transplant recipients despite antiviral prophylaxis. J Clin Microbiol. 2007;45(6):1804–10.
28. Gorzer I, Kerschner H, Jaksch P, Bauer C, Seebacher G, Klepetko W, et al. Virus load dynamics of individual CMV-genotypes in lung transplant recipients with mixed-genotype infections. J Med Virol. 2008;80(8):1405–14.
29. Ljungman P, Singh N. Human herpesvirus-6 infection in solid organ and stem cell transplant recipients. J Clin Virol. 2006;37 Suppl 1:S87–91.
30. Cone RW, Hackman RC, Huang ML, Bowden RA, Meyers JD, Metcalf M, et al. Human herpesvirus 6 in lung tissue from patients with pneumonitis after bone marrow transplantation. N Engl J Med. 1993;329(3):156–61.
31. Neurohr C, Huppmann P, Leuchte H, Schwaiblmair M, Bittmann I, Jaeger G, et al. Human herpesvirus 6 in bronchalveolar lavage fluid after lung transplantation: a risk factor for bronchiolitis obliterans syndrome? Am J Transplant. 2005;5(12):2982–91.
32. Ross DJ, Chan RC, Kubak B, Ardehali A, Laks H, Nichols WS. Bronchiolitis obliterans with organizing pneumonia: possible association with human herpes virus-7 infection after lung transplantation. J Heart Lung Transplant. 2001;20(2):171.
33. Engelmann I, Welte T, Fuhner T, Simon AR, Mattner F, Hoy L, et al. Detection of Epstein-Barr virus DNA in peripheral blood is associated with the development of bronchiolitis obliterans syndrome after lung transplantation. J Clin Virol. 2009;45(1):47–53.
34. Krams SM, Martinez OM. Epstein-Barr virus, rapamycin, and host immune responses. Curr Opin Organ Transplant. 2008;13(6):563–8.
35. Manuel O, Kumar D, Moussa G, Chen MH, Pilewski J, McCurry KR, et al. Lack of association between beta-herpesvirus infection and bronchiolitis obliterans syndrome in lung transplant recipients in the era of antiviral prophylaxis. Transplantation. 2009;87(5):719–25.
36. Kaiser L, Aubert JD, Pache JC, Deffernez C, Rochat T, Garbino J, et al. Chronic rhinoviral infection in lung transplant recipients. Am J Respir Crit Care Med. 2006;174(12):1392–9.
37. Weigt SS, Derhovanessian A, Liao E, Hu S, Gregson AL, Kubak BM, et al. CXCR3 chemokine ligands during respiratory viral infections predict lung allograft dysfunction. Am J Transplant. 2012;12(2):477–84.
38. Kumar D, Erdman D, Keshavjee S, Peret T, Tellier R, Hadjiliadis D, et al. Clinical impact of community-acquired respiratory viruses on bronchiolitis obliterans after lung transplant. Am J Transplant. 2005;5(8):2031–6.
39. Kumar D, Husain S, Chen MH, Moussa G, Himsworth D, Manuel O, et al. A prospective molecular surveillance study evaluating the clinical impact of community-acquired respiratory viruses in lung transplant recipients. Transplantation. 2010;89(8):1028–33.
40. Gottlieb J, Schulz TF, Welte T, Fuehner T, Dierich M, Simon AR, et al. Community-acquired respiratory viral infections in lung transplant recipients: a single season cohort study. Transplantation. 2009;87(10):1530–7.
41. Khalifah AP, Hachem RR, Chakinala MM, Schechtman KB, Patterson GA, Schuster DP, et al. Respiratory viral infections are a distinct risk for bronchiolitis obliterans syndrome and death. Am J Respir Crit Care Med. 2004;170(2):181–7.
42. Vilchez RA, Dauber J, McCurry K, Iacono A, Kusne S. Parainfluenza virus infection in adult lung transplant recipients: an emergent clinical syndrome with implications on allograft function. Am J Transplant. 2003;3(2):116–20.

43. Liu M, Mallory GB, Schecter MG, Worley S, Arrigain S, Robertson J, et al. Long-term impact of respiratory viral infection after pediatric lung transplantation. Pediatr Transplant. 2010;14(3):431–6.
44. Liu M, Worley S, Arrigain S, Aurora P, Ballmann M, Boyer D, et al. Respiratory viral infections within one year after pediatric lung transplant. Transpl Infect Dis. 2009;11(4):304–12.
45. Milstone AP, Brumble LM, Barnes J, Estes W, Loyd JE, Pierson 3rd RN, et al. A single-season prospective study of respiratory viral infections in lung transplant recipients. Eur Respir J. 2006;28(1):131–7.
46. Soccal PM, Aubert JD, Bridevaux PO, Garbino J, Thomas Y, Rochat T, et al. Upper and lower respiratory tract viral infections and acute graft rejection in lung transplant recipients. Clin Infect Dis. 2010;51(2):163–70.
47. Vu DL, Bridevaux PO, Aubert JD, Soccal PM, Kaiser L. Respiratory viruses in lung transplant recipients: a critical review and pooled analysis of clinical studies. Am J Transplant. 2011;11(5):1071–8.
48. Speich R, van der Bij W. Epidemiology and management of infections after lung transplantation. Clin Infect Dis. 2001;33 Suppl 1:S58–65.
49. Girgis RE, Tu I, Berry GJ, Reichenspurner H, Valentine VG, Conte JV, et al. Risk factors for the development of obliterative bronchiolitis after lung transplantation. J Heart Lung Transplant. 1996;15(12):1200–8.
50. Vos R, Vanaudenaerde BM, De Vleeschauwer SI, Van Raemdonck DE, Dupont LJ, Verleden GM. De novo or persistent pseudomonal airway colonization after lung transplantation: importance for bronchiolitis obliterans syndrome? Transplantation 2008;86(4):624–5; author reply 635–6.
51. Flume PA, Egan TM, Paradowski LJ, Detterbeck FC, Thompson JT, Yankaskas JR. Infectious complications of lung transplantation. Impact of cystic fibrosis. Am J Respir Crit Care Med. 1994;149(6):1601–7.
52. Nunley DR, Grgurich W, Iacono AT, Yousem S, Ohori NP, Keenan RJ, et al. Allograft colonization and infections with pseudomonas in cystic fibrosis lung transplant recipients. Chest. 1998;113(5):1235–43.
53. Botha P, Archer L, Anderson RL, Lordan J, Dark JH, Corris PA, et al. Pseudomonas aeruginosa colonization of the allograft after lung transplantation and the risk of bronchiolitis obliterans syndrome. Transplantation. 2008;85(5):771–4.
54. Gottlieb J, Mattner F, Weissbrodt H, Dierich M, Fuehner T, Strueber M, et al. Impact of graft colonization with gram-negative bacteria after lung transplantation on the development of bronchiolitis obliterans syndrome in recipients with cystic fibrosis. Respir Med. 2009;103(5):743–9.
55. Gupta MR, Valentine VG, Walker Jr JE, Lombard GA, LaPlace SG, Seoane L, et al. Clinical spectrum of gram-positive infections in lung transplantation. Transpl Infect Dis. 2009;11(5):424–31.
56. Huang HC, Weigt SS, Derhovanessian A, Palchevskiy V, Ardehali A, Saggar R, et al. Non-tuberculous mycobacterium infection after lung transplantation is associated with increased mortality. J Heart Lung Transplant. 2011;30(7):790–8.
57. Singh N, Paterson DL. Mycobacterium tuberculosis infection in solid-organ transplant recipients: impact and implications for management. Clin Infect Dis. 1998;27(5):1266–77.
58. Charpin JM, Stern M, Lebrun G, Aubin P, Grenet D, Israel-Biet D. Increased endothelin-1 associated with bacterial infection in lung transplant recipients. Transplantation. 2001;71(12):1840–7.
59. Borthwick LA, Sunny SS, Oliphant V, Perry J, Brodlie M, Johnson GE, et al. Pseudomonas aeruginosa accentuates epithelial-to-mesenchymal transition in the airway. Eur Respir J. 2011;37(5):1237–47.
60. Vos R, Blondeau K, Vanaudenaerde BM, Mertens V, Van Raemdonck DE, Sifrim D, et al. Airway colonization and gastric aspiration after lung transplantation: do birds of a feather flock together? J Heart Lung Transplant. 2008;27(8):843–9.

61. Glanville AR, Gencay M, Tamm M, Chhajed P, Plit M, Hopkins P, et al. Chlamydia pneumoniae infection after lung transplantation. J Heart Lung Transplant. 2005;24(2):131–6.
62. Kotsimbos TC, Snell GI, Levvey B, Spelman DW, Fuller AJ, Wesselingh SL, et al. Chlamydia pneumoniae serology in donors and recipients and the risk of bronchiolitis obliterans syndrome after lung transplantation. Transplantation. 2005;79(3):269–75.
63. Husain S, Kahane S, Friedman MG, Paterson DL, Studer S, McCurry KR, et al. Simkania negevensis in bronchoalveolar lavage of lung transplant recipients: a possible association with acute rejection. Transplantation. 2007;83(2):138–43.
64. Gunderson CC, Gupta MR, Lopez F, Lombard GA, LaPlace SG, Taylor DE, et al. Clostridium difficile colitis in lung transplantation. Transpl Infect Dis. 2008;10(4):245–51.
65. Nunley DR, Ohori P, Grgurich WF, Iacono AT, Williams PA, Keenan RJ, et al. Pulmonary aspergillosis in cystic fibrosis lung transplant recipients. Chest. 1998;114(5):1321–9.
66. Weigt SS, Elashoff RM, Huang C, Ardehali A, Gregson AL, Kubak B, et al. Aspergillus colonization of the lung allograft is a risk factor for bronchiolitis obliterans syndrome. Am J Transplant. 2009;9(8):1903–11.
67. Liu M, Worley S, Mallory Jr GB, Arrigain S, Robertson J, Schecter MG, et al. Fungal infections in pediatric lung transplant recipients: colonization and invasive disease. J Heart Lung Transplant. 2009;28(11):1226–30.
68. Danziger-Isakov LA, Worley S, Arrigain S, Aurora P, Ballmann M, Boyer D, et al. Increased mortality after pulmonary fungal infection within the first year after pediatric lung transplantation. J Heart Lung Transplant. 2008;27(6):655–61.
69. Husain S, Zaldonis D, Kusne S, Kwak EJ, Paterson DL, McCurry KR. Variation in antifungal prophylaxis strategies in lung transplantation. Transpl Infect Dis. 2006;8(4):213–8.
70. Neoh CF, Snell GI, Kotsimbos T, Levvey B, Morrissey CO, Slavin MA, et al. Antifungal prophylaxis in lung transplantation—a world-wide survey. Am J Transplant. 2011;11(2):361–6.
71. Drew RH, Dodds Ashley E, Benjamin Jr DK, Duane Davis R, Palmer SM, Perfect JR. Comparative safety of amphotericin B lipid complex and amphotericin B deoxycholate as aerosolized antifungal prophylaxis in lung-transplant recipients. Transplantation. 2004;77(2):232–7.
72. Husain S, Capitano B, Corcoran T, Studer SM, Crespo M, Johnson B, et al. Intrapulmonary disposition of amphotericin B after aerosolized delivery of amphotericin B lipid complex (Abelcet; ABLC) in lung transplant recipients. Transplantation. 2010;90(11):1215–9.
73. Griffiths PD, Stanton A, McCarrell E, Smith C, Osman M, Harber M, et al. Cytomegalovirus glycoprotein-B vaccine with MF59 adjuvant in transplant recipients: a phase 2 randomised placebo-controlled trial. Lancet. 2011;377(9773):1256–63.
74. Kumar D, Blumberg EA, Danziger-Isakov L, Kotton CN, Halasa NB, Ison MG, et al. Influenza vaccination in the organ transplant recipient: review and summary recommendations. Am J Transplant. 2011;11(10):2020–30.
75. Kumar D, Michaels MG, Morris MI, Green M, Avery RK, Liu C, et al. Outcomes from pandemic influenza A H1N1 infection in recipients of solid-organ transplants: a multicentre cohort study. Lancet Infect Dis. 2010;10(8):521–6.
76. Hynicka LM, Ensor CR. Prophylaxis and treatment of respiratory syncytial virus in adult immunocompromised patients. Ann Pharmacother. 2012;46(4):558–66.
77. Fuehner T, Dierich M, Duesberg C, DeWall C, Welte T, Haverich A, et al. Single-centre experience with oral ribavirin in lung transplant recipients with paramyxovirus infections. Antivir Ther. 2011;16(5):733–40.
78. Raza K, Ismailjee SB, Crespo M, Studer SM, Sanghavi S, Paterson DL, et al. Successful outcome of human metapneumovirus (hMPV) pneumonia in a lung transplant recipient treated with intravenous ribavirin. J Heart Lung Transplant. 2007;26(8):862–4.
79. Glanville AR, Scott AI, Morton JM, Aboyoun CL, Plit ML, Carter IW, et al. Intravenous ribavirin is a safe and cost-effective treatment for respiratory syncytial virus infection after lung transplantation. J Heart Lung Transplant. 2005;24(12):2114–9.

80. Pelaez A, Lyon GM, Force SD, Ramirez AM, Neujahr DC, Foster M, et al. Efficacy of oral ribavirin in lung transplant patients with respiratory syncytial virus lower respiratory tract infection. J Heart Lung Transplant. 2009;28(1):67–71.
81. Zamora MR, Budev M, Rolfe M, Gottlieb J, Humar A, Devincenzo J, et al. RNA interference therapy in lung transplant patients infected with respiratory syncytial virus. Am J Respir Crit Care Med. 2011;183(4):531–8.
82. Danzinger-Isakov L, Kumar D. Guidelines for vaccination of solid organ transplant candidates and recipients. Am J Transplant. 2009;9 Suppl 4:S258–62.
83. Jain R, Hachem RR, Morrell MR, Trulock EP, Chakinala MM, Yusen RD, et al. Azithromycin is associated with increased survival in lung transplant recipients with bronchiolitis obliterans syndrome. J Heart Lung Transplant. 2010;29(5):531–7.
84. Vos R, Vanaudenaerde BM, Verleden SE, Van Raemdonck DE, Dupont LJ, Verleden GM. Azithromycin in posttransplant bronchiolitis obliterans syndrome. Chest 2011;139(5):1246; author reply 1247.
85. Avery RK, Michaels MG. Strategies for safe living following solid organ transplantation. Am J Transplant. 2009;9 Suppl 4:S252–7.
86. Gordon SM, LaRosa SP, Kalmadi S, Arroliga AC, Avery RK, Truesdell-LaRosa L, et al. Should prophylaxis for Pneumocystis carinii pneumonia in solid organ transplant recipients ever be discontinued? Clin Infect Dis. 1999;28(2):240–6.
87. Nakajima T, Palchevsky V, Perkins DL, Belperio JA, Finn PW. Lung transplantation: infection, inflammation, and the microbiome. Semin Immunopathol. 2011;33(2):135–56.
88. Sharples LD, Tamm M, McNeil K, Higenbottam TW, Stewart S, Wallwork J. Development of bronchiolitis obliterans syndrome in recipients of heart-lung transplantation—early risk factors. Transplantation. 1996;61(4):560–6.
89. Gutierrez CA, Chaparro C, Krajden M, Winton T, Kesten S. Cytomegalovirus viremia in lung transplant recipients receiving ganciclovir and immune globulin. Chest. 1998;113(4): 924–32.
90. Smith MA, Sundaresan S, Mohanakumar T, Trulock EP, Lynch JP, Phelan DL, et al. Effect of development of antibodies to HLA and cytomegalovirus mismatch on lung transplantation survival and development of bronchiolitis obliterans syndrome. J Thorac Cardiovasc Surg. 1998;116(5):812–20.
91. Speich R, Thurnheer R, Gaspert A, Weder W, Boehler A. Efficacy and cost effectiveness of oral ganciclovir in the prevention of cytomegalovirus disease after lung transplantation. Transplantation. 1999;67(2):315–20.
92. Schulman LL, Weinberg AD, McGregor CC, Suciu-Foca NM, Itescu S. Influence of donor and recipient HLA locus mismatching on development of obliterative bronchiolitis after lung transplantation. Am J Respir Crit Care Med. 2001;163(2):437–42.
93. Fiser SM, Tribble CG, Long SM, Kaza AK, Kern JA, Jones DR, et al. Ischemia-reperfusion injury after lung transplantation increases risk of late bronchiolitis obliterans syndrome. Ann Thorac Surg 2002;73(4):1041–7; discussion 1047–8.
94. Jackson CH, Sharples LD, McNeil K, Stewart S, Wallwork J. Acute and chronic onset of bronchiolitis obliterans syndrome (BOS): are they different entities? J Heart Lung Transplant. 2002;21(6):658–66.
95. Luckraz H, Sharples L, McNeil K, Wreghitt T, Wallwork J. Cytomegalovirus antibody status of donor/recipient does not influence the incidence of bronchiolitis obliterans syndrome in lung transplantation. J Heart Lung Transplant. 2003;22(3):287–91.
96. Westall GP, Michaelides A, Williams TJ, Snell GI, Kotsimbos TC. Bronchiolitis obliterans syndrome and early human cytomegalovirus DNAaemia dynamics after lung transplantation. Transplantation. 2003;75(12):2064–8.
97. Hachem RR, Chakinala MM, Yusen RD, Lynch JP, Aloush AA, Patterson GA, et al. A comparison of basiliximab and anti-thymocyte globulin as induction agents after lung transplantation. J Heart Lung Transplant. 2005;24(9):1320–6.
98. Perreas KG, McNeil K, Charman S, Sharples LD, Wreghitt T, Wallwork J. Extended ganciclovir prophylaxis in lung transplantation. J Heart Lung Transplant. 2005;24(5):583–7.

99. Moffatt-Bruce SD, Karamichalis J, Robbins RC, Whyte RI, Theodore J, Reitz BA. Are heart-lung transplant recipients protected from developing bronchiolitis obliterans syndrome? Ann Thorac Surg 2006;81(1):286–91; discussion 291.
100. Ruttmann E, Geltner C, Bucher B, Ulmer H, Hofer D, Hangler HB, et al. Combined CMV prophylaxis improves outcome and reduces the risk for bronchiolitis obliterans syndrome (BOS) after lung transplantation. Transplantation. 2006;81(10):1415–20.
101. Chmiel C, Speich R, Hofer M, Michel D, Mertens T, Weder W, et al. Ganciclovir/valganciclovir prophylaxis decreases cytomegalovirus-related events and bronchiolitis obliterans syndrome after lung transplantation. Clin Infect Dis. 2008;46(6):831–9.
102. Kwakkel-van Erp JM, van de Graaf EA, Paantjens AW, van Ginkel WG, Schellekens J, van Kessel DA, et al. The killer immunoglobulin-like receptor (KIR) group A haplotype is associated with bronchiolitis obliterans syndrome after lung transplantation. J Heart Lung Transplant. 2008;27(9):995–1001.
103. Solidoro P, Libertucci D, Delsedime L, Ruffini E, Bosco M, Costa C, et al. Combined cytomegalovirus prophylaxis in lung transplantation: effects on acute rejection, lymphocytic bronchitis/bronchiolitis, and herpesvirus infections. Transplant Proc. 2008;40(6):2013–4.
104. Ranganathan K, Worley S, Michaels MG, Arrigan S, Aurora P, Ballmann M, et al. Cytomegalovirus immunoglobulin decreases the risk of cytomegalovirus infection but not disease after pediatric lung transplantation. J Heart Lung Transplant. 2009;28(10):1050–6.
105. Paraskeva M, Bailey M, Levvey BJ, Griffiths AP, Kotsimbos TC, Williams TP, et al. Cytomegalovirus replication within the lung allograft is associated with bronchiolitis obliterans syndrome. Am J Transplant. 2011;11(10):2190–6.
106. Kwakkel-van Erp JM, Paantjens AW, van Kessel DA, Grutters JC, van den Bosch JM, van de Graaf EA, et al. Mannose-binding lectin deficiency linked to cytomegalovirus (CMV) reactivation and survival in lung transplantation. Clin Exp Immunol. 2011;165(3):410–6.

Chapter 12
Gastroesophageal Reflux and Aspiration in Chronic Lung Allograft Dysfunction and Bronchiolitis Obliterans Syndrome: Detection and Treatment

Frank D'Ovidio and Beatrice Aramini

Abstract The role of gastroesophageal reflux (GER) as a risk factor in chronic lung allograft dysfunction (CLAD) and/or bronchiolitis obliterans syndrome (BOS) is strongly supported by the cumulative evidence collected to date. Proximal gastrointestinal tract motility studies and pH/impedance testing can be used to diagnose motility abnormalities and GER and to determine whether reflux is acid or nonacid. However, a true gold standard methodology for detecting penetrance of refluxed duodeno-gastric secretions into the lung is lacking, and a definitive marker of GER combined with microaspiration that identifies patients at significant risk for associated allograft injury and dysfunction needs to be determined. Prospective, multicenter, adequately powered clinical trials should be performed to better understand the role of GER in CLAD and to identify appropriate criteria for patient selection for possible surgical correction of GER.

Keywords Lung transplantation • Gastroesophageal reflux • Nonacid reflux • Chronic lung allograft dysfunction • Bronchiolitis obliterans syndrome

---

F. D'Ovidio, M.D., Ph.D. (✉)
Department of Surgery, New York-Presbyterian Hospital, Columbia University Medical Centre, 622 West 168th Street, PH14-108, New York, NY 10032, USA
e-mail: fd2133@columbia.edu

B. Aramini, M.D., Ph.D.
Dipartimento di Scienze Mediche e Chirurgiche Materno-Infantili e dell'Adulto, Azienda Ospedaliero-Universitaria Policlinico di Modena, Via del Pozzo 71, Modena 41100, Italy
e-mail: beatrice.aramini@gmail.com

K.C. Meyer and A.R. Glanville (eds.), *Bronchiolitis Obliterans Syndrome in Lung Transplantation*, Respiratory Medicine 8, DOI 10.1007/978-1-4614-7636-8_12,

Introduction

Over the last 3 decades, lung transplantation has become an accepted therapeutic option for patients with end-stage lung disease. A major limitation to long-term survival after lung transplantation is the development of chronic lung allograft dysfunction (CLAD), which is largely due to obliterative bronchiolitis (OB), a process of fibrous obliteration of the small airways that leads to progressive airflow obstruction. The clinical correlate of OB, bronchiolitis obliterans syndrome (BOS), is defined as persistent drop in FEV_1 to <80 % of a defined FEV_1 baseline of the mean of the two best FEV_1 values taken at least 3 weeks apart following transplantation. Alloimmune-mediated injury directed against endothelial and epithelial structures has been thought to be the underlying cause of OB. However, non-alloimmune inflammation including viral infections or ischemic injury also appears to play a role in its pathogenesis [1]. Retrograde aspiration secondary to gastroesophageal reflux (GER) has been implicated as a potential contributor to lung allograft dysfunction and, in particular, to development of CLAD and BOS [2–12]. Two forms of OB have been identified in the transplanted lung: (1) a relatively acellular, concentric fibrosing process limited to the terminal bronchioles, and (2) a focal cellular process extending into the distal alveolar spaces that is associated with aspirated material and foreign body-type giant cells [13]. The latter pathological finding is supportive of a role for GER in the development of BOS.

Pathophysiology of GER and Lung Disease

The potential of GER to cause pulmonary complications is underappreciated, although it has been recognized for a long time [14–20]. William Osler first described the relationship between asthma and GER in 1892 [14]. GER can affect the lungs via an esophago-tracheo-bronchial vagal reflex that can be associated with chronic cough and asthma, and GER with micro- or macro-aspiration has been linked to laryngitis, pneumonia, lung abscess, fibrosis, acute and chronic bronchitis and bronchiectasis.

The pathophysiology of gastro-esophageal reflux disease (GERD) is determined by a combination of factors that include decreased salivation, impaired esophageal clearance of refluxed secretions, impaired tissue resistance to potentially injurious components of refluxate, decreased resting tone of the lower esophageal sphincter (LES), the presence of hiatus hernia with a deranged anatomical relationship between the diaphragmatic hiatus and the LES, transient LES relaxations, and delayed gastric emptying. The role of the resting tone of the LES in GER is promoted by (1) increased gastric volume (e.g., large meals or increased gastric secretions) or (2) increased intra-abdominal pressure, which can be tonic (e.g., obesity, ascites, tight clothing, slouching posture) or phasic (e.g., contraction of the stomach, contraction of somatic muscles, cough, sneeze, wheeze, and strain). The LES tone is reduced or augmented by a number of substances, as given in Table 12.1.

Table 12.1 Modulators of lower esophageal sphincter (LES) tone

Agent	Decrease LES tone	Increase LES tone
Hormones	Secretin	Gastrin
	Cholecystokinin	Motilin
	Glucagon	Substance P
	Gastric inhibitory polypeptide (GIP)	
	Vasoactive intestinal peptide (VIP)	
	Progesterone	
Neuroactive agents	Alpha-adrenergic antagonists	Alpha-adrenergic agonists
	Beta-adrenergic agonists	Beta-adrenergic antagonists
	Cholinergic antagonists	Cholinergic agonists
	Serotonin	
Medications	Nitrates	Metoclopramide
	Calcium channel blockers	Domperidone
	Theophylline	Prostaglandin F
	Morphine	Cisapride
	Meperidine	
	Diazepam	
	Barbiturates	
Foods	Fat	Proteins
	Chocolate	
	Ethanol	
	Peppermint	

Transient LES relaxations are prolonged in time and not induced by swallowing, but LES relaxations can be triggered by distension of the gastric fundus and are considered the primary mechanism of non-pathologic reflux in healthy individuals as well as in patients who develop GERD. Delayed gastric emptying, which consequently causes distention of the gastric fundus, has been identified as a potent stimulus for transient LES relaxations [21, 22].

The anatomical relationship between the LES and the diaphragmatic hiatus is of importance to maintain the synergistic effect of the intrinsic LES tone and the extrinsic LES component that is provided by the diaphragmatic hiatus [23]. The importance of this anatomic relationship is well documented in the context of hiatus hernia complicated by esophageal shortening [24]. In severely advanced, end-stage lung disease, whether obstructive (as in advanced emphysema and cystic fibrosis, which are characterized by flattened or concave diaphragms) or restrictive (as in pulmonary fibrosis with severe cupping of the diaphragm) the anatomical relationship between the diaphragmatic hiatus (the extrinsic LES) and the intrinsic LES is likely stressed. The synergistic relationship between the intrinsic and extrinsic mechanisms is possibly less efficient in pulmonary fibrosis, which may especially be the case when intra-abdominal pressures change during the respiratory phases, cough, sneeze, wheeze, and strain.

The upper esophageal sphincter (UES) has no baseline tone during sleep and lacks the reflex capability to augment pressure in response to reflux; therefore, retrograde micro- or macro-aspirations are facilitated in the context of proximal GER [25]. Interestingly, impedance pH testing in normal individuals showed episodes of reflux that can be either distal or proximal, and the vast majority of such episodes are acid in the distal esophagus and nonacid when they reach the proximal esophagus [26].

GER has been shown to be prevalent in patients with a variety of lung diseases that include asthma, cystic fibrosis, idiopathic pulmonary fibrosis (IPF), and chronic obstructive pulmonary disease (COPD), and it has also been associated with the development of bronchiolitis obliterans organizing pneumonia (BOOP) a term that has been superseded by organizing pneumonia (OP) [27–37]. In a prospective study of consecutive lung transplant candidates, the LES tone was reduced in over 70 % of patient with end-stage COPD or advanced CF-associated lung disease, and in 54 % of patients with end-stage interstitial lung disease (ILD). Esophageal peristalsis may also be reduced, thus impairing esophageal clearance, as seen in 20–30 % of all end-stage lung disease patients [38]. Similar findings have been reported in other retrospective studies [39], and delayed gastric emptying has been observed in over 40 % of lung transplant candidates [38].

Proximal and distal esophagus 24-h pH testing in patients with end-stage lung disease who are candidates for lung transplantation showed that distal esophageal acid reflux (DeMeester score) was abnormal in 20 % of patients with COPD, 60 % with CF, and 32 % with ILD. Additionally, and likely more importantly, abnormal proximal esophageal acid exposure during the supine portion of the 24-h pH monitoring period was noted in 30 % of patients with COPD, 40 % with CF, and 16 % with IPF [38].

Lung defense mechanisms, including cough reflexes and mucociliary clearance, are markedly impaired in lung transplant recipients, and mucociliary clearance has been measured at less than 15 % of normal clearance time in transplanted lungs [2–7]. It is also conceivable that a prolonged contact time of aspirated gastric contents with respiratory mucosae may lead to substantially greater lung parenchymal injury. While GER may cause direct lung injury, it is also possible that it may alter innate immune responses and augment alloimmune responses by creating an up-regulated local inflammatory environment.

Diagnosis of GER in Lung Transplantation

Based on the assumption that acid reflux might be an important cause of CLAD and BOS, lung transplant patients commonly receive proton pump inhibitor (PPI) therapy. This pharmacologic therapy suppress gastric acid secretion and changes the pH of the refluxate from acid to nonacid, which may alleviate the classic GER-related symptoms from prolonged exposure of the esophageal mucosa to acid reflux, but it does not appear to reduce the quantity and or the frequency of reflux episodes. This has been demonstrated by studying GER using impedance pH monitoring with patients both on and off PPI medication [40]. Indeed, it is now well recognized that gastric secretions can still gain access to the esophagus and that such refluxate may not be acidic enough to be detected by pH monitoring such that symptoms classically associated with reflux are not evoked. Combined impedance and pH monitoring allow the detection of both acid and nonacid reflux and can determine the proximal extent to which refluxed secretions penetrate into the esophagus [41].

It should be noted that classic GER symptoms are absent in 57–94 % of patients with laryngeal manifestations of GER, in 43–73 % of patients with GER-related chronic cough, and in 40–60 % of patients with GER-related asthma [42, 43]. Moreover, a substantial number of lung transplant recipients have been found to be asymptomatic when abnormal GER is objectively documented [44–46].

Several methods have been studied that can document the relationship between lung disease and GER. These include scintigraphic monitoring, 24-h esophageal pH testing, assays for pepsin in saliva and sputum, and detection of lipid-laden macrophages, pepsin, or bile acids in bronchoalveolar lavage (BAL) [47–55]. Of note Hartwig et al. documented that chronic aspiration of acid gastric fluid accelerates the development of pulmonary allograft dysfunction in a rat model of lung transplantation [56]. The injurious agent may be gastric acid or other components of the gastroduodenal juices (bile, pepsin, trypsin, and others) rather than the acid reflux per se. In fact, chronic silent aspiration of acidic secretions alone may not be as injurious [57, 58] as aspiration of other components of the duodenal and gastric juice refluxate such as pepsin, trypsin, and bile acids. It should be noted that the bronchoalveolar environment has a pH that favors the activity of the duodeno-pancreatic agents rather than just the acidic gastric juice. Additionally, what has been considered standard pH testing does not test for the presence of alkaline ($pH > 7$) or weakly acid ($4 < pH < 7$) refluxate [59]. Multichannel intraluminal pH-impedance monitoring (in contrast to pH monitoring alone) allows monitoring of reflux episodes that are nonacid in quality, and such monitoring can discriminate between fluid and gas reflux regardless of pH, estimate the size of a refluxed secretion bolus and measure the proximal extent of GER into the esophagus while differentiating acid from nonacid reflux [41, 60–62]. This methodology is likely the best tool to investigate for significant GER in the context of lung transplantation. To date, however, the only apparatus with acceptable sensitivity for detecting the presence of duodeno-gastroesophageal refluxate remains the Bilitec 2000 (Medtronic); this spectrophotometric testing probe, which is calibrated for the detection of bilirubin, has not been widely adopted clinically due to its limited specificity, and it remains predominantly a clinical research tool [63].

GER and Chronic Lung Allograft Dysfunction

Retrospective studies with standard single-channel distal esophageal pH recordings have indicated an increased esophageal acid exposure in up to 70 % of lung transplant recipients [64, 65]. The prevalence and severity of GER following lung transplantation was found to be increased [64, 66], and the detection of GER is associated with worse pulmonary function test results. Therefore, it has been advocated that all lung transplant recipients should be screened for GER [64]. At the time of this study, 60 % of patients had BOS and 77 % of those patients who had developed BOS had abnormal esophageal pH testing as compared with 58 % of patients who had not developed BOS [64]. The frequency and severity of reflux, especially the upright contact time, was associated with the presence chronic allograft dysfunction [64]. The Toronto group reported [67] a prospective study that used 2-channel esophageal pH monitoring (proximal 5 cm below UES, and distal 5 cm above LES, implemented according to standard criteria) and showed that 30 % of lung transplant candidates (66/218 patients) had elevated distal esophageal pH findings (high DeMeester score), and proximal esophageal pH testing was abnormal in 19 % (41/218 patients) [67]. pH testing was also prospectively performed in the same patients at 3 and 12 months post-transplant, and DeMeester scores were observed in 35 % (16/46 patients) and 31 % (10/32 patients) at the two time points, respectively. Interestingly 64 % of patients with a high DeMeester score before transplant had normal testing at 3 months, but 34 % of patients with normal pre-transplant DeMeester scores had newly detected distal esophageal acid reflux at 3 months post-transplant. Similarly, 77 % of patients with abnormal proximal esophageal acid exposure before transplant had normal testing 3 months after transplantation, and similar findings were noted when comparing pre-transplant test results to those at 12 months post-transplant. Of particular interest is the observation that when results of testing at 3 months were compared to test results at 12 months post-transplant, the DeMeester score normalized in 36 %, but acid reflux was newly diagnosed in 30 %. In addition, abnormal proximal pH testing, if detected at 3 months, was found to be normal in 100 % esophageal acid reflux was noted in 15 % [67]. Therefore, simple acid ($pH<4$) detection by esophageal pH testing only could either overestimate or underestimate the true role of GER in the development of CLAD and BOS. These findings suggest that acid pH testing is likely not the most appropriate way to investigate GER and retrograde aspiration or to guide treatment post-transplant.

GER and retrograde aspiration are promoted by gastroparesis via the stimulation of inappropriate transient LES relaxations. Gastroparesis is a common disorder in lung transplant recipients and has been linked to the induction of BOS [10, 68, 69]. Gastroparesis has been attributed to preexisting lung disease [38, 70–74], vagal nerve injury or other intra-operative damage, or medications (especially calcineurin inhibitors) [75, 76]. In addition, the presence of other conditions, including weight loss [70], acute stress, diabetes mellitus, and uremia, may worsen gastroparesis before or after transplantation [77, 78]. Of note, the American Gastroenterology Association has included lung and heart-lung transplantation as one of the causes of delayed gastric emptying [79].

Gastric dysmotility after heart-lung transplantation has been shown to be present in nearly one-third of recipients [4]. In another study, one-third of patients with post-transplant GER had delayed gastric emptying, and 13 % had incomplete relaxation of the LES [80]. Similar findings were reported in a prospective study wherein 36 % of patients had abnormal liquid emptying at 3 months and 71 % at 12 months post-transplant [10–12]. Prolonged gastric emptying for solids was observed in

91 % of patients at 3 months after transplantation, and 80 % still had prolonged gastric emptying at 12 months [10–12].

In the context of delayed gastric emptying and considering that higher levels of bile acids are found in the stomach during the night [81], the likelihood of having nocturnal nonacid reflux is high when patients are given PPI therapy. Aspiration of nonacid gastric components during the night is facilitated by reduced protective reflexes (e.g., swallowing and coughing) [82]. Such factors might explain the association between nocturnal weakly acidic reflux and bile acid aspiration [83].

Acid and nonacid reflux may affect the allograft via two different mechanisms. Aspiration of refluxed acidic gastric juice may provoke lung inflammation, but patients treated with acid-suppression therapy (PPI) may aspirate nonacid refluxate that contains active pancreatic enzymes and bacterial substances such as lipopolysaccharides, which can also trigger significant bronchial inflammatory reaction [84].

Recently it has been demonstrated that 48 % of lung transplant patients have reflux at 1 year post-transplant, and nearly one-third of these patients exclusively had nonacid reflux as detected by pH/impedance testing [83]. Moreover, the presence of nonacid reflux as measured by pH/impedance testing increased the risk for developing BOS nearly threefold, while risk was not significantly associated with the presence of acid reflux [85]. Although abnormal acid GER can be detected via esophageal pH probe monitoring and nonacid reflux can be detected via pH/impedance monitoring, the detection of abnormal GER does not objectively identify microaspiration of refluxed gastroduodenal secretions, and a mild degree of GER can be observed in normal subjects and considered normal.

Single-center studies have used the detection of constituents of gastric juice (pepsin and bile acids) in BAL fluid of transplant recipients as a biomarker for retrograde aspiration associated with GER that is independent from the pH quality of the refluxate [10, 46, 86–88].

Pepsin in BAL fluid has been identified as a marker of GER and aspiration [87, 89, 90], and BAL pepsin levels were shown to be higher in the transplanted population when compared with normals, suggesting aspiration of gastric juice [46, 87]. Another study showed that pepsin levels in BAL were increased in lung transplant recipients without evidence of the presence of BOS, showing that pepsin can be present without airflow limitation. Interestingly, higher pepsin levels were associated with acute allograft rejection [88], which suggests that interactions between alloimmune and non-allo-immune-mediated allograft damage may occur [88]. However, others [87] have found that pepsin levels in BAL fluid did not correlate with FEV_1, while the presence of bile acids correlated with risk for developing BOS. This finding agrees with the correlation of high bile acid levels with the development of BOS that was initially reported by the Toronto group [10, 12]. They explored and described a link between GER and aspiration of bile acids in patients with BOS. Their findings suggested a role for duodeno-gastroesophageal refluxate, irrespective of the pH, retrograde aspiration of with investigations performed at a time when impedance testing was not yet widely available. Bile acids were detected in BAL fluid from 71 of 107 recipients who underwent surveillance bronchoscopies at 6 months after lung transplantation, and total bile acids were significantly increased in patients with BOS (stages 0–p and 1–3), but this increase was essentially limited to patients who developed BOS early (within 12 months after lung transplantation) vs. those with late BOS. Additionally, high levels of bile acids in BAL fluid correlated positively with BAL IL-8 and neutrophil levels, and the presence of bile acids was associated with significantly depressed levels of surfactant protein-A, surfactant protein-D, and dipalmitoylphosphatidylcholine, which led to the suggestion that one effect of aspirated bile acids may be depression of innate immune function in the lung allograft [12].

The lung transplant group in Leuven [46] also evaluated a cohort of lung transplant recipients and detected abnormal acid and nonacid GER in 22 of 45 patients and measured bile acids and pepsin in BAL fluid. All lung transplant recipients had detectable levels of pepsin in BAL, but levels of pepsin were 23-fold increased over that of control subjects. Twenty-two lung transplant recipients had bile acids detected in BAL fluid, and although pepsin levels showed no correlation with FEV_1 values, bile acids were significantly increased in patients with BOS stages 1–3. An additional, interesting aspect of this study was the persistence of abnormal GER, especially weakly acidic GER, in patients on PPI therapy (7 of 18 patients, five with weakly acid reflux), although esophageal acid exposure and acid reflux events were significantly reduced for patients on PPI when compared to a cohort of patients studied off PPI therapy. Vos et al. [91] found a significant association of allograft colonization by *Pseudomonas aeruginosa* with the presence of bile acid aspiration in a matched lung transplant recipient cohort of 24 subjects. Indeed, taken together, these investigations suggest that bile acids aspirated into the lower respiratory tract in the transplanted lung may be particularly injurious to respiratory mucosa and induce airway injury and dysfunction that can lead to chronic infection and/or BOS.

Various biomarkers of GER have been investigated in exhaled breath condensate in order to noninvasively detect reflux and microaspiration of gastroduodenal secretions [92–97]. However, this attractive methodology does not appear to be useful as a diagnostic technique using currently available technology. To date, no correlation of biomarker levels in BAL fluid with levels measured in exhaled breath condensate has been observed.

The presence of bile acids in BAL is considered to reflect duodeno-gastroesophageal reflux and aspiration [10, 83, 98], and bile acid aspiration into the lung has been associated with severe pulmonary injury [66, 83] and BOS. Bile acids are cytotoxic, disrupt cellular membranes, damage type II pneumocytes [99], which are responsible for surfactant protein and phospholipid production and homeostasis [10, 12, 68], and down-regulate innate immunity by affecting receptors on monocytes and macrophages [12, 68]. Althouph, todste the role of bile acids in reflux-related lung damage remains somewhat unclear, which is partly due to the fact that bile acid concentrations are difficult to accurately measure in the lung. Additionally, there is discordance between the presence of bile acids in BAL fluid and abnormal pH findings in lung transplant patients.

The uncertain cause and effect relationship between gastric aspiration, the detection of gastric juice constituents in BAL fluid, and the ultimate development of graft failure have been investigated in animal and in vitro models. A single lung transplant model has been developed in rats that demonstrates the harmful effects of gastric aspiration on airways. Recipients of major histocompatibility complex-mismatched grafts were exposed to repetitive airway stimulation with gastric contents via tracheal instillation. A significant increase in pulmonary infiltrates rich in CD8+ and CD68+ cells was observed in animals exposed to gastric contents, indicating a role for cytotoxic T cells and monocytes, which were associated with areas of acute airway fibrosis. Additionally, an increase in circulating levels of transforming growth factor-beta (TGF-β) was observed [100, 101]. Bile acids may alter innate immune responses by dampening the release of the lung collectins, surfactant protein-A, and surfactant protein-D, which play a key role in orchestrating the ability of lung macrophages to clear microbes [12]. Additionally, a receptor for bile acids, TGR5, that is expressed abundantly on human monocytes and macrophages has been identified, and this discovery has led to experiments that have confirmed the direct inhibitory effect of these bile acids on macrophages. The effect of bile acids on innate immune responses appears to be largely immunosuppressive, whereas other constituents of gastric juice appear to have the opposite effect and stimulate innate immune responses.

Additional studies correlating BAL markers of microaspiration with the presence of abnormal gastroesophageal GER with CLAD and/or BOS are needed to validate the predictive capability of such measurements. The combination of BAL biomarkers of aspiration with pH/impedance and proximal foregut motility studies may facilitate the accurate selection of recipients at risk for allograft dysfunction due to retrograde microaspiration from GER and facilitate the identification of lung transplant recipients who begin to display manifestations that are consistent with the onset of CLAD for more effective interventions to prevent reflux such as antireflux surgery.

Treatment Options for GER After Lung Transplantation

It is clear that GER that leads to aspiration of refluxed secretions is a significant risk factor for graft loss after lung transplantation. Therefore, one must ask what treatments or interventions can mitigate this risk, and when should such interventions be instituted. Because airway epithelia lack the defenses that protect gastric mucosae from foregut secretions, airways can be expected to be more vulnerable to aspiration injury. Therefore, treatments of gastroesophageal GER may prevent or attenuate BOS by reducing retrograde nocturnal reflux and microaspiration, which would prevent or lessen the epithelial injury and epithelial-mesenchymal transition that can lead to OB and BOS.

Acid suppression (e.g., PPI administration) is usually first-line therapy for GER and can improve classic GER symptoms, but lung transplant recipients may remain at risk to develop BOS because such therapy may only convert acid reflux into asymptomatic nonacid reflux, and gastroesophageal aspiration of bile acids may not reduced in patients on PPI therapy [46]. Lifestyle changes (avoiding late evening meals, not lying in bed for the first 2–3 h after dinner, avoiding snacks or drinks after the evening meal, elevating the head of the bed during sleep) may reduce the amount of nocturnal reflux and, thus, may help to prevent nocturnal GER and aspiration.

Prokinetic drugs, which may improve esophageal motility and accelerate gastric emptying, have been used either alone or in combination with PPIs for the treatment of GER [102–104]. Macrolide antibiotics (e.g., erythromycin) have a significant prokinetic effect on the gastrointestinal tract and have also been proposed for the treatment of GER [105], and the neomacrolide/azalide, azithromycin, has been shown to reduce GER and gastroesophageal bile acid aspiration in lung transplant recipients [106]. On the basis of these observations, it could be hypothesized that the beneficial effect of azithromycin, which is frequently used in lung transplant recipients, is not only due to its anti-inflammatory properties but might be further potentiated by an anti-reflux effect due to its prokinetic properties on esophageal and gastric motility. Baclofen, a GABA receptor agonist, has been shown to reduce episodes of transient LES relaxation and thereby might reduce both acid and non-acid GER, but most patients experience intolerable side effects [107, 108].

Surgical fundoplication for treatment of GER in lung transplant recipients has been shown to prevent BOS and improve patient survival. Laparoscopic Nissen fundoplication can be performed with reasonable safety on lung transplant candidates with advanced lung disease prior to lung transplant [45, 109, 110], and prophylactic fundoplication may decrease the incidence of post-transplant allograft dysfunction and BOS [8, 9, 111]. Potential benefits of anti-GER surgery prior to transplant include decreased risk of perioperative aspiration and immediate protection from microaspiration of gastroduodenal secretions that increase the risk of post-transplant allograft dysfunction [109]. However, as suggested by the Toronto group, transplantation itself may resolve pre-transplant acid GER by restoring the anatomic relationship between the diaphragmatic and LES [67].

In lung transplant recipients, lung function might be improved by anti-reflux surgery and freedom from developing BOS may be enhanced [46, 86–92]. A number of investigations, both retrospective and prospective, undertaken by the lung transplant group at Duke University have repeatedly supported benefit of laparoscopic Nissen fundoplication in preventing BOS [8, 9, 111–113], particularly if adopted early after lung transplantation [8]. Similarly, other investigators have shown that anti-reflux surgery is both safe and effective [45, 114], and that it can reduce pepsin levels in BAL fluid [115].

Laparoscopic Nissen fundoplication is the favored technique in the lung transplant candidate or recipient, and it is the anti-reflux surgical procedure of choice, unless esophageal dysmotility is present [8, 113]. Caution should prevail if esophageal dysmotility is present, because a complete wrap may obstruct passage of ingested food from esophagus to stomach and lead to dysphagia [113, 116]. Partial fundoplication can be performed for such patients as an alternative to the Nissen 360-degree wrap using the techniques described by Dor and Toupet [117–119].

In lung transplant recipients with severely delayed gastric emptying, the implantation of a gastric stimulator has been suggested, although the true role of this device in this patient population has not been explored [120–124]. Gastric emptying may improve following Nissen fundoplication and obviate the need for such a device.

Conclusion

The evidence collected to date strongly supports the role of GER as a risk factor for CLAD and/or BOS. Proximal gastrointestinal tract motility studies and pH/impedance testing can be used to diagnose motility abnormalities and GER (and determine whether refluxate is acid and/or nonacid), respectively. Unfortunately, a true gold standard for detecting aspiration of refluxed secretions into the lung is lacking, and a definitive marker of GER combined with microaspiration that identifies patients at significant risk for GER-associated allograft injury and dysfunction needs to be determined. Indications for anti-reflux surgery will most likely need to be based on reasonably stringent criteria, given that not all the patients with GER are likely to experience silent, retrograde aspiration of gastroduodenal contents into the lungs. Furthermore, GER that is identified pre-transplant may not persist following transplantation if the anatomical relationship of the gastroesophageal junction high-pressure zone is restored.

Prospective studies to determine the most effective approach to prevent reflux-related lung injury in lung transplant patients are needed, as only retrospective studies have linked prophylactic fundoplication for recipients with GER to improved post-transplant outcomes and decreased incidence and/or severity of CLAD and/or BOS. Future research should seek to identify the most effective protocols that can detect susceptibility to GER and microaspiration in lung transplant candidates and recipients. The optimal timing of diagnostic testing needs to be determined.

Prospective, multicenter, adequately powered clinical trials are needed to better understand the role of GER in CLAD and to establish appropriate criteria to select patients for anti-reflux surgery.

References

1. Estenne M, Maurer JR, Boehler A, Egan JJ, Frost A, Hertz M, et al. Bronchiolitis obliterans syndrome 2001: an update of the diagnostic criteria. J Heart Lung Transplant. 2002;21:297–310.
2. Reid KR, McKenzie FN, Menkis AH, Novick RJ, Pflugfelder PW, Kostuk WJ, et al. Importance of chronic aspiration in recipients of heart-lung transplants. Lancet. 1990;336: 206–8.
3. Kirk AJ, Colquhoun IW, Corris PA, Hilton CJ, Dark JH. Impaired gastrointestinal motility in pulmonary transplantation. Lancet. 1990;336:752.
4. Au J, Hawkins T, Venables C, Morritt G, Scott CD, Gascoigne AD, et al. Upper gastrointestinal dysmotility in heart-lung transplant recipients. Ann Thorac Surg. 1993;55:94–7.

5. Rinaldi M, Martinelli L, Volpato G, Pederzolli C, Silvestri M, Pederzolli N, et al. Gastroesophageal reflux as cause of obliterative bronchiolitis: a case report. Transplant Proc. 1995;27:2006–7.
6. Lubetkin EI, Lipson DA, Palevsky HI, Kotloff R, Morris J, Berry GT, et al. GI complications after lung transplantation. Am J Gastroenterol. 1996;91:2382–90.
7. Berkowitz H, Schulman LL, McGregor C, Markowitz D. Gastroparesis after lung transplantation-potential role in postoperative respiratory complications. Chest. 1995;108: 1062–607.
8. Cantu III E, Appel III JZ, Hartwig MG, Woreta H, Green C, Messier R, et al. Early fundoplication prevents chronic allograft dysfunction in patients with gastroesophageal reflux disease. Ann Thorac Surg. 2004;78:1142–51.
9. Davis Jr RD, Lau CL, Eubanks S, Messier RH, Hadjiliadis D, Steele MP, et al. Improved lung allograft function after fundoplication in patients with gastroesophageal reflux disease undergoing lung transplantation. J Thorac Cardiovasc Surg. 2003;125:533–42.
10. D'Ovidio F, Mura M, Tsang M, Waddell TK, Hutcheon MA, Singer LG, et al. Bile acid aspiration and the development of bronchiolitis obliterans after lung transplantation. J Thorac Cardiovasc Surg. 2005;129:1144–52.
11. D'Ovidio F, Mura M, Waddell TK, Pierre A, Hutcheon M, Hadjiliadis D, et al. Bile acids in bronchoalveolar lavage after lung transplantation as a marker of pulmonary aspiration associated with alveolar neutrophilia. J Heart Lung Transplant. 2004;23(2 Suppl 1):42.
12. D'Ovidio F, Mura M, Ridsdale R, Takahashi H, Waddell TK, Hutcheon M, et al. The effect of reflux and bile acid aspiration on the lung allograft and its surfactant and innate immunity molecules SP-A and SP-D. Am J Transplant. 2006;6:1930–8.
13. Abernathy EC, Hruban RH, Baumgartner WA, Reitz BA, Hutchins GM, et al. The two forms of bronchiolitis obliterans in heart-lung transplant recipients. Hum Pathol. 1991;22:1102–10.
14. Osler WB. Bronchial asthma. The principles and practice of medicine. New York: Appleton; 1892. p. 497–501.
15. Pearson JEG, Wilson RSE. Diffuse pulmonary fibrosis and hiatus hernia. Thorax. 1971;26: 300–5.
16. Belsey R. The pulmonary complications of dysphagia. Thorax. 1948;4:44–56.
17. Davis MV. Evolving concepts regarding hiatus hernia and gastroesophageal reflux. Ann Thorac Surg. 1969;7:120–33.
18. Paulson DL. Reflux respiratory threat called unappreciated. US Med. 1972;4:32.
19. Orringer MB, Skinner DB, Belsey RHR. Long-term results of the Mark IV operation for hiatal hernia and analysis of recurrences and their treatment. J Thorac Cardiovasc Surg. 1972;63:25–31.
20. Sadoun D, Valeyre D, Cargill J, Volter F, Amouroux J, Battesti JP. Bronchiolitis obliterans with cryptogenetic-like organizing pneumonia. Demonstration of gastroesophageal reflux in 5 cases. Presse Med. 1988;17:2383–5.
21. Holloway RH, HongoPalmer SM, Miralles AP, Howell DN, et al. Gastric distention: a mechanism for postprandial gastroesophageal reflux. Gastroenterology. 1985;118:1214–7.
22. Franzi SJ, Martin CJ, Cox MR, Dent J. Response of canine lower esophageal sphincter to gastric distention. Am J Physiol. 1990;259:G380–5.
23. Mittal RK, Balaban DH. The esophagogastric junction. N Engl J Med. 1997;336(13): 924–32.
24. Mattioli S, D'Ovidio F, Di Simone MP, Bassi F, Brusori S, Pilotti V, et al. Clinical and surgical relevance of the progressive phases of intrathoracic migration of the gastroesophageal junction in gastroesophageal reflux disease. J Thorac Cardiovasc Surg. 1998;116:267–75.
25. Kahrilas PJ, Dodds WJ, Dent J, Haeberle B, Hogan WJ, Arndorfer RC. Effect of sleep, spontaneous gastroesophageal reflux, and meal on upper esophageal sphincter pressure in normal human volunteers. Gastroenterology. 1987;92:466–71.
26. Oelschlager BK, Quiroga E, Isch JA, Cuenca-Abente F. Gastroesophageal and pharyngeal reflux detection using impedance and 24-hour pH monitoring in asymptomatic subjects: defining the normal environment. J Gastrointest Surg. 2006;10(1):54–62.

27. Mays EE, Dubois JJ, Hamilton GB. Pulmonary fibrosis with tracheobronchial aspiration. Chest. 1976;69:512–5.
28. Feigelson J, Girault F, Pecau Y. Gastro-oesophageal reflux and esophagitis in cystic fibrosis. Acta Paediatr Scand. 1987;76:989–90.
29. Tobin RW, Pope 2nd CE, Pellegrini CA, Emond MJ, Sillery J, Raghu G. Increased prevalence of gastroesophageal reflux in patients with idiopathic pulmonary fibrosis. Am J Respir Crit Care Med. 1998;158:1804–8.
30. Raghu G, Freudenberger TD, Yang S, Freudenberger TD, Yang S, Curtis JR, et al. High prevalence of abnormal acid gastro-oesophageal reflux in idiopathic pulmonary fibrosis. Eur Respir J. 2006;27:136–42.
31. Ahrens P, Weimer B, Hofmann D. Severe interstitial lung disease from pathologic gastro-esophageal reflux in children. Pneumologie. 1999;53:569–72.
32. Bibi H, Khvolis E, Shoseyov D, Ohaly M, Ben Dor D, London D, et al. The prevalence of gastroesophageal reflux in children with tracheomalacia and laryngomalacia. Chest. 2001;119:409–13.
33. Ing AJ. Interstitial lung disease and gastroesophageal reflux. Am J Med. 2001;111:41s–4.
34. Herbst JJ, Minton SD, Book LS. Gastroesophageal reflux causing respiratory distress and apnea in newborn infants. J Pediatr. 1979;95:763.
35. Hills BA, Chen Y, Masters IB, Hills Y. Raised bile acid concentration in SIDS lungs at necroscopy. Arch Dis Child. 1997;77:120–3.
36. Matsuse T, Oka T, Kida K, Fukuchi Y. Importance of diffuse aspiration bronchiolitis caused by chronic occult aspiration in the elderly. Chest. 1996;110:1289–93.
37. Sontag SJ, Schnell TG, Miller Q, Khandelwal S, O'Connell S, Chejfec G, et al. Prevalence of oesophagitis in asthmatics. Gut. 1992;33:872–6.
38. D'Ovidio F, Singer LG, Hadijiliadis D, Pierre A, Waddell TK, de Perrot M, et al. Prevalence of gastroesophageal reflux in end-stage lung disease candidates for lung transplant. Ann Thorac Surg. 2005;80:1254.
39. Sweet MP, Herbella FA, Leard L, Hoopes C, Golden J, Hays S, et al. The prevalence of distal and proximal gastroesophageal reflux in patients awaiting lung transplantation. Ann Surg. 2006;244:491–7.
40. Tamhankar AP, Peters JH, Portale G, Hsieh CC, Hagen JA, Bremner CG, et al. Omeprazole does not reduce gastroesophageal reflux: new insights using multichannel intraluminal impedance technology. J Gastrointest Surg. 2004;8:888–96.
41. Emerenziani S, Sifrim D. New developments in detection of gastroesophageal reflux. Curr Opin Gastroenterol. 2005;21:450–3.
42. Irwin RS, Richter JE. Gastroesophageal reflux and chronic cough. Am J Gastroenterol. 2000;95:S9–14.
43. Irwin RS, Curley FJ, French CL. Chronic cough. The spectrum and frequency of causes, key components of the diagnostic evaluation, and outcome of specific therapy. Am Rev Respir Dis. 1990;141:640–7.
44. Sweet MP, Patti MG, Leard LE, Golden JA, Hays SR, Hoopes C, et al. Gastroesophageal reflux in patients with idiopathic pulmonary fibrosis referred for lung transplantation. J Thorac Cardiovasc Surg. 2007;133:1078–84.
45. Hoppo T, Jarido V, Pennathur A, Morrell M, Crespo M, Shigemura N, et al. Antireflux surgery preserves lung function in patients with gastroesophageal reflux disease and end-stage lung disease before and after lung transplantation. Arch Surg. 2011;146:1041–7.
46. Blondeau K, Mertens V, Vanaudenaerde BA, Verleden GM, Van Raemdonck DE, Sifrim D, et al. Gastro-oesophageal reflux and gastric aspiration in lung transplant patients with or without chronic rejection. Eur Respir J. 2008;31:707–13.
47. Ghaed N, Stein M. Assessment of a technique for scintigrafic monitoring of pulmonary aspiration of gastric contents in asthmatics with gastroesophageal reflux. Ann Allergy. 1979;42:306.
48. Patti MG, Debas HT, Pellegrini CA. Esophageal manometry and 24-hour pH monitoring in the diagnosis of pulmonary aspiration secondary to gastroesophageal reflux. Am J Surg. 1992;163:401–6.

49. Potluri S, Friedenberg F, Parkman HP, Chang A, MacNeal R, Manus C, et al. Comparison of a salivary/sputum pepsin assay with 24-hour esophageal pH monitoring for detection of gastric reflux into the proximal esophagus, oropharynx and lung. Dig Dis Sci. 2003;48:1813–7.
50. Reich SB, Earley WC, Ravin TH, Goodman M, Spector S, Stein MR. Evaluation of gastropulmonary aspiration by a radioactive technique. J Nucl Med. 1977;18:1079.
51. Gleeson K, Eggli DF, Maxwell SL. Quantitative aspiration during sleep in normal subjects. Chest. 1997;111:1266–72.
52. Chernow B, Johnson LF, Janowitz WR, Castell DO. Pulmonary aspiration as a consequence of gastroesophageal reflux: a diagnostic approach. Dig Dis Sci. 1979;24:839–44.
53. Metheny NA, Chang YH, Song J, Edwards SJ, Defer J, Dahms TE, et al. Pepsin as a marker for pulmonary aspiration. Am J Crit Care. 2002;11:150–4.
54. Corwin RW, Irwin RS. The lipid laden alveolar macrophage as a marker of aspiration in parenchymal lung disease. Am Rev Respir Dis. 1985;132:576.
55. Nussbaum E, Maggi JC, Mathis R, Galant SP. Association of lipid-laden alveolar macrophages and gastroesophageal reflux in children. J Pediatr. 1987;110:190.
56. Hartwig MG, Appel JZ, Li B, Hsieh CC, Yoon YH, Lin SS, et al. Chronic aspiration of gastric fluid accelerates pulmonary allograft dysfunction in a rat model of lung transplantation. J Thorac Cardiovasc Surg. 2005;131:209–17.
57. Effros R, Jacobs ER, Schapira RM, Biller J. Response of the lungs to aspiration. Am J Med. 2001;111:15S–9.
58. Effros RM, Hogan G, Hoagland KW, Olson L, Lin W. Protection of the lungs from acid during aspiration. Am J Med. 2001;111:56S–9.
59. Mattioli S, Felice V, Pastina M, Pilotti V, D'Ovidio F, Bacchi ML, et al. Duodenogastric and non acid gastro-oesophageal reflux in patients with reflux oesophagitis. Hepatogastroenterology. 1995;42:360–6.
60. Oelschlager BK, Chang L, Pope 2nd CE, Pellegrini CA. Typical GERD symptoms and esophageal pH monitoring are not enough to diagnose pharyngeal reflux. J Surg Res. 2005;128:55–60.
61. Tutuian R. Update in the diagnosis of gastroesophageal reflux disease. J Gastrointestin Liver Dis. 2006;15:243–7.
62. Kahrilas PJ, Sifrim D. High-resolution manometry and impedance-pH/manometry: valuable tools in clinical and investigational esophagology. Gastroenterology. 2008;135:756–69.
63. Vaezi MF, Richter JE. Duodenogastroesophageal reflux and methods to monitor nonacidic reflux. Am J Med. 2001;111(8A):160S–8.
64. Hadjiliadis D, Duane Davis R, Steele MP, Messier RH, Lau CL, Eubanks SS, et al. Gastroesophageal reflux disease in lung transplant recipients. Clin Transplant. 2003;17:363–8.
65. Benden C, Aurora P, Curry J, Whitmore P, Priestley L, Elliott MJ, et al. High prevalence of gastroesophageal reflux in children after lung transplantation. Pediatr Pulmonol. 2005;40:68–71.
66. Halsey KD, Wald A, Meyer KC, Torrealba JR, Gaumnitz EA. Non-acidic supraesophageal reflux associated with diffuse alveolar damage and allograft dysfunction after lung transplantation: a case report. J Heart Lung Transplant. 2008;27:564–7.
67. D'Ovidio F, Waddell T, Singer LG, Pierre A, De Perrot M, Chaparro C, et al. Spontaneous reversal of acid GER after lung transplantation. J Heart Lung Transplant. 2008;27(2S):S109.
68. D'Ovidio F, Keshavjee S. Gastroesophageal reflux and lung transplantation. Dis Esophagus. 2006;19:315–20.
69. Raviv Y, D'Ovidio F, Pierre A, Chaparro C, Freeman M, Keshavjee S, et al. Prevalence of gastroparesis before and after lung transplantation and its association with lung allograft outcomes. Clin Transplant. 2012;26(1):133–42.
70. Bodet-Milin C, Querellou S, Oudoux A, Haloun A, Horeau-Llanglard D, Carlier T, et al. Delayed gastric emptying scintigraphy in cystic fibrosis patients before and after lung transplantation. J Heart Lung Transplant. 2006;25:1077.

71. Marie I, Levesque H, Ducrotte P, Denis P, Hellot MF, Benichou J, et al. Gastric involvement in systemic sclerosis: a prospective study. Am J Gastroenterol. 2001;96:77.
72. Harding SM. Nocturnal asthma: role of gastroesophageal reflux. Chronobiol Int. 1999;16:641.
73. Schiller LR. Upper gastrointestinal motility disorders and respiratory symptoms. Am J Health Syst Pharm. 1996;53(22 Suppl 3):S13.
74. Fisher RS. Gastroduodenal motility disturbances in man. Scand J Gastroenterol Suppl. 1985;109:59.
75. Maes BO, Vanawalleghem J, Kuypers D, Ghoose Y, Rtgeerts PJ, Vanrenterghem YF. Differences in gastric motor activity in renal transplant recipients treated with FK-506 versus cyclosporine. Transplantation. 1999;68:1482.
76. Verleden GM, Besse T, Maes B. Successful conversion from cyclosporine to tacrolimus for gastric emptying motor dysfunction in lung transplant recipient. Transplantation. 1974;2002:73.
77. Samson M, Vermeijden JR, Smout AJ. Prevalence of delayed gastric emptying in diabetic patients and relationship to dyspeptic symptoms: a prospective study in unselected diabetic patients. Diabetes Care. 2003;26:116.
78. Samson M, Akkermans LM, Jebbink RJ, Van Isselt H, Van Berge-Henegouwen GP, Smout AJ. Gastrointestinal motor mechanisms in hyperglycemia induced delayed gastric emptying type I diabetes mellitus. Gut. 1997;40:641.
79. Parkman HP, Hasler WL, Fisher RS. American Gastroenterological Association technical review on the diagnosis and treatment of gastroparesis. Gastroenterology 2004;127: 1592–1622.
80. Young LR, Hadjiliadis D, Davis RD, Palmer SM. Lung transplantation exacerbates gastroesophageal reflux disease. Chest. 2003;124:1689–93.
81. Gotley DC, Morgan AP, Ball D, Owen RW, Cooper MJ. Composition of gastrooesophageal refluxate. Gut. 1991;32:1093–9.
82. Fass R, Achem SR, Harding S, Mittal RK, Quigley E. Review article: supraoesophageal manifestations of gastro-oesophageal reflux disease and the role of night-time gastro-oesophageal reflux. Aliment Pharmacol Ther. 2004;20 Suppl 9:26–38.
83. Blondeau K, Mertens V, Vanaudenaerde BA, Verleden GM, Van Raemdonck DE, Sifrim D, et al. Nocturnal weakly acidic reflux promotes aspiration of bile acids in lung transplant recipients. J Heart Lung Transplant. 2009;28:141–8.
84. Mertens V, Blondeau K, Pauwels A, Blondeau G, Sifrim D, Dupont LJ. Effect of gastric juice from patients "on" acid suppressive therapy (PPI) on human bronchial epithelial cells. J Heart Lung Transplant. 2009;28:S212.
85. King BJ, Iyer H, Leidi AA, Carby MR. Gastroesophageal reflux in bronchiolitis obliterans syndrome: a new perspective. J Heart Lung Transplant. 2009;28:870–5.
86. Hopkins PM, Kermeen F, Duhig E, Fletcher L, Gradwell J, Whitfield L, et al. Oil red O stain of alveolar macrophages is an effective screening test for gastroesophageal reflux disease in lung transplant recipients. J Heart Lung Transplant. 2010;29:859–64.
87. Ward C, Forrest IA, Brownlee IA, Johnson GE, Murphy DM, Pearson JP, et al. Pepsin like activity in bronchoalveolar lavage fluid is suggestive of gastric aspiration in lung allografts. Thorax. 2005;60:872–4.
88. Stovold R, Forrest IA, Corris PA, Murphy DM, Smith JA, Decalmer S, et al. Pepsin, a biomarker of gastric aspiration in lung allografts: a putative association with rejection. Am J Respir Crit Care Med. 2007;175:1298–303.
89. Tasker A, Dettmar PW, Panetti M, Koufman JA, Birchall JP, Pearson JP. Reflux of gastric juice and glue ear in children. Lancet. 2002;359:493.
90. Ufberg JW, Bushra JS, Patel D, Wong E, Karras DJ, Kueppers F. A new pepsin assay to detect pulmonary aspiration of gastric contents among newly intubated patients. Am J Emerg Med. 2004;22:612–4.
91. Vos R, Blondeau K, Vanaudenaerde BM, Mertens V, Van Raemdonck DE, Sifrim D, et al. Airway colonization and gastric aspiration after lung transplantation: do birds of a feather flock together? J Heart Lung Transplant. 2008;27:843–9.

92. Shimizu Y, Dobashi K, Nagoshi A, Kawamura O, Mori M. Assessment of airway inflammation by exhaled breath condensate and impedance due to gastroesophageal reflux disease (GERD). Inflamm Allergy Drug Targets. 2009;8:292–6.
93. Davis CS, Gagermeier J, Dilling D, Alex C, Lowery E, Kovacs EJ, et al. A review of the potential applications and controversies of non-invasive testing for biomarkers of aspiration in the lung transplant population. Clin Transplant. 2010;24:E54–61.
94. Yates DH, Krishnan A, Chow S, Thomas PS. Non-invasive assessment of exhaled biomarkers in lung transplantation. J Breath Res. 2011;5:024001.
95. Jackson AS, Sandrini A, Campbell C, Chow S, Thomas PS, Yates DH. Comparison of biomarkers in exhaled breath condensate and bronchoalveolar lavage. Am J Respir Crit Care Med. 2007;175:222–7.
96. Dupont LJ, Dewandeleer Y, Vanaudenaerde BM, Van Raemdonck DE, Verleden GM. The pH of exhaled breath condensate of patients with allograft rejection after lung transplantation. Am J Transplant. 2006;6:1486–92.
97. Soter S, Kelemen K, Barta I, Valyon M, Csiszer E, Antus B. Exhaled breath condensate pH in lung transplant recipients with bronchiolitis obliterans syndrome. Transplantation. 2011;91:793–7.
98. Gautam A. Gastrointestinal complications following transplantation. Surg Clin North Am. 2006;86:1195–206.
99. Oelberg DG, Downey SA, Flynn MM, Oelberg DG, Downey SA, Flynn MM. Bile salt-induced intracellular Ca^{++} accumulation in type II pneumocytes. Lung. 1990;168:297–308.
100. Li B, Hartwig MG, Appel JZ, Bush EL, Balsara KR, Holzknecht ZE, et al. Chronic aspiration of gastric fluid induces the development of obliterative bronchiolitis in rat lung transplants. Am J Transplant. 2008;8:1614–21.
101. Jarmuz T, Roser S, Rivera H, Gal A, Roman J. Transforming growth factor-beta1, myofibroblasts, and tissue remodeling in the pathogenesis of tracheal injury: potential role of gastroesophageal reflux. Ann Otol Rhinol Laryngol. 2004;113:488–97.
102. Fink SM, Lange RC, McCallum RW. Effect of metoclopramide on normal and delayed gastric emptying in gastroesophageal reflux patients. Dig Dis Sci. 1983;28:1057–61.
103. Mansi C, Borro P, Giacomini M, Biagini R, Mele MR, Pandolfo N, et al. Comparative effects of levosulpiride and cisapride on gastric emptying and symptoms in patients with functional dyspepsia and gastroparesis. Aliment Pharmacol Ther. 2000;14:561–9.
104. Takeda T, Konomi H, Naritomi G, Yoshida J, Matsunaga H, Akazawa K, et al. Single oral dose of cisapride accelerates gastric antral emptying in healthy humans: an ultrasonographic study. J Gastroenterol. 1996;31:323–8.
105. Netzer P, Schmitt B, Inauen W. Effects of ABT-229, a motilin agonist, on acid reflux, oesophageal motility and gastric emptying in patients with gastro-oesophageal reflux disease. Aliment Pharmacol Ther. 2002;16:1481–90.
106. Mertens V, Blondeau K, Pauwels A, Farre R, Vanaudenaerde B, Vos R, et al. Azithromycin reduces gastroesophageal reflux and aspiration in lung transplant recipients. Dig Dis Sci. 2009;54:972–9.
107. Vela MF, Tutuian R, Katz PO, Castell DO. Baclofen decreases acid and non-acid post-prandial gastro-oesophageal reflux measured by combined multichannel intraluminal impedance and pH. Aliment Pharmacol Ther. 2003;17:243–51.
108. Koek GH, Sifrim D, Lerut T, Janssens J, Tack J. Effect of the GABA(B) agonist baclofen in patients with symptoms and duodeno-gastrooesophageal reflux refractory to proton pump inhibitors. Gut. 2003;52:1397–402.
109. Linden PA, Gilbert RJ, Yeap BY, Boyle K, Deykin A, Jaklitsch MT, et al. Laparoscopic fundoplication in patients with end-stage lung disease awaiting transplantation. J Thorac Cardiovasc Surg. 2006;131:438–46.
110. Gasper WJ, Sweet MP, Hoopes C, Leard LE, Kleinhenz ME, Hays SR, et al. Antireflux surgery for patients with end-stage lung disease before and after lung transplantation. Surg Endosc. 2008;22:495–500.

111. Lau CL, Palmer SM, Howell DN, McMahon R, Hadjiliadis D, Gaca J, et al. Laparoscopic antireflux surgery in the lung transplant population. Surg Endosc. 2002;16:1674–8.
112. O'Halloran EK, Reynolds JD, Lau CL, Manson RJ, Davis RD, Palmer SM, et al. Laparoscopic Nissen fundoplication for treating reflux in lung transplant recipients. J Gastrointest Surg. 2004;8:132–7.
113. Hartwig MG, Anderson DJ, Onaitis MW, Reddy S, Snyder LD, Lin SS, et al. Fundoplication after lung transplantation prevents the allograft dysfunction associated with reflux. Ann Thorac Surg. 2011;92:462–8.
114. Burton PR, Button B, Brown W, Lee M, Roberts S, Hassen S, et al. Medium-term outcome of fundoplication after lung transplantation. Dis Esophagus. 2009;22:642–8.
115. Fisichella PM, Davis CS, Lundberg PW, Lowery E, Burnham EL, Alex CG, et al. The protective role of laparoscopic antireflux surgery against aspiration of pepsin after lung transplantation. Surgery. 2011;150:598–606.
116. Darling G, Deschamps C. Technical controversies in fundoplication surgery. Thorac Surg Clin. 2005;15:437–44.
117. Broeders JA, Bredenoord AJ, Hazebroek EJ, Broeders IA, Gooszen HG, Smout AJ. Reflux and belching after 270 degree versus 360 degree laparoscopic posterior fundoplication. Ann Surg. 2012;255:59–65.
118. Ramos RF, Lustosa SA, Almeida CA, Silva CP, Matos D. Surgical treatment of gastroesophageal reflux disease: total or partial fundoplication? Systematic review and meta-analysis. Arq Gastroenterol. 2011;48:252–60.
119. Del Genio G, Tolone S, Del Genio F, Dalessandro A, Brusciano L, Aggarwal R, et al. Impact of total fundoplication on esophageal transit: analysis by combined multichannel intraluminal impedance and manometry. J Clin Gastroenterol. 2012;46:e1–5.
120. Yiannopoulos A, Shafazand S, Ziedalski T, Berry GJ, Robbins RC, Theodore J, et al. Gastric pacing for severe gastroparesis in a heart-lung transplant recipient. J Heart Lung Transplant. 2004;23(3):371–4.
121. Morgan KG, Szurszewski JH. Mechanisms of phasic and tonic actions of pentagastrin on canine gastric smooth muscle. J Physiol. 1980;301:229–42.
122. Forster J, Sarosiek I, Delcore R, Lin Z, Raju GS, McCallum RW. Gastric pacing is a new surgical treatment for gastroparesis. Am J Surg. 2001;182:676–81.
123. Olufemi AA, Faul LJ, Vierra M, Triadafilopoulos G, Theodore J. The surgical management of severe gastroparesis in heart/lung transplant recipients. Chest. 2000;111:907–10.
124. Weinkauf JG, Yiannopoulos A, Faul JL. Transcutaneous electrical nerve stimulation for severe gastroparesis after lung transplantation. J Heart Lung Transplant. 2005;24(9):1444.

Chapter 13
Bronchiolitis Obliterans Syndrome in Children

Paul D. Robinson and Paul Aurora

Abstract Extrapolation of adult-based evidence into pediatric management decisions is often unavoidable owing to a lack of sufficiently powered, suitably designed pediatric studies. Pediatric data are emerging but are challenged by the lower numbers of lung and heart–lung transplants performed annually as compared to adult transplantation. Pediatric data are further diluted by the relatively large number of centers that perform pediatric transplants internationally. This chapter will discuss available pediatric data to illustrate the similarities that exist between pediatric and adult subjects with respect to incidence, risk factors, diagnosis, and management of bronchiolitis obliterans (BO). Although the pediatric lung transplant literature generally supports the use of data that are extrapolated from lung transplantation in adults, specific challenges also exist that are unique to the pediatric age range, and the resultant differences in approach are outlined.

Keywords Pediatric • Extrapolation • Lung function • Diagnosis • Risk factors • Management

P.D. Robinson, M.B.Ch.B., M.R.C.P.C.H., F.R.A.C.P., Ph.D. (✉)
Portex Respiratory Unit, UCL Institute of Child Health, London, UK

Department of Pediatric Respiratory Medicine, The Children's Hospital at Westmead, Locked Bag 4001, Westmead, Sydney, NSW 2145, Australia
e-mail: paul.robinson1@health.nsw.gov.au; dr.pdrobinson@gmail.com

P. Aurora, M.B.B.S., M.R.C.P., Ph.D.
Department of Paediatric Respiratory Medicine, Great Ormond Street Hospital for Children, Great Ormond Street, London, UK

K.C. Meyer and A.R. Glanville (eds.), *Bronchiolitis Obliterans Syndrome in Lung Transplantation*, Respiratory Medicine 8, DOI 10.1007/978-1-4614-7636-8_13,

Introduction

As with many areas of pediatric medicine, evidence-based management is challenged by a lack of sufficiently powered, suitably designed studies. Extrapolation from adult studies is not ideal, as children should not be thought of as simply "small adults," but such extrapolation is often unavoidable. This chapter will discuss similarities between the two different age groups, which may in part support this extrapolated approach. However, we will also outline how the approach to risk factors, surveillance, and management of bronchiolitis obliterans (BO) may differ in pediatric lung and heart–lung transplant recipients as compared to their adult counterparts.

Overview of Pediatric Lung Transplantation

The following is an overview of pediatric lung and heart–lung transplants based on data contained in the last official report of the ISHLT in 2011 [1]. The number of centers performing pediatric lung and heart–lung transplantation is growing steadily and has now reached almost 50 centers worldwide, but the majority continue to perform relatively small numbers per year, with over 50 % of centers performing fewer than five procedures annually. Approximately 130 pediatric transplants occur globally each year, based on data reported to the registry, but this total is recognized to be an underestimate of true numbers. The most common indications for transplant are idiopathic pulmonary hypertension in preschoolers (aged <6 years) and cystic fibrosis in older children. Single lung transplantation, heart–lung transplantation, and living related lobar lung transplantation are now rarely performed.

Peri- and post-transplant immunosuppression regimens are similar to those employed in adults. The most common regimen involves induction therapy (approximately 60 % of cases), followed by triple-agent maintenance immunosuppression with tacrolimus, the preferred calcineurin inhibitor (CNI); mycophenolate mofetil (MMF), the preferred cell-cycle inhibitor (78 % and 65 % of cases at 1 year post-transplant, respectively); and prednisolone. Almost all children continue to receive prednisolone at 5 years post-transplant, in contrast to almost all other solid organ recipient groups.

Overall survival in pediatric subjects appears comparable to adult recipients, with a median survival of 5.5 and 5.4 years, respectively, but longer-term survival appears to be greater in pediatric subjects (Fig. 13.1). In addition, pediatric survival appears to be improving over time [2]. Within the pediatric age range, the best survival rates are seen in children aged 1–11 years, and while infants (aged <1 year) have the lowest short-term survival, subsequent long-term outcomes are comparable. The adolescent age range has the poorest long-term survival of the pediatric age range, and this is attributed to factors including treatment compliance issues [3, 4].

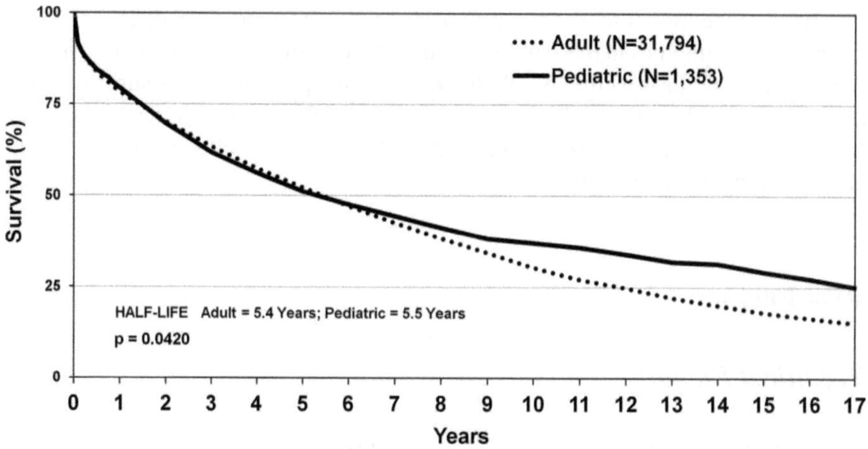

Fig. 13.1 Kaplan–Meier survival in pediatric and adult recipients of lung and heart–lung transplant between 1990 and 2009 [1]. Reprinted from The Journal of Heart and Lung Transplantation, 30/10, Benden C, Aurora P, Edwards LB, Kucheryavaya AY, Christie JD, Dobbels F, et al., The registry of the International Society for Heart and Lung Transplantation: Fourteenth Pediatric Lung and Heart-Lung Transplantation Report—2011, 1123–1132, Copyright 2011, with permission from Elsevier

Incidence of BOS

Current registry data provides the best available estimate of the incidence of BOS in pediatric recipients, and the incidence appears to be similar to that seen in adults: It is the second most common morbidity within 5 years post-transplantation and reported in 56 % of recipients [2] vs. 49 % of adults [5]. Interestingly, an age effect did appear in a recent analysis that was based on incidence at 4 years post-transplantation. Incidence is lowest in the youngest transplant recipients (31 % in those transplanted in the first year of life compared to 44 % of recipients aged 1–11 years and 54 % of children aged ≥12 years at the time of transplantation). Lower rates are also reported in living related lobar transplant recipients [6]. It is important to note that registry data are based on fulfilling BOS grade 1, not the expanded criteria including the earlier grade 0p; therefore, true incidence may be underestimated.

These lower rates in infants are intriguing and match similar reduced rejection rates seen in infant recipients of cardiac or liver grafts. This may reflect the potential benefit of transplantation early in life during a period of relative immune system immaturity. The explanation for this lower incidence of chronic rejection has yet to be fully understood, but successful ABO-incompatible heart (and subsequently lung) transplantation has also been demonstrated in this age group. ABO-incompatible infant heart transplantation is now an established procedure across multiple centers, and survival outcomes are comparable to those achieved in ABO-compatible subjects [7]. The first ABO-incompatible infant lung transplant described in the literature was recently performed in Toronto, Canada [8]. The lack of anti-graft antibodies in these infants is thought to be due to several factors, including acquired donor-specific B-cell tolerance from persistent exposure to donor antigens during this immunological window [9], development of graft cellular resistance to humoral injury [10], or reduced antibody-binding effectiveness to donor cells allowing accommodation [11].

Risk Factors

Technical Factors

Although the transplant procedure used in children is very similar to that used in adults, one notable difference is that cardiopulmonary bypass (CPB) is more commonly used in children [12]. CPB has been reported to be an independent risk factor for primary graft dysfunction (PGD) [13]. However, direct comparison of PGD incidence between adult and pediatric cohorts at a single center failed to document a significant difference [14], and the significance of this increased use of CPB remains unclear. BOS incidence is recognized to increase with PGD severity [15]. Nonetheless, despite the greater technical challenge of performing the operation in smaller children and infants, the authors are not aware of any data suggesting that ischemia time is longer in the pediatric and infant age range than it is in adults.

Acute Rejection Episodes

Adult data have demonstrated that a single episode of minimal acute cellular rejection (grade A1) is a significant independent predictor of BOS at 3 years post-transplant [16, 17], but this is not reflected in the pediatric data that are available to date. In a retrospective multicenter analysis of 383 subjects across 14 European and North American sites (age less than 21 years), Benden et al. found no documented increase in the early risk of BOS (within the first year post-transplant) in subjects suffering either a single or repeat A1 episode. However, a single A2 episode doubled subsequent early BOS risk [18].

Gastroesophageal Reflux Disease

Adult series have shown that gastroesophageal reflux disease (GERD) is common in recipients and associated with both increased frequency and earlier onset of acute rejection [19] as well as lower subsequent lung function [20]. Additionally, GERD has been shown to be a significant independent risk factor for BO, especially if nonacid reflux is present [21]. In a series of 59 adult transplant recipients screened for GERD using impedance/pH monitoring, 65 % had abnormal acid reflux and 27 % had abnormal nonacid reflux with a hazard ratio of 2.8 between nonacid reflux and BOS. Initial published pediatric data suggest that GERD is a significant issue post-transplantation in children as well. A protocol has been in place at our hospital since 2002 to screen all pediatric lung transplant recipients within the first 3–6 months for GERD, initially using pH studies and more recently by including impedance monitoring. In a small case series published in 2005, asymptomatic abnormal acid reflux was found in a high proportion of children (nine of ten cases screened) and tended to be moderate to severe in intensity (seven of nine cases) [22]. Of these ten cases, three had episodes of acute rejection, and all three of these children had moderate to severe GERD on pH probe screening.

Increased Role of Viral Infections

Community-acquired respiratory viral infections (CARV) such as respiratory syncytial virus (RSV), human metapneumovirus, parainfluenza, and influenza are risk factors for acute rejection, development of BOS, and death from BOS in adult lung transplant cohorts [23, 24]. CARV are common in the pediatric age range, especially during the infant and preschool years. In a recent multicenter study of 576 pediatric lung transplant recipients between 1988 and 2005 across 14 centers in the United States and Europe, younger age was associated with shorter time to an episode of CARV, and the occurrence of CARVs was independently associated with decreased 1-year survival (hazard ratio 2.6, 95 % confidence interval 1.6–4.4) [25]. No association with acute rejection episodes was demonstrated within this large pediatric cohort. The relative impact of CARV on pediatric lung transplant outcomes is now the focus of a prospective, current National Institutes of Health (NIH)-funded multicenter study, and the results of this investigation are eagerly awaited.

The lower incidence of recipient CMV exposure in the pediatric age range increases the risk of CMV mismatch at the time of transplant. CMV is the most common opportunistic infection encountered post-lung transplantation and is a well-recognized risk factor for chronic graft dysfunction [26]. CMV prophylaxis has been shown to reduce the incidence of BOS in adults in the first year post-transplantation [27]. Recently, chronic EBV viremia has been linked with BOS development within a lung transplant cohort [28]. Previous EBV exposure at the time of transplantation is less common in the pediatric population, with half of all 5-year-old children having been exposed compared to 90–95 % of adults in the United States [29].

Age of Donor

Almost two-thirds of pediatric transplant recipients (based on collated data over a 15-year period between 1986 and 2010) received organs from pediatric donors, although geographical variation exists, ranging from 45 % in Europe to 64 % in

North America. Only 6 % of children received organs from donors aged over 50 years over the same time period [1]. Survival benefits may be present if pediatric donors are used, and decreased survival has been suggested with increasing donor age. In a study of 37 pediatric lung transplant recipients by Cano et al., survival rates were worse in those receiving a graft from a donor aged over 16 years: 1-, 3-, 5-, and 10-year survival was 33 %, 25 %, 12.5 %, and 12.5 % compared to 76 %, 67 %, 56 %, and 49 %, respectively, in those receiving organs from donors aged less than 16 years ($p=0.005$) [30]. Adult studies have tended to focus on the survival impact of much older donors, and lower rates of survival (16 % vs. 39 % at 10 years, $p=0.07$) and higher relative BOS rates (65 % vs. 34 % at 10 years, $p=0.01$) have been described in adult cohorts with use of organs from donors aged over 60 years as compared to donors aged less than 60 [31].

Diagnostic Challenges of Bronchiolitis Obliterans in Children

Transbronchial Biopsy

Regular bronchoscopy with transbronchial biopsy is an integral component of surveillance of lung transplant recipients, as it can detect both acute rejection and respiratory infection. When suspicious symptoms are present, this investigation is clinically indicated and uncontroversial, but the optimal frequency and duration of surveillance bronchoscopy (i.e., in asymptomatic individuals) remains unclear. At Great Ormond Street Hospital, surveillance biopsies are performed at 1 week and at 1, 3, 6, and 12 months post-transplantation. An evaluation of this approach was published by Benden et al. in 2007, and, in our opinion, the use of surveillance bronchoscopy is supported. Asymptomatic rejection (≥A2) and symptomatic rejection were detected in 4 % and 12 % of biopsies, respectively. In addition, potential pathogens were detected in 29 % of asymptomatic and 69 % of symptomatic children, and the overall diagnostic yield was 35 % for asymptomatic children and 85 % for children with respiratory symptoms [32]. Detection of clinically silent acute cellular rejection (ACR) in the initial post-lung transplant period has also been described in other pediatric populations [33].

Challenges specific to pediatric subjects relate to the size of instruments that can be used for transbronchial biopsy and the challenge of getting adequate samples for processing and grading. Broadly speaking, there are two different transbronchial biopsy forcep options for use in the pediatric age range: radial jaw forceps with a cup volume of 2.0 μL, which can fit down a 2-mm working channel; and smooth oval cup forceps with a cup volume of 0.5 μL, which can be used with a 1.2-mm working channel. The smallest flexible bronchoscopes currently available with 2.0- and 1.2-mm working channels have an outer diameter of 4.0 mm and 2.8 mm, respectively, although actual diameter of a 4.0-mm scope is 4.4 mm beyond the tip. Flexible bronchoscopes can also vary significantly from the manufacturers specifications [34]. Obtaining adequate samples is challenging with smaller instruments. In a retrospective analysis at one institution, adequate samples were obtained in 97 % and 84 % of specimens collected with the radial and oval cup forcep equipment set-ups, respectively, defined as a minimum of five alveolar tissue fragments or if a specific diagnosis (i.e., treatable grade of ACR or infection) was possible [35]. The presence of bronchial tissue for B grading of biopsies for ACR was not assessed in this study. The overall complication rate (bleeding >150 mL, bleeding that required a transfusion, pneumothorax, or septicemia) was 2 %, which is consistent with complication rates quoted in the adult literature.

The actual number of biopsies taken in each patient to obtain at least five adequate samples was not outlined, but studies in adult recipients have shown that taking 10–12 tissue fragments via transbronchial biopsy yields an average of six acceptable fragments of alveolated lung parenchyma, which meets the Lung Rejection Study Group recommendations of retrieving at least five pieces of lung 98 % of the time (with only 3.6 % of subjects not having adequate bronchial wall for histological staging of bronchial inflammation) [36]. The reported complication rate was 6 %, although the pediatric complication rate is felt to be lower, which may reflect that, in general, fewer biopsies are taken in pediatric recipients (typically five to six per subject at our center).

The earlier practice of performing bronchoscopy and transbronchial biopsy under heavy sedation with midazolam and fentanyl plus topical lidocaine [35] is now far less common. The majority of centers (including our own) now perform these procedures under general anesthesia with fluoroscopic guidance. In cases where transbronchial biopsy is not felt to be adequate, either open lung biopsy or video-assisted thoracoscopic surgical (VATS) lung biopsy is considered. However, even open lung biopsy may not be 100 % diagnostic [37]. It should be noted that transbronchial biopsy cannot be employed to diagnose BO. If histological confirmation of this diagnosis is required, a more invasive procedure is mandated.

Diagnosis of Bronchiolitis Obliterans Syndrome

As outlined elsewhere in this book, clinical diagnostic criteria for chronic allograft dysfunction have been developed due to the patchiness of the disease process and the relative insensitivity of transbronchial biopsy. Although raw (or actual) values for spirometry test results are commonly used for adults, this is inappropriate in children. Specifically, the challenge within the pediatric population is that somatic growth is an ongoing process, and measures of lung function need to take account of concurrent changes in lung volume and airway caliber.

The issue of whether transplanted lungs will continue to grow in proportion to ongoing somatic growth is unique to pediatrics, and the question remains unanswered. The available evidence suggests that the transplantation of immature or mature lungs into children allows continued growth and alveolarization in line with somatic growth. Infant lung function studies and studies using CT scanning to directly measure airway dimensions suggest that transplanted lungs continue to grow over time. However, while increases in forced expiratory volume values provide information about increase in lung size (and probably airway size), whether continuing alveolarization actually occurs remains unclear. Data from transplantation of mature single lobes from living related donors into pediatric recipients suggest that increase in lung size occurs by alveolar distension rather than increase in alveolar numbers [38].

For physiological monitoring of lung allograft function in the pediatric age range, it is recommended that all spirometry outcomes be converted to percent predicted values or standard deviation scores using recognized reference equations. This was recommended in the 2001 update to the BOS diagnosis guidelines [39], but, anecdotally, this recommendation is not universally applied, particularly in adult institutions that primarily perform transplants on adult patients but also care for a smaller number of pediatric patients (who are typically in the adolescent age range). The impact of using percent predicted values (instead of raw values) for the baseline lung function (maximum post-transplant FEV_1 value) achieved and for establishing the subsequent incidence and time to detection of BOS remains unclear. Baseline lung function in the growing child may take a number of years to be achieved, in contrast to adults, where baseline values are typically reached within the first year. A large number of reference equations are available for use in the pediatric age range, but many are based on cohorts measured a number of decades ago and may no longer represent contemporary values that are predictive of normal lung function. Additionally, due to varying numbers of subjects at outlying ages included in these data, these predicted values may not be accurate in younger children. Recently "all age" reference equations have been produced by collating a number of these data sets together to produce optimized reference data that are applicable down to age 4 years [40, 41]. However, the lack of appropriate reference data for infant lung function remains a concern, and until this is addressed, the clinical utility of lung function in this age range remains unclear [42].

Further difficulty may be encountered due to variable lung function technique, and the majority of pediatric lung function laboratories may not establish adequately reproducible techniques until age 6–7 years. Spirometry in the preschool age range has excellent feasibility in specialty centers, but this requires modification of existing quality control criteria. These include use of $FEV_{0.5}$ rather than FEV_1, volume of back extrapolation to determine start of test, and repeatability criteria of two FVCs within 10 % of each other. Feasibility rates of 75 % have been reported amongst preschoolers [43]. However effort-dependent measures such as peak expiratory flow rate are not used for monitoring purposes in the pediatric age range.

The recent incorporation of FEF_{25-75} criteria into early BOS (BOS 0p) appears to be applicable to recipients in the pediatric age range as well, with initial data supporting a role in earlier detection. Woo et al. reviewed the post-transplant lung function changes in 18 pediatric subjects (aged 14.1 ± 3.7 years) who subsequently met the current BOS 1 criteria (FEV_1 decrease of 20 % from baseline) and found that when compared to changes in other parameters such as FEF_{25-75} and V_{max} at 60 %, 70 %, and 80 % from post-transplant baseline, FEV_1 was the first abnormality detected in only 39 %, while a decline in FEF_{25-75} of >30 % was the primary abnormality in 78 % [44].

Other potential markers for chronic allograft dysfunction exist, but clinical utility has yet to be established. Tidal breathing lung function tests, such as the forced oscillation technique and inert gas washout [45], have strong feasibility across the pediatric age range but have not been systematically evaluated to date. Air trapping or mosaic pattern on expiratory slice HRCT is a marker of small airway disease, but studies have yet to demonstrate strong clinical utility in BOS surveillance due to poor specificity despite reports of good sensitivity [46]. Concerns about the cumulative radiation dose associated with surveillance CT scanning protocols are less relevant in a population with shortened life expectancy. However, relative radiation risk is inversely proportional to age and highest in infancy [47]. Therefore, risk of cumulative radiation exposure needs to be taken into account. Ventilation perfusion (V/Q) scans are also feasible in children and have some evidence for utility in monitoring lung disease in conditions such as cystic fibrosis (CF) [48], but utility of V/Q scanning in monitoring for BO following lung transplantation is unclear. KL-6, a glycoprotein expressed on type 2 pneumocytes, is detectable in higher concentrations in the serum of pediatric BOS subjects ($n=9$ mean [SD] KL-6 596 [309] vs. $n=36$ non-BOS KL-6 352 [140] U/mL [$p=0.05$]) [49], and the relative sensitivity to detect BOS if a threshold of 200 U/mL elevation from baseline was 67 % with a specificity of 95 %. No increases in KL-6 were seen during acute rejection episodes. Although the authors felt that KL-6 was a relatively specific marker of BOS, further studies are warranted, and use of KL-6 as a biomarker of BOS remains a research tool at present.

Exhaled nitric oxide (eNO) has been proposed as a sensitive measure of acute post-transplant complications, such as acute rejection [50] and infection. However, the evidence for utility of eNO for detection of BOS in adults is conflicting. Although Silkoff et al. found no elevation in eNO levels, a subsequent study by Verleden et al. described increased eNO levels in BOS and potential utility of eNO as an early diagnostic measure due to the observation that eNO was elevated mean (SD) 263 (169) days before a formal diagnosis of BOS was made using the FEV_1 diagnostic criteria for BOS stage 1 [51]. No pediatric-based biomarker studies have been published to date.

Management

Management of pediatric BOS is extrapolated from adult data, and there is no current evidence to suggest that the underlying disease process fundamentally differs from that seen in the adult transplant population.

Augmentation of immunosuppression is controversial and should only be attempted if there is evidence of under-immunosuppression (e.g., through repeated ACR episodes), because the disadvantage of increased infections is likely to outweigh any benefit. Experience with sirolimus or everolimus is increasing, but use of these agents within the pediatric population remains limited according to registry data. Azithromycin is well tolerated within the pediatric population, and it tends to be started once children fulfill BOS diagnostic criteria due to the beneficial results that have been described in adult transplant BOS populations. The characteristics of pediatric responders have not been described to date, and it is unknown whether the benefits of early commencement of azithromycin therapy during BOS stage 0p [52] or in those with neutrophilic airway inflammation are also present in younger subjects. Montelukast, which has been suggested to be beneficial in recipients with BOS stage 2 who lack significant BAL neutrophilia (either on or off azithromycin therapy) [53], is also readily available for administration to recipients in the pediatric age range, both as granules for children aged less than 2 years and as chewable tablets for older children.

Increased use of statins in pediatric patients has been triggered by adult data describing an association with reduced acute rejection rates [54] and delayed progression to chronic kidney disease [55]. Statins are generally well tolerated by recipients in the pediatric age range, although pediatric-specific data showing benefit are lacking. Pediatric guidelines for familial hyperlipidemia recommend that statins should not be used in children until they have attained Tanner stage II or higher in pubertal development [56].

Other therapeutic options include fundoplication and total lymphoid irradiation (TLI), and gastric fundoplication has been shown to improve lung function in adult cohorts when GERD is present [57]. Although fundoplication is feasible in children, it is unclear from currently available, published pediatric data whether fundoplication can lead to improved pulmonary outcomes and lower BOS rates [58]. Published experience with TLI is limited to the adult transplant literature, although TLI has been used at our own center in children with BOS with varying success.

Outcomes for re-transplantation for pediatric BOS were analyzed in the ISHLT registry report in 2011. Half of the 105 pediatric re-transplantation procedures were for BOS, and almost three-quarters were performed in older pediatric subjects (aged ≥12 years). Re-transplantation is slightly more common in North American transplant centers, but it still only accounts for 3–7 % of annual pediatric transplants. Overall survival is inferior to that for first-time transplants, with 1- and 5-year survival at only 63 % and 38 %, respectively, and it does not differ when re-transplant is performed for BOS vs. non-BOS indications [1]. The ethics of re-transplantation in a climate of limited availability of suitable pediatric donor organs, given the inferior survival statistics, will continue to be debated.

Preventative measures include screening for GERD at an early stage post-transplantation, early commencement of azithromycin once diagnostic criteria for BOS are fulfilled, and avoidance of associated risk factors such as viral and bacterial infections. Recipients are asked to avoid day-care facilities when respiratory viral infection rates are high and should have annual flu vaccination. A causative role for bacterial infection in development of BO remains controversial, but the two often coexist, and most centers treat bacterial infections aggressively. Post-transplant treatment of CF paranasal sinus disease to decrease contamination of the lower airways has been described. Initial data suggest that a reduced incidence of BOS may be possible, but adequately powered studies need to be performed before it can be accepted as an essential component of routine management.

Conclusion

Most aspects of prevention, detection, and treatment of BO in children are the same as for adults. Given the small number of children transplanted every year, extrapolation from adult practice to pediatric practice is inevitable and appropriate. Modifications to monitoring protocols, particularly with regard to lung function and bronchoscopic biopsy, are required.

References

1. Benden C, Aurora P, Edwards LB, Kucheryavaya AY, Christie JD, Dobbels F, et al. The Registry of the International Society for Heart and Lung Transplantation: Fourteenth pediatric lung and heart-lung transplantation report–2011. J Heart Lung Transplant. 2011;30(10):1123–32.
2. Aurora P, Edwards LB, Kucheryavaya AY, Christie JD, Dobbels F, Kirk R, et al. The Registry of the International Society for Heart and Lung Transplantation: Thirteenth official pediatric lung and heart-lung transplantation report–2010. J Heart Lung Transplant. 2010;29(10):1129–41.
3. Nevins TE. Non-compliance and its management in teenagers. Pediatr Transplant. 2002;6(6): 475–9.
4. Shellmer DA, Dabbs AD, Dew MA. Medical adherence in pediatric organ transplantation: what are the next steps? Curr Opin Organ Transplant. 2011;16(5):509–14.
5. Christie JD, Edwards LB, Kucheryavaya AY, Benden C, Dobbels F, Kirk R, et al. The registry of the International Society for Heart and Lung Transplantation: Twenty-eighth adult lung and heart-lung transplant report–2011. J Heart Lung Transplant. 2011;30(10):1104–22.
6. Woo MS, MacLaughlin EF, Horn MV, Szmuszkovicz JR, Barr ML, Starnes VA. Bronchiolitis obliterans is not the primary cause of death in pediatric living donor lobar lung transplant recipients. J Heart Lung Transplant. 2001;20(5):491–6.
7. Dipchand AI, Pollock BarZiv SM, Manlhiot C, West LJ, VanderVliet M, et al. Equivalent outcomes for pediatric heart transplantation recipients: ABO-blood group incompatible versus ABO-compatible. Am J Transplant. 2010;10(2):389–97.
8. Grasemann H, de Perrot M, Bendiak GN, Cox P, van Arsdell GS, Keshavjee S, et al. ABO-incompatible lung transplantation in an infant. Am J Transplant. 2012;12(3):779–81.
9. Fan X, Ang A, Pollock-Barziv SM, Dipchand AI, Ruiz P, Wilson G, et al. Donor-specific B-cell tolerance after ABO-incompatible infant heart transplantation. Nat Med. 2004;10(11): 1227–33.
10. Takahashi K. Accommodation in ABO-incompatible kidney transplantation: why do kidney grafts survive? Transplant Proc. 2004;36(2 Suppl):193S–6.
11. Ishida H, Tanabe K, Ishizuka T, Furusawa M, Miyamoto N, Ishikawa N, et al. The mechanism responsible for accommodation after living-related kidney transplantations across the blood barrier. Transpl Int. 2005;18(6):716–20.
12. Sweet SC. Pediatric lung transplantation. Proc Am Thorac Soc. 2009;6(1):122–7.
13. Barr ML, Kawut SM, Whelan TP, Girgis R, Bottcher H, Sonett J, et al. Report of the ISHLT Working Group on primary lung graft dysfunction part IV: recipient-related risk factors and markers. J Heart Lung Transplant. 2005;24(10):1468–82.
14. Meyers BF, de la Morena M, Sweet SC, Trulock EP, Guthrie TJ, Mendeloff EN, et al. Primary graft dysfunction and other selected complications of lung transplantation: a single-center experience of 983 patients. J Thorac Cardiovasc Surg. 2005;129(6):1421–9.
15. Daud SA, Yusen RD, Meyers BF, Chakinala MM, Walter MJ, Aloush AA, et al. Impact of immediate primary lung allograft dysfunction on bronchiolitis obliterans syndrome. Am J Respir Crit Care Med. 2007;175(5):507–13.

16. Hachem RR, Khalifah AP, Chakinala MM, Yusen RD, Aloush AA, Mohanakumar T, et al. The significance of a single episode of minimal acute rejection after lung transplantation. Transplantation. 2005;80(10):1406–13.
17. Hopkins PM, Aboyoun CL, Chhajed PN, Malouf MA, Plit ML, Rainer SP, et al. Association of minimal rejection in lung transplant recipients with obliterative bronchiolitis. Am J Respir Crit Care Med. 2004;170(9):1022–6.
18. Benden C, Faro A, Worley S, Arrigain S, Aurora P, Ballmann M, et al. Minimal acute rejection in pediatric lung transplantation–does it matter? Pediatr Transplant. 2010;14(4):534–9.
19. Shah N, Force SD, Mitchell PO, Lin E, Lawrence EC, Easley K, et al. Gastroesophageal reflux disease is associated with an increased rate of acute rejection in lung transplant allografts. Transplant Proc. 2010;42(7):2702–6.
20. Hadjiliadis D, Duane Davis R, Steele MP, Messier RH, Lau CL, Eubanks SS, et al. Gastroesophageal reflux disease in lung transplant recipients. Clin Transplant. 2003;17(4): 363–8.
21. King BJ, Iyer H, Leidi AA, Carby MR. Gastroesophageal reflux in bronchiolitis obliterans syndrome: a new perspective. J Heart Lung Transplant. 2009;28(9):870–5.
22. Benden C, Aurora P, Curry J, Whitmore P, Priestley L, Elliott MJ. High prevalence of gastroesophageal reflux in children after lung transplantation. Pediatr Pulmonol. 2005;40(1):68–71.
23. Khalifah AP, Hachem RR, Chakinala MM, Schechtman KB, Patterson GA, Schuster DP, et al. Respiratory viral infections are a distinct risk for bronchiolitis obliterans syndrome and death. Am J Respir Crit Care Med. 2004;170(2):181–7.
24. Kumar D, Erdman D, Keshavjee S, Peret T, Tellier R, Hadjiliadis D, et al. Clinical impact of community-acquired respiratory viruses on bronchiolitis obliterans after lung transplant. Am J Transplant. 2005;5(8):2031–6.
25. Liu M, Worley S, Arrigain S, Aurora P, Ballmann M, Boyer D, et al. Respiratory viral infections within one year after pediatric lung transplant. Transpl Infect Dis. 2009;11(4):304–12.
26. Patel N, Snyder LD, Finlen-Copeland A, Palmer SM. Is prevention the best treatment? CMV after lung transplantation. Am J Transplant. 2012;12(3):539–44.
27. Duncan SR, Grgurich WF, Iacono AT, Burckart GJ, Yousem SA, Paradis IL, et al. A comparison of ganciclovir and acyclovir to prevent cytomegalovirus after lung transplantation. Am J Respir Crit Care Med. 1994;150(1):146–52.
28. Engelmann I, Welte T, Fuhner T, Simon AR, Mattner F, Hoy L, et al. Detection of Epstein-Barr virus DNA in peripheral blood is associated with the development of bronchiolitis obliterans syndrome after lung transplantation. J Clin Virol. 2009;45(1):47–53.
29. Epstein-Barr Virus and Infectious Mononucleosis. National Center for Infectious Diseases [1st May 2012]. http://www.cdc.gov/ncidod/diseases/ebv.htm.
30. Cano JR, Cerezo F, Algar FJ, Alvarez A, Espinosa D, Moreno P, et al. Prognostic factors influencing survival rates in children following lung transplantation. Transplant Proc. 2008;40(9):3070–2.
31. De Perrot M, Waddell TK, Shargall Y, Pierre AF, Fadel E, Uy K, et al. Impact of donors aged 60 years or more on outcome after lung transplantation: results of an 11-year single-center experience. J Thorac Cardiovasc Surg. 2007;133(2):525–31.
32. Benden C, Harpur-Sinclair O, Ranasinghe AS, Hartley JC, Elliott MJ, Aurora P. Surveillance bronchoscopy in children during the first year after lung transplantation: is it worth it? Thorax. 2007;62(1):57–61.
33. Faro A, Visner G. The use of multiple transbronchial biopsies as the standard approach to evaluate lung allograft rejection. Pediatr Transplant. 2004;8(4):322–8.
34. Linnane B, Hafen GM, Ranganathan SC. Diameter of pediatric sized flexible bronchoscopes: when size matters. Pediatr Pulmonol. 2006;41(8):787–9.
35. Visner GA, Faro A, Zander DS. Role of transbronchial biopsies in pediatric lung diseases. Chest. 2004;126(1):273–80.
36. Hopkins PM, Aboyoun CL, Chhajed PN, Malouf MA, Plit ML, Rainer SP, et al. Prospective analysis of 1,235 transbronchial lung biopsies in lung transplant recipients. J Heart Lung Transplant. 2002;21(10):1062–7.

37. Weill D, McGiffin DC, Zorn Jr GL, Alexander CB, Early LJ, Kirklin JK, et al. The utility of open lung biopsy following lung transplantation. J Heart Lung Transplant. 2000;19(9):852–7.
38. Sritippayawan S, Keens TG, Horn MV, MacLaughlin EF, Barr ML, Starnes VA, et al. Does lung growth occur when mature lobes are transplanted into children? Pediatr Transplant. 2002;6(6):500–4.
39. Estenne M, Maurer JR, Boehler A, Egan JJ, Frost A, Hertz M, et al. Bronchiolitis obliterans syndrome 2001: an update of the diagnostic criteria. J Heart Lung Transplant. 2002;21(3):297–310.
40. Stanojevic S, Wade A, Cole TJ, Lum S, Custovic A, Silverman M, et al. Spirometry centile charts for young Caucasian children: the asthma UK collaborative initiative. Am J Respir Crit Care Med. 2009;180(6):547–52.
41. Stanojevic S, Wade A, Stocks J, Hankinson J, Coates AL, Pan H, et al. Reference ranges for spirometry across all ages: a new approach. Am J Respir Crit Care Med. 2008;177(3):253–60.
42. Stocks J, Modi N, Tepper R. Need for healthy control subjects when assessing lung function in infants with respiratory disease. Am J Respir Crit Care Med. 2010;182(11):1340–2.
43. Aurora P, Stocks J, Oliver C, Saunders C, Castle R, Chaziparasidis G, et al. Quality control for spirometry in preschool children with and without lung disease. Am J Respir Crit Care Med. 2004;169(10):1152–9.
44. Sritippayawan S, Keens TG, Horn MV, Starnes VA, Woo MS. What are the best pulmonary function test parameters for early detection of post-lung transplant bronchiolitis obliterans syndrome in children? Pediatr Transplant. 2003;7(3):200–3.
45. Beydon N, Davis SD, Lombardi E, Allen JL, Arets HG, Aurora P, et al. An official American thoracic society/European respiratory society statement: pulmonary function testing in preschool children. Am J Respir Crit Care Med. 2007;175(12):1304–45.
46. Cook RC, Fradet G, Muller NL, Worsely DF, Ostrow D, Levy RD. Noninvasive investigations for the early detection of chronic airways dysfunction following lung transplantation. Can Respir J. 2003;10(2):76–83.
47. Brenner DJ, Hall EJ. Computed tomography: an increasing source of radiation exposure. N Engl J Med. 2007;357(22):2277–84.
48. Jaffe A, Hamutcu R, Dhawan RT, Adler B, Rosenthal M, Bush A. Routine ventilation scans in children with cystic fibrosis: diagnostic usefulness and prognostic value. Eur J Nucl Med. 2001;28(9):1313–8.
49. Haberman B, Doan ML, Smith EO, Schecter MG, Mallory GB, Elidemir O. Serum KL-6 level and the development of bronchiolitis obliterans syndrome in lung transplant recipients. Pediatr Transplant. 2010;14(7):903–8.
50. Silkoff PE, Caramori M, Tremblay L, McClean P, Chaparro C, Kesten S, et al. Exhaled nitric oxide in human lung transplantation. A noninvasive marker of acute rejection. Am J Respir Crit Care Med. 1998;157(6 Pt 1):1822–8.
51. Verleden GM, Dupont LJ, Van Raemdonck DE, Vanhaecke J. Accuracy of exhaled nitric oxide measurements for the diagnosis of bronchiolitis obliterans syndrome after lung transplantation. Transplantation. 2004;78(5):730–3.
52. Federica M, Nadia S, Monica M, Alessandro C, Tiberio O, Francesco B, et al. Clinical and immunological evaluation of 12-month azithromycin therapy in chronic lung allograft rejection. Clin Transplant. 2011;25(4):E381–9.
53. Verleden GM, Verleden SE, Vos R, De Vleeschauwer SI, Dupont LJ, Van Raemdonck DE, et al. Montelukast for bronchiolitis obliterans syndrome after lung transplantation: a pilot study. Transpl Int. 2011;24(7):651–6.
54. Johnson BA, Iacono AT, Zeevi A, McCurry KR, Duncan SR. Statin use is associated with improved function and survival of lung allografts. Am J Respir Crit Care Med. 2003;167(9):1271–8.
55. Fried LF, Orchard TJ, Kasiske BL. Effect of lipid reduction on the progression of renal disease: a meta-analysis. Kidney Int. 2001;59(1):260–9.

56. McCrindle BW, Urbina EM, Dennison BA, Jacobson MS, Steinberger J, Rocchini AP, et al. Drug therapy of high-risk lipid abnormalities in children and adolescents: a scientific statement from the American Heart Association Atherosclerosis, Hypertension, and Obesity in Youth Committee, Council of Cardiovascular Disease in the young, with the Council on Cardiovascular Nursing. Circulation. 2007;115(14):1948–67.
57. Davis Jr RD, Lau CL, Eubanks S, Messier RH, Hadjiliadis D, Steele MP, et al. Improved lung allograft function after fundoplication in patients with gastroesophageal reflux disease undergoing lung transplantation. J Thorac Cardiovasc Surg. 2003;125(3):533–42.
58. Zheng C, Kane TD, Kurland G, Irlano K, Spahr J, Potoka DA, et al. Feasibility of laparoscopic Nissen fundoplication after pediatric lung or heart-lung transplantation: should this be the standard? Surg Endosc. 2011;25(1):249–54.

Chapter 14
Immunosuppression for the Prevention and Treatment of BOS

Sangeeta M. Bhorade

Abstract Over the past 3 decades, lung transplantation has evolved into a life-saving procedure for patients with end-stage lung disease. During this time, further development of biologic agents and newer immunosuppressive agents has continued to improve outcomes after transplantation. Although there is variability among centers regarding specific immunosuppressive medications, the overall approach to immunosuppressive regimens in lung transplantation is quite uniform and consists of a triple-drug immunosuppressive regimen that includes a calcineurin inhibitor, an antimetabolite, and corticosteroids (CS), with or without a biological agent as induction therapy. However, the discovery and continued development of new immunosuppressive agents that target novel immune pathways provide alternate therapeutic options for lung recipients with progressive decline in pulmonary function. The current goal of immunosuppression is to maintain allograft viability by preventing acute and chronic rejection while decreasing toxicities associated with immunosuppression. This chapter will review the current approach to immunosuppressive medications that are used in the maintenance of allograft stability and the prevention and treatment of bronchiolitis obliterans syndrome (BOS).

Keywords Cyclosporine • Tacrolimus • Azathioprine • Mycophenolate mofetil • Corticosteroids • Thymoglobulin • Basiliximab • Alemtuzumab • Rituximab • Bortezomib • Belatacept • Lung transplant • Bronchiolitis obliterans syndrome

S.M. Bhorade, M.D. (✉)
University of Chicago Medical Center, 5841 S. Maryland Ave., MC0999, Chicago, IL 60637, USA
e-mail: sbhorade@medicine.bsd.uchicago.edu

K.C. Meyer and A.R. Glanville (eds.), *Bronchiolitis Obliterans Syndrome in Lung Transplantation*, Respiratory Medicine 8, DOI 10.1007/978-1-4614-7636-8_14,

Introduction

Lung transplantation has evolved into a life-saving procedure for patients with advanced lung disease. Since the first lung transplant, which was performed in 1963 by Dr. James Hardy, the success of long-term survival after lung transplantation has been largely due to the discovery of more potent immunosuppressive medications. Corticosteroids (CS) and azathioprine (AZA) were the initial primary immunosuppressive agents that were used in lung transplantation between the 1960s until the 1980s. During this time, survival after lung transplantation was limited owing to poor bronchial anastomotic healing and persistent rejection with graft loss. The discovery of cyclosporine A (CsA) in the 1980s significantly improved success rates after lung transplantation. Over the past 3 decades, further development of biologic agents and newer immunosuppressive agents has continued to improve outcomes after transplantation.

The ultimate goal of immunosuppression is to enable the recipient's immune system to develop and maintain tolerance to the lung allograft. Unfortunately, this goal has not quite been attained, as can be seen by the high incidence of chronic rejection or bronchiolitis obliterans syndrome (BOS) after lung transplantation. As a result, the current goal of immunosuppression is to maintain allograft viability by preventing acute and chronic rejection while decreasing toxicities associated with immunosuppression. Current immunosuppressive therapies target multiple pathways involved in the alloimmune response to the allograft.

Although there is variability among centers regarding specific immunosuppressive medications, the overall approach to immunosuppressive regimens in lung transplantation is quite uniform. Specifically, a triple immunosuppressive drug regimen consisting of a calcineurin inhibitor, antimetabolite, and CS is administered life-long in lung transplant recipients. In addition, per the International Society of Heart and Lung Transplant (ISHLT) registry, approximately 55 % of lung transplant recipients receive induction therapy with a biological agent that is administered at the time of transplantation in order to augment immunosuppression early after transplantation [1]. This chapter will review the current approach to immunosuppressive medications that are used in the maintenance of allograft stability and the prevention and treatment of BOS.

Maintenance Immunosuppression

Calcineurin Inhibitors

Cyclosporine A

Cyclosporine A (CsA) is a natural, highly aliphatic cyclic compound that was initially isolated from the fungus *Trichoderma polysporum Rifai* in 1979 [2]. In 1983 Dr. Joel Cooper and his colleagues at the University of Toronto performed the first single-lung transplant with the use of a CsA-based immunosuppressive regimen. This patient survived 6 years and revolutionized the success of lung transplantation.

Cyclosporine A is a potent inhibitor of T-cell activation and proliferation. Cyclosporine A binds to cyclophilin, an immunophilin that engages and inhibits calcineurin, a calcium-dependent phosphatase. Calcineurin inhibition decreases activation of several transcription factors, including the nuclear factor of activated T cells (NFAT). Therefore, CsA arrests the lymphocyte cell cycle in the early phase of activation (G0–G1 phase). Inhibition of NFAT blocks transcription of other cytokine growth factors, including IL-2, as well as co-stimulatory molecules, including CD40 ligand. Decreased elaboration of cytokines and growth factors subsequently leads to decreased antigen recognition and decreased clonal expansion of lymphocytes [3].

The unique structure of CsA impacts upon its delivery system, its absorptive properties, and dosing regimens. The chemical structure of CsA, specifically its aqueous insolubility, has made reliable formulations and delivery systems of CsA more complicated. As a result, there is significant variability in intra- and interindividual absorption of CsA. Cyclosporine A is administered either orally or intravenously. The initial oral formulation was an oil-based formulation (Sandimmune, Novartis, New York, NY, USA) that resulted in variable absorption due to dependence on bile flow and the timing and nature of oral intake. In addition, certain patient populations, including cystic fibrosis patients, African Americans, and diabetics, tend to absorb this agent erratically. A newer microemulsion formulation, Neoral (Novartis, New York, NY, USA) has improved bioavailability with more rapid absorption [4, 5]. Given the variability in absorption, different CsA formulations should not be interchanged. If one formulation is substituted for another, careful monitoring of therapeutic drug levels is necessary to ensure appropriate dosing.

The efficacy and safety profile of CsA correlate best with the total drug exposure as measured by area under the curve (AUC). However, due to the cumbersome technique of obtaining AUC, most transplant programs previously measured 12-h trough levels. Unfortunately, trough levels have been shown to correlate poorly with systemic exposure to CsA [6]. Instead, CsA levels drawn at 2 or 3 h post-dose (C2 and C3, respectively) are highly predictive to estimate the exposure to CsA over time [7]. A recent study comparing 50 lung transplant recipients with C2 monitoring to a group of historical control patients with trough monitoring revealed lower rates of acute and chronic rejection and improved renal function in the C2 monitoring group [8].

Aerosolization of CsA was initially proposed in order to increase drug delivery directly to the lung parenchyma while minimizing systemic toxicity. Initial studies showed that the use of inhaled CsA improved refractory acute rejection and was associated with a trend toward improved survival [9, 10]. A single-center, randomized, double-blind, placebo-controlled trial compared the addition of inhaled CsA to placebo to standard immunosuppression in lung transplant recipients. The study showed no difference in acute rejection rates but did show an improvement in overall survival as well as chronic rejection-free survival at 3 years after transplantation. This study prompted a larger, randomized, placebo-controlled, multicenter trial in order to confirm these results. Two hundred eighty-four patients from 19 lung transplant centers were randomized to either inhaled CsA or placebo in addition to standard immunosuppression. Unfortunately, preliminary results from this study did not show a significant difference in BOS-free survival (hazard ratio (HR) = 1.32; confidence interval (CI): 0.86–2.04; $p = 0.23$) or all-cause mortality (HR = 1.39; CI: 0.73–2.65; $p = 0.42$) between the two groups [11].

Tacrolimus

Tacrolimus (TAC) (FK506, Prograf, Astellas Pharma US, Deerfield, IL, USA) is a macrolide antibiotic that was initially isolated from the soil microorganism *Streptomyces tsukubaensis* in Northern Japan in 1984. Tacrolimus was approved by the Food and Drug Administration (FDA) in 1994, and its use has now surpassed that of CsA in lung transplantation. The mechanism of action for TAC is very similar to that of CsA. Tacrolimus binds intracellularly with cytoplasmic immunophilin, FK binding protein (FKBP). The TAC-FKBP complex then engages and inhibits calcineurin, a calcium-dependent phosphatase. Calcineurin inhibition prevents the dephosphorylation of NFAT, thereby inhibiting the transcription of several T-cell growth cytokines. Tacrolimus is approximately 100 times more potent than CsA. However, when administered to provide equivalent levels of calcineurin inhibition, the efficacy of the two drugs is similar [12].

Tacrolimus is administered orally, sublingually, or intravenously. Like CsA, TAC has poor oral absorption, variable bioavailability, and a narrow therapeutic window. A fatty meal (46 % fat) will reduce the rate and extent of absorption of TAC by up to 37 %. It is recommended that patients take the drug on an empty stomach or 2 h after a meal. Similar to CsA, absorption of TAC is quite variable, and trough levels have shown poor correlation with overall exposure to TAC over time [13]. Recent data suggest that 3-h post-dose concentrations may more accurately reflect AUC exposure to TAC [14].

Drug Interactions with Calcineurin Inhibitors

Both CsA and TAC are metabolized via the hepatic cytochrome P-450 system. Therefore, any alteration of the P-450 system, either by medications or hepatic dysfunction, will result in variable trough levels. Several medications may interact with the P-450 system and result in variability in CsA or TAC levels (Table 14.1). Careful monitoring of calcineurin inhibitor levels is warranted if any of these medications are added to a patient's regimen. Dosing of calcineurin inhibitors should be adjusted for renal dysfunction.

Toxicities Associated with Calcineurin Inhibitors

Several side effects and toxicities are associated with both CsA and TAC. The most significant side effect is nephrotoxicity. In general, there appear to be three forms of

Table 14.1 Drugs that affect the cytochrome P450 system

Drugs that inhibit cytochrome P450 (increase levels of calcineurin inhibitors)	Drugs that induce cytochrome P450 (decrease levels of calcineurin inhibitors)
Calcium channel blockers	*Anticonvulsants*
Diltiazem	Carbamazepine
Nifedipine	Phenobarbital
Nicardipine	Phenytoin
Verapamil	
Amlodipine	
Macrolides	*Antibiotics*
Erythromycin	Nafcillin
Clarithromycin (not azithromycin)	Rifampin
	Rifampicin
	Rifabutin
Antifungals	*Other agents*
Itraconazole	Octreotide
Ketoconazole	Ticlodipine
Fluconazole	Orlistat
Clotrimazole	St. John's wort
Prokinetic agents	
Cisapride	
Metoclopramide	
GI agents	
Cimetidine	
Lansoprazole	
Rabeprazole	
Anti-gout agents	
Colchicine	
Allopurinol	
Other agents	
Chloroquine	
Sertraline	
Danazole	
Grapefruit juice	

renal injury, including (1) an acute renal dysfunction due to vasoconstriction of the afferent arteriole, (2) a thrombotic microangiopathy that leads to thrombotic thrombocytopenic purpura and hemolytic uremic syndrome, and (3) chronic interstitial fibrosis and arteriolar sclerosis associated with persistent deterioration of renal function [5].

Other common side effects include hypertension, hyperkalemia, hyperglycemia, and hyperlipidemia. Neurological side effects are well described and range from mild tremor to frank delerium and seizures. Posterior reversible encephalopathy syndrome (PRES) has been associated with the calcineurin inhibitors, most commonly in the critical care setting in the presence of systemic hypertension. Hirsutism and gingival hypertrophy are associated with CsA use. Neurological complications and post-transplant diabetes are more strongly associated with TAC. Toxicity is clearly associated with higher trough levels and may be treated with dose adjustments.

Clinical Trials Comparing CsA and TAC

There are now four randomized controlled studies that have compared CsA to TAC in lung transplantation. Although results from these studies are somewhat conflicting, taken altogether, the studies suggest that TAC may be more effective than CsA in lung transplantation. The first single-center study of 133 patients compared CsA and TAC in combination with AZA and CS. The study showed a statistically significant reduction in the incidence of obliterative bronchiolitis and a trend toward decreased acute rejection episodes and improved survival with TAC [15, 16]. In a second study comparing CsA and TAC in conjunction with mycophenolate mofetil (MMF) and CS, there was a trend toward decreased acute rejection episodes with TAC, but this did not reach statistical significance [17]. In a third study that compared 90 patients who received either CsA or TAC in combination with AZA and CS, TAC was associated with significant reduction in cumulative acute cellular rejection and lymphocytic bronchiolitis with a median follow-up period of 2 years [18]. Recently, a large, multicenter, randomized study compared de novo TAC to CsA in combination with MMF and CS. This study showed a statistically significant decrease in the 3-year incidence of BOS with TAC compared to CsA (11.6 % vs. 21.3 %, respectively). There was no significant difference in acute rejection rates or survival between the two groups. In total, these results suggest that TAC may result in decreased alloreactivity and overall improved allograft function [19]. Per the ISHLT registry, TAC is used in approximately 80 % of all lung transplant recipients, while CsA is used in less than 20 % of all lung transplant recipients [1].

Antimetabolites

Azathioprine

Developed in the 1960s, azathioprine (AZA) in combination with CS transformed organ transplantation from an experimental science to an acceptable therapy for a number of inflammatory disorders. Azathioprine is an imidazole-derivated prodrug that is metabolized by glutathione to 6-mercaptopurine (6-MP) and inactivated by the enzyme thiopurine *S*-methyltransferase (TPMT). 6-mercaptopurine interferes with de novo purine synthesis and inhibits DNA replication. As a result, AZA inhibits the proliferation of T and B lymphocytes, and reduces the number of circulating monocytes [20].

Azathioprine is available in both oral and intravenous formulations. It is rapidly but incompletely absorbed with an oral bioavailability of 40 %. Given the longer half-life of its metabolites, AZA is typically dosed at 2 mg/kg once daily. It is important to note that approximately 10 % of the population has polymorphisms of the enzyme TPMT that reduce the enzyme's activity and enhance the myelosuppressive effects of AZA [21]. As a result, some transplant centers routinely screen lung transplant candidates for TPMT deficiency and consider either dose reduction or use of an alternative agent in patients with low TPMT levels.

Drug levels of AZA are not routinely monitored. However, accumulation of its active metabolites may occur in renal insufficiency. There are fewer drug interactions associated with AZA compared to the calcineurin inhibitors. However, one important drug interaction includes allopurinol. Allopurinol inhibits metabolism of 6-MP, resulting in a fivefold increase in 6-MP levels. Therefore, AZA and allopurinol should not be used together. If necessary, the AZA dose should be lowered by one-fourth of the normal dose. The main adverse effects related to AZA are bone marrow suppression, gastrointestinal symptoms, including nausea, diarrhea, and anorexia, pancreatitis, and cholestatic hepatic damage. Hepatic dysfunction can improve with discontinuation of AZA. Increased risk of malignancy has also been described with the use of AZA.

Mycophenolate Mofetil

MMF is the prodrug of its active component, mycophenolic acid (MPA), which was initially isolated as a fermentation product of *Penicillium brevicompactum*. However, MPA did not surface as an immunosuppressive agent until the early 1990s. Development of the drug was based on the principle that defects of the de novo purine biosynthesis pathway lead to immunosuppression without affecting other tissues. MMF was FDA-approved for the prevention of renal allograft rejection in 1995. Immunosuppression by MMF occurs when its active metabolite, MPA, blocks inosine monophosphate dehydrogenase (IMPDH), the rate-limiting enzyme in the de novo synthesis of guanosine monophosphate (GMP). While resting lymphocytes and otherproliferating tissues can rely on the salvage pathway for purine biosynthesis alone, T and B lymphocytes depend on both the salvage and the de novo pathway for proliferation. Therefore, by blocking the de novo pathway for GMP production, T and B lymphocyte clonal expansion is selectively inhibited [22].

MMF is available via both oral and intravenous formulation and is usually administered at 1 g twice daily. While drug levels of MPA are monitored, recommendations regarding ideal drug levels have not been established for lung transplantation. Drug interactions with MMF are relatively uncommon. Antacids and cholestyramine have been demonstrated to reduce levels of MMF. In addition, CsA may also reduce MMF levels by 50 % by interfering with enterohepatic recirculation. The most common side effects associated with MMF include gastrointestinal symptoms (most notably diarrhea) and bone marrow suppression. A new enteric-coated formulation of MMF was developed to decrease the adverse gastrointestinal effects of MMF. Clinical trials in renal and heart transplantation have shown comparable efficacy to the previous formulation of MMF [23, 24].

Clinical Trials Comparing AZA and MMF

There have been several clinical trials in heart and renal transplantation that have suggested that MMF is superior to AZA in decreasing acute rejection rates and improving survival [25–27]. Similarly, several small, single-center, retrospective studies have also suggested a potential benefit of MMF in reducing the incidence of acute rejection and BOS in lung transplantation [28–30]. However, two large, prospective, randomized studies in lung transplantation have not shown similar results. Palmer and colleagues initially performed a randomized study comparing MMF to AZA in a CsA-based regimen. They found no difference in 6-month acute rejection rates between the two groups [31]. In a subsequent multicenter, prospective, randomized, controlled study, MMF was compared to AZA in a CsA-based regimen with anti-thymocyte globulin induction. No significant difference in 3-year acute rejection rates, incidence of BOS, or survival was detected between the two groups. In addition, there was no difference in infection rates or malignancy between the two groups. Importantly, there was an increased number of withdrawals in the AZA group, primarily due to lack of efficacy [32]. Per the ISHLT registry, approximately 60 % of lung transplant recipients receive MMF, and 30 % receive AZA [1].

Corticosteroids

Corticosteroids have been an integral aspect of immunosuppression in solid organ transplantation since the inception of renal transplantation in the late 1950s. While CS remain a mainstay of immunosuppression in lung transplantation, several transplant centers have minimized the dose of CS in order to attenuate the toxicities of steroid use. Although there have been a few reports of successful steroid withdrawal in lung transplantation, in general, complete steroid withdrawal is not advocated in lung transplantation due to the high risk of developing acute and/or chronic rejection.

Corticosteroids have both immunosuppressive and anti-inflammatory properties, and they may affect the immune system by a myriad of pathways, most of which remain to be adequately elucidated. Corticosteroids bind to specific glucocorticoid receptors and inhibit transcription factors, including nuclear factor kappa B (NFκB). In addition, CS are potent anti-inflammatory agents, as manifested by inhibition of leukotrienes and prostaglandins via a variety of different pathways [33].

The most common steroid preparations in transplantation include oral prednisone, oral prednisolone, intravenous methylprednisolone, or intravenous hydrocortisone. In general, many transplant centers will use steroid induction therapy (methylprednisolone, 500–1,000 mg intravenously) intraoperatively prior to implantation of the lung. This dose is usually followed by a prednisone taper to 5 mg/day by 3 months after transplantation.

Corticosteroids continue to be the most important first-line agent in the treatment of acute rejection. In general, once the diagnosis of acute rejection is confirmed, methylprednisolone with daily dosing of 500–1,000 mg is typically administered intravenously for 3 days. This dose is usually followed by a rapid prednisone taper to the previous maintenance dose of CS. In cases of milder rejection, high-dose prednisone (80–100 mg/day) may be considered for approximately 7–10 days followed by a rapid steroid taper. In general, sustained, high-dose CS is not recommended for the treatment of BOS due to lack of efficacy.

The side effects of CS are numerous and are associated with considerable morbidity. Corticosteroids have been associated with Cushingoid features (acne, moon facies, buffalo hump, truncal obesity), weight gain, fluid retention, diabetes mellitus, peptic ulcer disease, hypertension, cataracts, emotion lability, osteoporosis, poor wound healing, and growth retardation in children. The side effects associated with CS are dose-related and may be attenuated by decreasing the dose of CS whenever possible.

Mammalian Target of Rapamycin Inhibitors

Sirolimus

Sirolimus, a macrocyclic lactone produced by the actinomycete, *Streptomyces hygroscopicus*, was discovered in the soil of Easter Island in 1975. It was initially evaluated as an antifungal medication. However, due to its effects on lymphoid tissue further research into its antifungal properties was abandoned [34]. Sirolimus was FDA-approved for the prevention of renal allograft rejection in 1999. Although sirolimus is structurally similar to tacrolimus and binds to FKBP, this sirolimus:FKBP complex does not inhibit calcineurin. Instead, sirolimus exerts its effects by binding to and inhibiting the activation of the mammalian target of rapamycin (mTOR), a critical regulatory kinase of the cell cycle. This inhibition prevents T-cell proliferation by inhibiting cell cycle progression from the G1 to the S phase. In addition to inhibiting T-cell proliferation, sirolimus also inhibits B cells as well as the proliferation of vascular smooth muscle cells, fibroblasts, and endothelial cells [35–39].

Sirolimus is a highly lipophilic agent with a half-life of approximately 60 h. Consequently, it is administered as a once-daily oral agent initiated at 2 mg/day. Sirolimus is often used in conjunction with the calcineurin inhibitors. Given the synergistic effect of the mTOR inhibitors and the calcineurin inhibitors, levels of both agents should be decreased. The calcineurin inhibitors should be reduced by a third to a half of their usual dosing. In addition, it is important to note that there is a pharmacokinetic interaction between CsA and sirolimus. Therefore, sirolimus should not be administered within 4 h of CsA [39, 40]. Therapeutic trough levels of sirolimus are generally between 5 and 10 ng/mL if combined with calcineurin inhibitors and between 10 and 15 ng/mL when used without calcineurin inhibitors. In addition, sirolimus is metabolized in the liver by the cytochrome P-450 system (CYP3A4). Consequently, sirolimus should be used with caution in the presence of hepatic dysfunction, and levels should be carefully monitored when these medications are added to the patient's regimen. Given this concern, a black box warning was issued for the concomitant use of sirolimus and voriconazole. Sirolimus is not removed by hemodialysis, and no dose adjustment is required in the presence of renal insufficiency.

Everolimus

Everolimus is a synthetic derivative of sirolimus that is designed to have greater bioavailability than that of sirolimus. Everolimus recently received FDA approval for use in renal transplantation. Its mechanism of action is similar to that of sirolimus, but it has a shorter half-life than sirolimus, and dosing is often initiated at 1.5 mg twice daily. Similar to sirolimus, everolimus often acts synergistically with the calcineurin inhibitors, and dosing should be adjusted in a similar fashion. Target trough levels for everolimus are between 3 and 12 ng/mL when used in conjunction with the calcineurin inhibitors [41, 42].

Toxicities Associated with mTOR Inhibitors

Several toxicities associated with the mTOR inhibitors often limit their effectiveness in lung transplantation. One of the most concerning toxicities is impaired wound healing, and bronchial anastomotic dehiscence may occur if mTOR inhibitors are given peri-operatively. Two case series have associated the administration of sirolimus with the development of fatal bronchial anastomotic dehiscence when sirolimus was initiated at the time of transplantation. Therefore, if mTOR inhibitors are used, such therapy is generally not initiated until 6–12 weeks after transplantation [43, 44].

Other toxicities associated with mTOR inhibitors include myelosuppression, dyslipidemia, venous thromboembolic disease, gastrointestinal side effects, and pulmonary toxicities, which include interstital pneumonitis, lymphocytic alveolitis, organizing pneumonia, and diffuse alveolar hemorrhage. Thrombotic thrombocytopenia and hemolytic uremic syndrome have also been described with mTOR inhibitors when used in combination with the calcineurin inhibitors. Other non-life-threatening toxicities that often lead to discontinuation of mTOR inhibitors include apthous ulcers, acneiform rash, pedal edema, and excessive bleeding [45–49].

Of note, mTOR inhibitors are not independently nephrotoxic but may potentitate calcineurin inhibitor nephrotoxicity. In contrast, substitution of the calcineurin inhibitor by an mTOR inhibitor has been shown to improve renal function in lung transplant receipients with renal insufficiency [50].

Clinical Trials with mTOR Inhibitors

Given the prominent antiproliferative effects of the mTOR inhibitors, there was much promise that these agents may be able to decrease the incidence of BOS.

There are two published, randomized, multicenter clinical trials comparing the mTOR inhibitors to the antimetabolites. The initial study of mTOR inhibitors in lung transplantation was a randomized, double-blind, placebo-controlled trial that compared everolimus to MMF in a CsA-based immunosuppressive regimen. The investigators randomized stable patients between 3 and 12 months post-transplantation. At 24-month follow-up, there was no significant difference in the primary endpoints, which included FEV_1 decline >15 % of baseline, death, or graft loss. Interestingly, although there was a significant reduction in the incidence of acute rejection with everolimus, there was no significant difference in the rate of BOS. Additionally, an increase in adverse events with everolimus compared to MMF was observed [49].

In a recent prospective, randomized, open-label, multicenter study, 181 lung transplant recipients were randomized to either sirolimus or AZA with a tacrolimus-based immunosuppressive regimen. Patients were randomized at 3 months post-transplantation to avoid the complications of bronchial anastomotic dehiscence and followed to 3 years post-transplant. There was no significant difference in the incidence of acute rejection episodes, BOS, or survival between the two groups. There was a higher rate of early discontinuation of sirolimus due to poor tolerance of the drug. Interestingly, while there was no significant difference in the incidence of all infections, there was a lower rate of CMV events with sirolimus [48].

Two recent clinical trials have been presented in abstract form at the recent ISHLT meeeting in Prague (April 2012). The first of these studies is an Australian/European multicenter study that compared everolimus to enteric-coated mycophenolate sodium in a CsA-based regimen where CsA was monitored by C2 levels. One hundred and sixty-four patients were randomized at 12 weeks post-transplant to avoid the risk of bronchial anastomotic dehiscence. There was no significant difference in the incidence of BOS or survival at 3 years post-transplant. However, there were an increased number of adverse events associated with mycophenolate, which included leukopenia, diarrhea, and the incidence of CMV infection [51]. The second study is a prospective, randomized, single-center study comparing everolimus to MMF in a CsA-based regimen. Randomization occurred at 6 weeks post-transplant. In contrast to the previous studies, preliminary analyses found an increase in the 2-year BOS-free survival in the everolimus group. The study also showed an increase in 2-year CMV-free survival with everolimus compared to MMF [52]. Nonetheless, the results of these studies do not unequivocally prove that mTOR inhibitors are more beneficial than other antimetabolites when used in combination with the calcineurin inhibitors for post-transplant immunosuppression, and the use of the mTOR inhibitors is often limited by their tolerability. According to the ISHLT registry, less than 20 % of lung transplant recipients receive mTOR inhibitors in their maintenance immunosuppressive regimen [1].

Table 14.2 presents a list of drugs used for maintenance immunosuppression in lung transplantation.

Table 14.2 Maintenance immunosuppression following lung transplantation

Drug	Mechanism of action	Suggested dose	Drug monitoring	Interactions with other medications	Common major adverse effects	Comments
Calcineurin inhibitors						
Cyclosporine	Prevents T-cell activation and proliferation by inhibiting the production of interleukins and other cytokines	3 mg/kg/day intravenously immediately postoperatively Maintenance oral dose: 3–5 mg/kg twice per day, adjusted according to trough or C2 concentration	Adjust dose to target trough levels of 250–350 ng/mL and 2-h post-dose (C2) concentration of 900–1,200 ng/mL	Metabolized by cytochrome P450 enzyme system Cytochrome P450 (3A4) substrate/inhibitor, p-glycoprotein substrate/inhibitor Please see Table 14.1 for common drug interactions	Renal dysfunction Hypertension Hyperlipidemia Hyperglycemia Gingival hyperplasia Neurotoxicity (tremor, headache) Hirsutism	High inter- and intra-individual absorption variability Monitor levels when changing doses or switching between different formulations
Tacrolimus	Prevents T-cell activation and proliferation by inhibiting the production of interleukins and other cytokines	0.05–0.1 mg/kg intravenously or sublingually immediately postoperatively Maintenance oral dose: 0.1–0.3 mg/kg twice daily taken on an empty stomach or 2 h after eating	Adjust dose to target trough levels of 8–15 ng/mL	Metabolized by cytochrome P450 enzyme system Cytochrome P450 (3A4) substrate Please see Table 14.1 for common drug interactions	Renal dysfunction Diabetes (more than cyclosporine) Hypertension (less than cyclosporine) Hyperlipidemia Neurotoxicity (more than cyclosporine) Electrolyte abnormalities (hyperkalemia, hypomagnesemia)	High inter- and intra-individual absorption variability Monitor levels when changing doses or switching between different formulations
Antimetabolites						
Azathioprine	Nucleotide blocking agent Inhibits T- and B-cell proliferation by blocking nucleotide synthesis	IV equivalent to oral Starting dose: 2 mg/kg daily and adjusted to prevent development of leukopenia	Monitor WBC Dose adjusted for leukopenia Monitor LFTs	Levels increased by: Allopurinol (preferably avoid coadministration; if coadministration is required, reduce azathioprine by up to 75 %) May diminish anticoagulant effects of warfarin	Nausea, vomiting Diarrhea Bone marrow suppression Hepatitis Pancreatitis	Requires TPMT enzyme for metabolism Individuals with profound initial side effects may be deficient in this enzyme

Mycophenolate mofetil	Nucleotide blocking agent Inhibits T-cell proliferation by blocking nucleotide synthesis	IV equivalent to oral Starting dose: 1,000 mg twice daily immediately postoperatively Enteric-coated mycophenolate dosing is 360–720 mg twice daily	Monitor WBC Dose adjusted for leukopenia	Levels decreased by: Magnesium Aluminum hydroxide Antacids Cholestyramine Cyclosporine (but not tacrolimus) Levels increased by: Probenecid Acyclovir	Nausea, vomiting Diarrhea Abdominal pain Myelosuppression Anemia	May inactivate protein-bound drugs, especially *oral contraceptives*
Glucocorticoids Methylprednisolone, prednisone	Inhibits humoral and cell-mediated immunity Binds with DNA sequences (±nuclear factor-κB) to inhibit production of inflammatory cytokines	At time of transplant: 500–1,000 mg methylprednisolone intravenously Maintenance oral prednisone dose: 0.5–1 mg/kg/day initially after transplant, with taper to a goal of 5–10 mg/day over several months to 1 year Protocols may vary by institution	N/A	Cytochrome P450 3A4 substrate; see Table 14.1	Diabetes GERD, PUD Osteoporosis Skeletal muscle wasting Hypertension Hyperlipidemia Weight gain	Do not stop abruptly; may be taken with food to reduce dyspepsia
mTOR inhibitors						
Sirolimus	Inhibits T-cell proliferation by cell cycle arrest in G1 phase	Sirolimus is initiated 6–12 weeks post-transplantation, due to effects on wound healing Starting dose: 2 mg orally per day and adjusted to target trough levels Administer sirolimus 4 h after cyclosporine	Adjust dose to target trough level 5–15 ng/mL	Metabolized by cytochrome P450 3A enzyme system Cytochrome P450 3A4 substrate, p-glycoprotein substrate Calcineurin inhibitors should be decreased by one-half to two-thirds when co-administered with sirolimus Please see Table 14.1 for common drug interactions	Fatal airway anastomotic dehiscence if administered early after lung transplantation Myelosuppression Hyperlipidemia Pulmonary toxicity Gastrointestinal side effects TTP-HUS (especially in combination with calcineurin inhibitors)	Do not administer until 6–12 weeks post-transplantation due to bronchial anastomotic dehiscence

(continued)

Table 14.2 (continued)

Drug	Mechanism of action	Suggested dose	Drug monitoring	Interactions with other medications	Common major adverse effects	Comments
Everolimus	Inhibits T-cell proliferation by cell cycle arrest in G1 phase	Everolimus is initiated 6–12 weeks post-transplantation, due to effects on wound healing Starting dose: 0.75–1.5 mg orally every 12 h and adjusted to target trough levels	Adjust dose to target trough level 3–12 ng/mL	Metabolized by cytochrome P450 3A enzyme system Cytochrome P450 3A4 substrate, p-glycoprotein substrate/inhibitor Calcineurin inhibitors should be decreased by one-half to two-thirds when co-administered with everolimus Numerous clinically relevant interactions in transplant patients; see Table 14.1	Fatal airway anastomotic dehiscence if administered early after lung transplantation Bone marrow suppression Hyperlipidemia Pulmonary toxicity Diarrhea Nausea TTP-HUS (especially in combination with calcineurin inhibitors)	Do not administer until 6–12 weeks post-transplantation due to bronchial anastomotic dehiscence

GERD gastroesophageal reflux disease, *PUD* peptic ulcer disease, *PO* oral, *WBC* white blood cell count, *CMV* cytomegalovirus, *LFT* liver function tests, *TPMT* thiopurine methyltransferase, *mTOR* mammalian target of rapamycin, *TTP-HUS* thrombotic thrombocytopenia-hemolytic uremic syndrome

Induction Therapy with Biologic Agents

The use of biologic agents for immunosuppression dates to the very beginnings of solid organ transplantation. These agents have been used as both induction agents and for treatment for refractory acute rejection in solid organ transplantation. In some cases, the biologic agents have been used in the early phase of BOS. Induction therapy in lung transplantation is most often used in the perioperative and early postoperative period to decrease early alloreactivity as well as to allow for the gradual introduction of the nephrotoxic calcineurin inhibitors. In general, induction therapies have been associated with increased infection and malignancy due to their potent effects upon lymphocytes [1]. Table 14.3 presents a list of drugs used for induction therapy following lung transplantation.

IL-2 Receptor Antagonist Antibodies

The IL-2 receptor antagonists or anti-CD25 monoclonal antibodies are the most commonly used agents in lung transplantation. Initially, two agents (basiliximab and daclizumab) were commercially available for use in transplantation. However, daclizumab (a humanized monoclonal antibody) is no longer being manufactured. As a result, basiliximab, a chimeric murine/human monoclonal antibody to the α (alpha) subunit (CD25) of the IL-2 receptor, is the only IL-2 receptor antagonist that is currently available for clinical use. These antibodies inhibit T-cell proliferation and differentiation by binding to the IL-2 receptor, but they do not cause T-cell depletion. Basiliximab has a half-life of approximately 13 days and is approved for a 20-mg dose on Day 0 and Day 4 post-transplant. Due to the chimeric nature of these antibodies, they are generally well tolerated and have few side effects. However, there have been a few case reports of pulmonary edema associated with basiliximab [53, 54].

Anti-thymocyte Globulin

The first induction agent used was anti-lymphocyte serum (ALS), created by immunizing animals with human lymphoid cells. This was a very nonspecific agent with low potency and significant toxicity, but it was refined into several purified anti-lymphocyte and anti-thymocyte immunoglobulin preparations that included anti-lymphocyte globulin (ALG), anti-thymocyte globulin (Atgam [horse], Thymoglobulin [rabbit]), and Minnesota anti-lymphoblast globulin (MALG). Currently, only Atgam (Pfizer, New York, NY, USA) and Thymoglobulin (Genzyme, Cambridge, MA, USA) are commercially available.

Table 14.3 Induction therapy following lung transplantation

Drug	Mechanism of action	Suggested dose	Drug monitoring	Adverse effects	Comments
IL-2 receptor antagonists Basiliximab Daclizumab (withdrawn from United States and other markets)	Chimeric monoclonal antibody binds with high affinity to CD25 on T cells to inhibit IL-2-mediated T-cell proliferation	Basiliximab: 20 mg on day 0 and day 4 after transplantation Daclizumab: 1 mg/kg on day of transplant, then every 2 weeks for a total of five doses	N/A	Low rate of adverse effects Few cases of pulmonary edema with basiliximab	Most commonly used induction agent Daclizumab is no longer being manufactured due to decreased market demands
Anti-thymocyte globulin Thymoglobulin Atgam	Polyclonal antibody that causes nonspecific T-cell depletion	Thymoglobulin (rabbit origin): 1.5 mg/kg over 6 h, then two additional doses given 24-h apart Atgam (horse origin): 7.5–15 mg/kg/day for 3–5 days post-transplant Induction protocols may vary by institution	Monitor CBC and lymphocyte subsets Monitor LFTs	Leukopenia Cytokine release syndrome Infusion reactions Thrombocytopenia Glomerulonephritis Serum sickness Hypersensitivity reactions	Premedication includes glucocorticoids (e.g., methylprednisolone 125 mg intravenously), antihistamines (e.g., diphenhydramine 50 mg orally or intravenously), and antipyretics (e.g., acetaminophen 1 g orally) 1 h prior to infusion
Muromonab-CD3 (withdrawn from United States and other markets)	Mouse monoclonal antibody that binds to the T-cell receptor-CD3 complex, causing depletion of T cells	2.5 mg/day for patients weighing <80 kg or 5 mg/day for patients ≥80 kg, given for 7–14 days after transplant	Monitor CBC and lymphocyte subsets	Cytokine release storm (e.g., fevers, rigors, vomiting, diarrhea, hemodynamic instability, pulmonary edema)	Patients will develop neutralizing antibodies to OKT3, limiting prolonged use and necessitating use of alternative drug if future augmentation of immunosuppression is needed Premedication includes glucocorticoids (e.g., methylprednisolone 125 mg intravenously), antihistamines (e.g., diphenhydramine 50 mg orally or intravenously), and antipyretics (e.g., acetaminophen 1 g orally) 1 h prior to infusion
Alemtuzumab (Campath-1H)	Monoclonal rat antibody directed at CD52 on T cells and B cells, causing depletion of these lymphocytes	30 mg IV intra-operatively infused over 2 h Induction protocols may vary by institution	Monitor CBC and lymphocyte subsets	Lymphopenia: T cells may remain depressed for up to 3 years B cells may be depressed for several months May cause cytokine release syndrome, but milder than compared to muromonab (OKT3)	Limited experience in induction therapy

CBC complete blood count, *LFT* liver function test

Polyclonal antibodies act by inducing profound generalized lymphocyte depletion. This nonspecific action is directed against a wide range of lymphocyte surface antigens and may induce either complement- or antibody-dependent cytolysis. When used as induction therapy, the first dose is given intra-operatively before implantation of the allograft. Atgam has a half-life of 2–7 days, and Thymoglobulin has a half-life of 30 days. In general, both agents are given daily to 14 days. Dosing is quite variable and often determined by individual center protocols along with lymphocyte subset studies [55–57].

The most significant toxicity of anti-thymocyte antibodies is a "cytokine release syndrome" that often results in fever, chills, diarrhea, nausea, and vomiting. In addition, increased vascular permeability can result in significant fluid shifts, causing pulmonary edema and hemodynamic instability. Appropriate prophylaxis with glucocorticoids, antihistamines, and antipyretics may attenuate this syndrome. In up to 30 % of cases, the recipient can form an immune response to the foreign antibodies that may reduce their effectiveness. Serum sickness, while rare, has also been associated with ATG administration [55–57].

Anti-CD3 Monoclonal Antibody

OKT3 is a murine monoclonal antibody that has been used as induction therapy since the 1980s. OKT3 targets the epsilon chain of the CD3 molecule in the CD3/TCR complex on T cells and can cause a profound depletion of circulating T cells. Immediately following administration, OKT3 paradoxically activates a large number of T cells, which releases massive amounts of cytokines. Often this "cytokine release syndrome" is more profound than that of anti-thymocyte globulin and may result in fevers, rigors, pulmonary edema, renal failure, encephalopathy, and hemodynamic instability. Like polyclonal antibodies, patients should be pretreated with glucocorticoids, antihistamines, and antipyretics. In addition, OKT3 has been associated with aseptic meningitis, pulmonary edema, elevated pulmonary artery pressures, and decreased oxygenation. Due to the intolerable side effects of this medication, OKT3 has largely fallen out of favor in clinical use [58].

Alemtuzumab

Alemtuzumab (Campath-1H, Genzyme, Cambridge, MA, USA) is a humanized monoclonal antibody to CD52 that is found on both T and B cells, natural killer cells, and monocytes. It was initially used in chronic lymphocytic leukemia (CLL), other lymphoid malignancies, graft-versus-host disease, and multiple sclerosis. By binding to CD52 surface antigen, alemtuzumab causes a profound depletion of mononuclear cells through multiple pathways, including complement-mediated and direct cellular toxicity. This prolonged depletion leads to delayed recovery of CD4 and CD8 T cells, often up to 3 years after administration of alemtuzumab. The effect of alemtuzumab on B cells is less prolonged, and recovery of B cells occurs in approximately 3 months [59, 60]. Due to the profound effects on all monocyte populations, the use of alemtuzumab has been associated with increased infections. A recent large study including 547 solid organ transplant recipients from the University of Pittsburgh showed that alemtuzumab was an independent risk factor for opportunistic infections [61]. Alemtuzumab is currently used in only a few lung transplant centers across the world [62, 63]. In one of the largest reports of the use of alemtuzumab in lung transplantation, the University of Pittsburgh group performed a retrospective single-center study comparing alemtuzumab to historical controls receiving either IL-2 receptor antagonist, Thymoglobulin, or no induction therapy. The results showed a greater freedom from acute rejection, lymphocytic bronchiolitis, obliterative bronchiolitis, and BOS with alemtuzumab. In addition, patients who received alemtuzumab had improved survival [62]. The study is limited by the single-center retrospective sequential study design and the absence of reporting of infections and other adverse events. Although the study is provocative, further investigations should be undertaken to confirm the benefits seen in this study.

Currently, dosing of alemtuzumab is variable and center-specific. Toxicities associated with alemtuzumab include a cytokine release syndrome, although this is milder than previously reported with OKT3. Consequently, when alemtuzumab is given, patients receive prophylaxis with steroids, antihistamines, and antipyretics. Not surprisingly, alemtuzumab is associated with profound and prolonged cytopenias. In addition, there have been case reports of diffuse alveolar hemorrhage and paroxysmal nocturnal hematuria with the use of alemtuzumab.

Clinical Trials with Induction Therapy

The use of induction therapy in lung transplantation remains controversial. Per the ISHLT registry, only 55 % of all lung transplant recipients receive induction therapy (37 % receive an IL-2 receptor antagonist, 13 % receive ATG, and 5 % receive alemtuzumab), highlighting the difference in opinions regarding the benefit of these agents among lung transplant physicians. Data from the ISHLT registry suggest that there is a small but significant improvement in survival with the use of induction therapy contingent upon survival to 14 days post-transplantation [1]. However, any benefit of induction therapy must be balanced by the increased risk of this therapy, including increased incidence of infections, other adverse events, and higher costs.

There have been numerous studies comparing the use of different biological agents to each other and/or to placebo in lung transplantation. Unfortunately, the data have been somewhat conflicting, due in part to the small single-center trial designs and registry reports. As a result, there is no consensus regarding the type of induction therapy or whether induction therapy is of benefit in lung transplantation [64–70]. Data from the ISHLT registry suggest that IL-2 receptor antagonists are associated with a decreased incidence of acute rejection compared to no induction therapy or ATG. A recent retrospective analysis of the ISHLT registry evaluated approximately 4,000 lung transplant recipients who received either an IL-2 receptor antagonist, ATG or no induction therapy. The study showed a decrease in rejection rates and an increase in 4-year survival in the patients who received the IL-2 receptor antagonist. Interestingly there was no difference among the groups in the incidence of BOS. However, there was a higher incidence of infection in patients who received induction therapy [71]. Several small single-center studies have shown variable results regarding the benefit of IL-2 receptor antagonist, ATG and OKT3 compared to no induction therapy. The majority of these studies suggest that these agents are beneficial in reducing early (<6 months) acute rejection. However, there did not appear to be a significant difference in BOS rate or survival. Comparisons among different agents have yielded conflicting results with respect to acute and chronic rejection primarily due to suboptimal study designs [64–70]. As a result, large, prospective, randomized, controlled studies are necessary to identify optimal induction therapies (if any) in lung transplantation.

Antihumoral Therapy

The majority of the therapies utilized as maintenance immunosuppression after lung transplantation primarily suppress T cells and cell-mediated rejection. Recently, there has been more evidence that antibodies may also play a role in lung allograft dysfunction. These antibodies, which are often specific for donor alloantigens (donor-specific antibodies [DSA]) may be present prior to transplantation (sensitized candidate) or may develop de novo after transplantation. In addition, DSA may be associated with histological findings of graft injury and physiological lung allograft dysfunction, also known as antibody-mediated rejection (AMR) [72]. There have been case reports of successful treatment of AMR with combinations of several agents, including CS, intravenous immunoglobulin, plasmapheresis, rituximab, and/or bortezomib in lung transplant recipients. However, further understanding of the pathogenesis of AMR is clearly needed in order to better evaluate the benefit of the immunosuppressive medications used to treat this condition [73].

Rituximab

Rituximab is a chimeric monoclonal antibody that is used in the treatment of lymphoma and rheumatoid arthritis. Rituximab binds to CD20 surface antigen present on early B cells (not mature plasma cells that produce antibodies) and depletes B cells by several mechanisms, including antibody- and/or complement-dependent cellular cytotoxicity as well as by inducing apoptosis. Pharmacodynamic studies have shown that B cells were eliminated from the peripheral blood within 1–2 days of treatment and remained suppressed for at least 1 year. There have been several anecdotal studies in lung, renal, and heart transplant that suggest potential benefit for rituximab when given in addition to other therapies in the treatment of AMR [73–76]. While the usual dose is 375 mg/m^2, the number of doses for the treatment of AMR has been variable. It should also be noted that most of these studies were often small, retrospective, and performed in combination with several other therapies for AMR. Consequently, further investigation of rituximab for the treatment of AMR is needed in order to confirm its benefit in lung transplantation. Adverse events associated with the use of rituximab include infusion reactions (which occurs most commonly with the first infusion) and cytopenia.

Bortezomib

Bortezomib is a proteasome inhibitor that has been approved for use in multiple myeloma. Bortezomib has been shown to cause apoptosis of mature plasma cells that produce antibodies, including DSA. Bortezomib is typically administered on days 1, 4, 8, and 11 in a 21-day cycle. There have been a few case reports of the use of bortezomib in combination with other agents that have shown a decrease in DSA, reversal of rejection, and stabilization of graft function in renal transplantation [77, 78]. In a single case report of refractory rejection in lung transplantation, one cycle of bortezomib allowed for recovery of graft function [79]. Side effects of bortezomib include gastrointestinal effects and peripheral neuropathy.

Belatacept

Belatacept is a humanized CTLA-4 fusion protein that prevents T-cell activation by binding to CD80 and CD86 on antigen-presenting cells. It is a selective costimulation blocker whose specificity was designed to provide effective immunosuppression while avoiding the toxicities of the calcineurin inhibitors. Belatacept was recently approved by the FDA for prophylaxis against acute rejection in renal transplantation. A large, multicenter, randomized, controlled study of renal transplant recipients compared belatacept to CsA. Six hundred and sixty-six renal transplant recipients were randomized to receive one of three immunosuppressive regimens: a more intensive regimen of belatacept (MI), a less intensive regimen of belatacept (LI), or CsA in combination with MMF and steroids. The study revealed similar patient and graft survival among all three arms and superior renal function and decreased metabolic complications (hypertension, hyperlipidemia, and diabetes mellitus) in both belatacept arms compared to the CsA arm. However, there was an increased rate of early (<1-year post-transplant) acute rejection and post-transplant lymphoproliferative disorder (PTLD) in the belatacept treatment arms. The risk of PTLD was highest in patients who were EBV serostatus negative and received the more intensive belatacept regimen. The authors concluded that belatacept may be beneficial for a select group of patients, but the risk:benefit ratio for each individual should be assessed [80, 81]. To date, there have been no reports of the use of belatacept in lung transplantation. However, the addition of the agent to the current immunosuppressives may allow clinicians to further tailor immunosuppressive medications to the individual patient.

Conclusion

Unfortunately, there is currently no panacea for BOS. As a result, there is no consensus regarding first-line therapies among expert clinicians regarding treatment for BOS [82]. In general, there are three main strategies regarding immunosuppression in BOS management, including (1) substituting one immunosuppressive agent for another, (2) augmenting the overall level of immunosuppression, and (3) adding other immunomodulating therapies, such as azithromycin, statins, photopheresis, or total lymphoid irradiation (these are discussed elsewhere). These strategies may be undertaken consecutively or simultaneously, depending upon the patient, the trajectory of decline in pulmonary function, and the clinician's experience. The majority of the data that support these strategies are from small, single-center, retrospective, uncontrolled studies; consequently, the evidence supporting these strategies is quite variable.

Conversion of baseline immunosuppression from one agent to another is often undertaken when the initial decline of pulmonary function is identified. There have been several small studies that have shown that the conversion from CsA to TAC has been associated with reversal or refractory acute rejection and have decreased the rate of decline of pulmonary function [83–85]. An international, retrospective, multicenter study also showed that conversion of CsA to TAC allowed for reversal of refractory acute rejection and short-term stabilization of pulmonary function [86]. Likewise, conversion of AZA to MMF or mTOR inhibitors has also been associated with stabilization of pulmonary function in patients diagnosed with BOS [28–30].

Augmentation of immunosuppression by the addition of biologic agents (IL-2 receptor antagonists, ATG, alemtuzumab) is another strategy that has been utilized to stabilize pulmonary function in patients with BOS. Some studies have documented treatment of refractory acute rejection and stabilization of pulmonary function with the use of these agents [63, 71, 87]. However, these studies are small, retrospective, and lack long-term follow-up. Therefore, these agents should be used with caution in the treatment of BOS, and the risk:benefit ratio must be carefully weighed prior to administration of these medications.

In conclusion, there has been a significant increase in the armamentarium of immunosuppressive medications used for solid organ transplantation over the past 3 decades. These new agents have enhanced the ability of clinicians to tailor immunosuppressive therapy to a given individual. Unfortunately, there is no specific immunosuppressive regimen that is superior to the others in the prevention or treatment of BOS. Further investigation into the pathophysiology of BOS may lead to the identification of molecular targets for future novel and innovative therapies. In addition, large, multicenter, randomized trials are necessary to identify new immunosuppressive agents that are truly beneficial in the prevention and treatment of BOS.

References

1. Christie JD, Edwards LB, Kucheryavaya AY, Benden C, Dobbels F, Kirk R, et al. The Registry of the International Society for Heart and Lung Transplantation: twenty-eighth adult lung and heart-lung transplant report—2011. J Heart Lung Transplant. 2011;30(10):1104–22.
2. Wenger RM. Structures of cyclosporine and its metabolites. Transplant Proc. 1990;22:1104–9.
3. Kahan BD. Cyclosporine. N Engl J Med. 1989;321:1725–38.
4. Kovarik JM, Mueller EA, van Bree JB, Tetzloff W, Kutz K. Reduced inter- and intraindividual variability in cyclosporine pharmacokinetics from a microemulsion formulation. J Pharm Sci. 1994;83:444–6.
5. Keown P, Landsberg D, Halloran P, Shoker A, Rush D, Jeffery J, et al. A randomized prospective multicenter pharmacoepidemiologic study of cyclosporine microemulsion in stable renal graft recipients. Report of the Canadian Neoral Renal Transplantation Study Group. Transplantation. 1996;62:1744–52.
6. Dunn CJ, Wagstaff AJ, Perry CM, Plosker GL, Goa KL. Cyclosporin: an updated review of the pharmacokinetic properties, clinical efficacy and tolerability of a microemulsion based formulation in organ transplantation. Drugs. 2001;61(13):1957–2016.
7. Levy G, Thervet E, Lake J, Uchida K. Consensus on Neoral C(2): Expert Review in Transplantation (CONCERT) Group. Patient management by neoral C(2) monitoring: an international consensus statement. Transplantation. 2002;73 Suppl 9:S12–8.
8. Glanville AR, Aboyoun CL, Morton JM, Plit M, Malouf MA. Cyclosporine C2 target levels and acute cellular rejection after lung transplantation. J Heart Lung Transplant. 2006;25(8):928–34.
9. Iacono AT, Keenan RJ, Duncan SR, Smaldone GC, Dauber JH, Paradis IL, et al. Aerosolized cyclosporine in lung recipients with refractory chronic rejection. Am J Respir Crit Care Med. 1996;153(4 Pt 1):1451–5.
10. Iacono AT, Johnson BA, Grgurich WF, Youssef JG, Corcoran TE, Seiler DA, et al. Randomized trial of inhaled cyclosporine in lung transplant recipients. N Engl J Med. 2006;354(2):141–50.
11. Johnson BA, Zamore MR, Budev MM, et al. Cyclosporine inhalation solution does not improve bronchiolitis obliterans syndrome-free survival following lung transplant: results from the CYCLIST Trial. J Heart Lung Transplant. 2012;31:S66.
12. Kino T, Hatanaka H, Miyata S, Inamura N, Nishiyama M, Yajima T, et al. FK-506, a novel immunosuppressant isolated from a Streptomyces. II. Immunosuppressive effect of FK-506 in vitro. J Antibiot. 1987;40:1256–65.
13. Briffa N, Morris RE. New immunosuppressive regimens in lung transplantation. Eur Respir J. 1997;10(11):2630–7.
14. Kahan BD, Keown P, Levy GA, Johnston A. Therapeutic drug monitoring of immuosuppressant drugs in clinical practice. Clin Ther. 2002;24:330–50.
15. Keenan RJ, Konishi H, Kawai A, Paradis IL, Nunley DR, Iacono AT, et al. Clinical trial of tacrolimus versus cyclosporine in lung transplantation. Ann Thorac Surg. 1995;60:580–5.
16. Keenan RJ, Dauber JH, Iacono AT, et al. Long-term follow-up clinical trial of tacrolimus versus cyclosporine in lung transplantation. J Heart Lung Transplant. 1998;17:59A.
17. Zuckermann A, Reichenspurner H, Birsan T, Treede H, Deviatko E, Reichart B, et al. Cyclosporine A versus tacrolimus in combination with mycophenolate mofetil and steroids as primary immunosuppression after lung transplantation: one-year results of a 2-center prospective randomized trial. J Thorac Cardiovasc Surg. 2003;125(4):891–900.
18. Hachem RR, Yusen RD, Chakinala MM, Meyers BF, Lynch JP, Aloush AA, et al. A randomized controlled trial of tacrolimus versus cyclosporine after lung transplantation. J Heart Lung Transplant. 2007;26(10):1012–8.
19. Treede H, Glanville AR, Klepetko W, Aboyoun C, Vettorazzi E, Lama R, European and Australian Investigators in Lung Transplantation. Tacrolimus and cyclosporine have differential effects on the risk of development of bronchiolitis obliterans syndrome: results of a prospective, randomized international trial in lung transplantation. J Heart Lung Transplant. 2012;31(8):797–804.

20. Maltzman JS, Koretzky GA. Azathioprine: old drug, new actions. J Clin Invest. 2003;111:1122–4.
21. Holme SA, Duley JA, Sanderson J, Routledge PA, Anstey AV. Erythrocyte thiopurine methyl transferase assessment prior to azathioprine use in the UK. QJM. 2002;95:439–44.
22. Allison AC, Eugui EM. Mechanisms of action of mycophenolate mofetil in preventing acute and chronic allograft rejection. Transplantation. 2005;80:S181–90.
23. Kobashigawa JA, Renlund DG, Gerosa G, Almenar L, Eisen HJ, Keogh AM, et al. Similar efficacy and safety of enteric coated mycophenolate sodium compare with mycophenolate mofetil in de novo heart transplant recipients: results of a 12-month, single-blind, randomized, parallel-group multicenter study. J Heart Lung Transplant. 2006;25:935–41.
24. Budde K, Curtis J, Knoll G, Chan L, Neumayer HH, Seifu Y, et al. Enteric-coated mycophenolate sodium can be safely administered in maintenance renal transplant patients: results of a 1 year study. Am J Transplant. 2004;4:237–43.
25. European Mycophenolate Mofetil Cooperative Study Group. Placebo controlled study of mycophenolate mofetil combined with cyclosporin and steroids for prevention of acute rejection. Lancet. 1995;345:1321–5.
26. The Tricontinental Mycophenolate Mofetil Renal Transplantation Study Group. A blinded, randomized clinical trial of mycophenolate mofetil for the prevention of acute rejection in cadaveric renal transplantation. Transplantation. 1996;61:1029–37.
27. Sollinger HW for the US Renal Transplant Mycophenolate Mofetil Study Group. Mycophenolate mofetil for the prevention of acute rejection in primary cadaveric renal allograft recipients. Transplantation. 1995;60:225–32.
28. Ross DJ, Waters PF, Levine M, Kramer M, Ruzevich S, Kass RM. Mycophenolate mofetil versus azathioprine immunosuppressive regimens after lung transplantation: preliminary experience. J Heart Lung Transplant. 1998;17:768–74.
29. Zuckermann A, Klepetko W, Birsan T, Taghavi S, Artemiou O, Wisser W, et al. Comparison between mycophenolate mofetil and azathioprine based immunosuppressions in clinical lung transplantation. J Heart Lung Transplant. 1999;18:423–40.
30. O'Hair DP, Cantu E, McGregor C, Jorgensen B, Gerow-Smith R, Galantowicz ME, et al. Preliminary experience with mycophenolate mofetil used after lung transplantation. J Heart Lung Transplant. 1998;17:864–8.
31. Palmer SM, Baz MA, Sanders L, Miralles AP, Lawrence CM, Rea JB, et al. Results of a randomized, prospective, multicenter trial of mycophenolate mofetil versus azathioprine in the prevention of acute lung allograft rejection. Transplantation. 2001;71:1772–6.
32. McNeil K, Glanville AR, Wahlers T, Knoop C, Speich R, Mamelok RD, et al. Comparison of mycophenolate mofetil and azathioprine for prevention of bronchiolitis obliterans syndrome in de novo lung transplant recipients. Transplantation. 2006;81(7):998–1003.
33. Schimmer BP, Parker KL. Adrenocorticotrophic hormone; adrenocortical steroids and their synthetic analogs; Inhibitors of the synthesis and actions of adrenocortical hormones. In: Hardman JG, Goodman Gilman A, Limbard LE, editors. Goodman and Gilman's the pharmacological basis of therapeutics. 9th ed. New York: McGraw Hill; 1996. p. 1459–85.
34. Calne RY, Collier DS, Lim S, Pollard SG, Samaan A, White DJ, et al. Rapamycin for immunosuppression in organ allografting. Lancet. 1989;2(8656):227.
35. Morris R, Meiser B. Identification of a new pharmacologic action for an old compound. Med Sci Res. 1989;17:609–10.
36. Cao W, Mohacsi P, Shorthouse R. Effects of rapamycin on growth factor-stimulated vascular smooth muscle cell DNA synthesis. Inhibition of basic fibroblast growth factor and platelet-derived growth factor action and antagonism of rapamycin by FK506. Transplantation. 1995;59(3):390–5.
37. Gregory CR, Huang X, Pratt RE, Dzau VJ, Shorthouse R, Billingham ME, et al. Treatment with rapamycin and mycophenolic acid reduces arterial intimal thickening produced by mechanical injury and allows endothelial replacement. Transplantation. 1995;59(5):655–61.
38. Lai JH, Tan TH. CD28 signaling causes a sustained down-regulation of I kappa B alpha which can be prevented by the immunosuppressant rapamycin. J Biol Chem. 1994;269(48): 30077–80.

39. Terada N, Lucas JJ, Szepsi A, Franklin RA, Domenico J, Gelfand EW. Rapamycin blocks cell cycle progression of activated T cells prior to events characteristic of the middle to late G1 phase of the cycle. J Cell Physiol. 1993;154:7–15.
40. Longoria J, Roberts RF, Marboe CC, Stouch BC, Starnes VA, Barr ML, et al. Sirolimus (rapamycin) potentiates cyclosporine in prevention of acute lung rejection. J Thorac Cardiovasc Surg. 1999;117(4):714–8.
41. Kovarik JM, Snell GI, Valentine V, Aris R, Chan CK, Schmidli H, et al. Everolimus in pulmonary transplantation: pharmacokinetics and exposure-response relationships. J Heart Lung Transplant. 2006;25(4):440–6.
42. Doyle RL, Hertz MI, Dunitz JM, Loyd JE, Stecenko AA, Wong RL, et al. RAD in stable lung and heart/lung transplant recipients: safety, tolerability, pharmacokinetics and impact of cystic fibrosis. J Heart Lung Transplant. 2001;20:330–9.
43. King-Biggs MB, Dunitz JM, Park SJ, Kay Savik S, Hertz MI. Airway anastomotic dehiscence associated with use of sirolimus immediately after lung transplantation. Transplantation. 2003;75(9):1437–43.
44. Groetzner J, Kur F, Spelsberg F, Behr J, Frey L, Bittmann I, et al. Airway anastomosis complications in de novo lung transplantation with sirolimus based immunosuppression. J Heart Lung Transplant. 2004;23:632–8.
45. McWilliams TJ, Levvey BJ, Russell PA, Milne DG, Snell GI. Interstitial pneumonitis associated with sirolimus: a dilemma for lung transplantation. J Heart Lung Transplant. 2003;22(2):210–3.
46. Ahya VN, McShane PJ, Baz MA, Valentine VG, Arcasoy SM, Love RB, et al. Increased risk of venous thromboembolism with a sirolimus based immunosuppression regimen in lung transplantation. J Heart Lung Transplant. 2011;30(2):175–81.
47. Champion L, Stern M, Israel-Iet D, Mamzer-Bruneel MF, Peraldi MN, Kreis H, et al. Brief communication: sirolimus associated pneumonitis: 24 cases in renal transplant recipients. Ann Intern Med. 2006;144(7):505–9.
48. Bhorade S, Ahya VN, Baz MA, Valentine VG, Arcasoy SM, Love RB, et al. Comparison of sirolimus to azathioprine in a tacrolimus based regimen in lung transplantation. Am J Respir Crit Care Med. 2011;183(3):379–87.
49. Snell GI, Valentine VG, Vitulo P, Glanville AR, McGiffin DC, Loyd JE, et al. Everolimus versus azathioprine in maintenance lung transplant recipients: an international, randomized, double-blind clinical trial. Am J Transplant. 2006;6(1):169–77.
50. Snell GI, Levvey BJ, Chin W, Kotsimbos T, Whitford H, Waters KN, et al. Sirolimus allows renal recovery in lung and heart transplant recipients with chronic renal impairment. J Heart Lung Transplant. 2002;21(5):540–6.
51. Glanville AR, Aboyoun C, Klepetko W, et al. 3-year results of the CeMyLungs study, a 3-year randomised, open label, multi-centre investigator driven study comparing de novo enteric coated mycophenolate sodium with delayed onset everolimus, both arms in combination with cyclosporin (using C2 monitoring) and corticosteroids for the prevention of bronchiolitis obliterans syndrome in heart-lung. Bilateral lung and single lung transplant recipients. J Heart Lung Transplant. 2012;31:S66.
52. Martin S, Thomas F, Gregor W, et al. Everolimus versus MMF in lung transplant recipients. J Heart Lung Transplant. 2012;31:S67.
53. Onrust SV, Wiseman LR. Basiliximab. Drugs. 1999;57:207–13.
54. Wiseman LR, Faulds D. Daclizumab: a review of its use in the prevention of acute rejection in renal transplant recipients. Drugs. 1999;58:1029–42.
55. Taniguchi Y, Frickhofen N, Raghavachar A, Digel W, Heimpel H. Antilymphocyte immunoglobulins stimulate peripheral blood lymphocytes to proliferate and release lymphokines. Eur J Haematol. 1990;44:244–51.
56. Carrier M, White M, Perrault LP, Pelletier GB, Pellerin M, Robitaille D, et al. A 10-year experience with intravenous thymoglobulin in induction of immunosuppression following heart transplantation. J Heart Lung Transplant. 1999;18:1218–23.
57. Brennan DC, Flavin K, Lowell JA, Howard TK, Shenoy S, Burgess S, et al. A randomized, double-blinded comparison of thymoglobulin versus ATGAM for induction immunosuppressive therapy in adult renal transplant recipients. Transplantation. 1999;67:1011–8.

58. Todd PA, Brogden RN. Muromonab CD3: a review of its pharmacology and therapeutic potential. Drugs. 1989;37:871–99.
59. Magliocca JF, Knechtle SJ. The evolving role of alemtuzumab (Campath-1H) for immunosuppressive therapy in organ transplantation. Transpl Int. 2006;19(9):705–14.
60. Weaver TA, Kirk AD. Alemtuzumab. Transplantation. 2007;84:1545–7.
61. Peleg AY, Husain S, Kwak EJ, Silveira FP, Ndirangu M, Tran J, et al. Opportunistic infections in 547 organ transplant recipients receiving alemtuzumab, a humanized monoclonal CD-52 antibody. Clin Infect Dis. 2007;44(2):204–12.
62. van Loenhout KC, Groves SC, Galazka M, Sherman B, Britt E, Garcia J, et al. Early outcomes using alemtuzumab induction in lung transplantation. Interact Cardiovasc Thorac Surg. 2010;10(2):190–4.
63. Shyu S, Dew MA, Pilewski JM, DeVito Dabbs AJ, Zaldonis DB, Studer SM, et al. Five year outcomes with alemtuzumab induction after lung transplantation. J Heart Lung Transplant. 2011;30(7):743–54.
64. Garrity Jr ER, Villanueva J, Bhorade S, Husain AN, Vigneswaran WT, et al. Low rate of acute lung allograft rejection after the use of daclizumab, an interleukin 2 receptor antibody. Transplantation. 2001;71(6):773–7.
65. Palmer SM, Miralles AP, Lawrence CM, Gaynor JW, Davis RD, Tapson VF, et al. Rabbit antithymocyte globulin decreases acute rejection after lung transplantation: results of a randomized, prospective study. Chest. 1999;116(1):127–33.
66. Hartwig MG, Snyder LD, Appel III JZ, Cantu III E, Lin SS, Palmer SM, et al. Rabbit antithymocyte globulin induction therapy does not prolong survival after lung transplantation. J Heart Lung Transplant. 2008;27(5):547–53.
67. Hachem RR, Chakinala MM, Yusen RD, Lynch JP, Aloush AA, Patterson GA, et al. A comparison of basiliximab and anti-thymocyte globulin as induction agents after lung transplantation. J Heart Lung Transplant. 2005;24(9):1320–6.
68. Burton CM, Andersen CB, Jensen AS, Iversen M, Milman N, Boesgaard S, et al. The incidence of acute cellular rejection after lung transplantation: a comparative study of antithymocyte globulin and daclizumab. J Heart Lung Transplant. 2006;25(6):638–47.
69. Mullen JC, Oreopoulos A, Lien DC, Bentley MJ, Modry DL, Stewart K, et al. A randomized, controlled trial of daclizumab vs. anti-thymocyte globulin induction for lung transplantation. J Heart Lung Transplant. 2007;26(5):504–10.
70. Brock MV, Borja MC, Ferber L, Orens JB, Anzcek RA, Krishnan J, et al. Induction therapy in lung transplantation: a prospective controlled clinical trial comparing OKT3, anti-thymocyte globulin, and daclizumab. J Heart Lung Transplant. 2001;20:1282–90.
71. Hachem RR, Edwards LB, Yusen RD, Chakinala MM, Alexander Patterson G, Trulock EP. The impact of induction on survival after lung transplantation: an analysis of the International Society for Heart and Lung Transplantation Registry. Clin Transplant. 2008;22(5):603–8.
72. Blume OR, Yost SE, Kaplan B. Antibody-mediated rejection: pathogenesis, prevention, treatment and outcomes. J Transplant. 2012;2012:201754.
73. Glanville AR. Antibody mediated rejection in lung transplantation: myth or reality? J Heart Lung Transplant. 2010;29(4):395–400.
74. Faguer S, Kama N, Guilbeaud-Frugier D, Fort M, Modesto A, Mari A, et al. Rituxmab therapy for acute humoral rejection after kidney transplantation. Transplantation. 2007;833:1277–80.
75. Kacmarek I, Deutsch MA, Sadoni S, Brenner P, Schmauss D, Daebritz SH, et al. Successful management of antibody-mediated cardiac allograft rejection with combined immunoadsorption and anti-CD20 monoclonal antibody treatment. Case report and literature review. J Heart Lung Transplant. 2007;26:511–5.
76. Hachem RR, Yusen RD, Meyers BF, Aloush AA, Mohanakumar T, Patterson GA, et al. Anti-human leukocyte antigen antibodies and preemptive antibody-directed therapy after lung transplantation. J Heart Lung Transplant. 2010;29(9):973–80.
77. Everly MJ. An update on antibody reduction and rejection reversal following bortezomib use: a report of 52 cases across 10 centers. Clin Transplant. 2010;353–62.
78. Trivedi HL, Terasaki PI, Feroz A, Everly MJ, Vanikar AV, Shankar V, et al. Abrogation of anti-HLA antibodies via proteasome inhibition. Transplantation. 2009;87(10):1555–61.

79. Neumann J, Tarrasconi H, Bortolotto A, Machuca T, Canabarro R, Sporleder H, et al. Acute humoral rejection in a lung recipient: reversion with bortezomib. Transplantation. 2010;89(1): 125–6.
80. Vincenti F, Charpentiier B, Vanrenterghem Y, Rostaing L, Bresnahan B, Darji P, et al. A phase III study of belatacept based immunosuppression regimens versus cyclosporine in renal transplant recipients (BENEFIT study). Am J Transplant. 2010;10:535–46.
81. Pestana JO, Grinyo JM, Vanrenterghem Y, Becker T, Campistol JM, Florman S, et al. Three-year outcomes from BENEFIT-EXT: a phase III study of belatacept versus cyclosporine in recipients of extended criteria donor kidneys. Am J Transplant. 2012;12:630–9.
82. Levine SM. A survey of clinical practice of lung transplantation in North America. Chest. 2004;125(4):1224–38.
83. Horning NR, Lynch JP, Sundaresan SR, Patterson GA, Trulock EP. Tacolimus therapy for persistent or recurrent acute rejection after lung transplantation. J Heart Lung Transplant. 1998;17:761–7.
84. Kesten S, Chaparro C, Scavuzzo M, Gutierrez C. Tacrolimus as rescue therapy for bronchiolitis obliterans syndrome. J Heart Lung Transplant. 1997;16:905–12.
85. Ross DJ, Lewis MI, Kramer M, Vo A, Kass RM. FK506 rescue immunosuppression for obliterative bronchiolitis after lung transplantation. Chest. 1997;112:1175–9.
86. Sarahrudi K, Estenne M, Corris P, Niedermayer J, Knoop C, Glanville A, et al. International experience with conversion from cyclosporine to tacrolimus for acute and chronic lung allograft rejection. J Thorac Cardiovasc Surg. 2004;127:1126–32.
87. Reams BD, Musselwhite LW, Zaas DW, Steele MP, Garantziotis S, Eu PC, et al. Alemtuzumab in the treatment of refractory acute rejection and bronchiolitis obliterans syndrome after human lung transplantation. Am J Transplant. 2007;7(12):2802–8.

Chapter 15
Macrolides for the Treatment and Prevention of BOS

Robin Vos, Stijn E. Verleden, David Ruttens, Bart M. Vanaudenaerde, and Geert M. Verleden

Abstract Chronic lung allograft rejection or its clinical correlate, the bronchiolitis obliterans syndrome (BOS), characterized by a persistent decline in forced expiratory volume in 1 s (FEV_1) from an established baseline, is the single most important cause of death in lung transplant recipients after the first postoperative year. BOS is thought to be the final common endpoint of various injuries to the pulmonary allograft, triggering different innate and adaptive immune responses. Most preventive and therapeutic strategies for BOS have thus far been largely unsuccessful. However, the introduction of macrolide antibiotics, such as clarithromycin or particularly azithromycin (AZI), in the field of lung transplantation (LTx) as of 2003 made it clear that some patients with established BOS might in fact benefit from such therapy due to its various anti-inflammatory and immunomodulatory properties, as summarized in this chapter. Particularly in patients with an increased bronchoalveolar lavage (BAL) neutrophilia, AZI treatment could result in an increase in FEV_1 of at least 10 %. More recently, it has become clear that prophylactic therapy with AZI actually may prevent BOS and improve FEV_1 after LTx. However, one should always be aware of possible adverse effects related to AZI when implementing this drug as prophylactic or long-term treatment. Even so, AZI therapy after LTx can generally be considered as safe.

Keywords Azithromycin • Bronchiolitis obliterans syndrome • Chronic lung allograft rejection • Macrolide • Lung transplantation • Obliterative bronchiolitis

---

R. Vos, M.D., Ph.D. (✉) • S.E. Verleden, M.Sc. • D. Ruttens, M.D.
B.M. Vanaudenaerde, Ph.D. • G.M. Verleden, M.D., Ph.D.
Lung Transplantation Unit, University Hospital Gasthuisberg,
49, Herestraat, Leuven 3000, Belgium
e-mail: robin.vos@uzleuven.be; stijn.verleden@med.kuleuven.be;
david.ruttens@med.kuleuven.be; bart.vanaudenaerde@med.kuleuven.be; geert.verleden@uzleuven.be

K.C. Meyer and A.R. Glanville (eds.), *Bronchiolitis Obliterans Syndrome in Lung Transplantation*, Respiratory Medicine 8, DOI 10.1007/978-1-4614-7636-8_15,

Pathophysiological Mechanisms Involved in Chronic Lung Allograft Rejection/BOS

Chronic lung allograft rejection/BOS is thought to be the final common endpoint of a multifactorial process of injuries to the pulmonary allograft in the context of recipient immune recognition, and this multifactorial process involves alloimmune, nonalloimmune, and (probably) autoimmune components [1, 2]. The most important alloimmune-dependent risk factors for chronic lung allograft rejection are undoubtedly early acute allograft rejection and late or recurrent/refractory acute rejection. Another alloimmune risk factor is lymphocytic bronchiolitis, with late-onset lymphocytic bronchiolitis posing a greater risk. Next, total human leukocyte antigen (HLA) mismatches and HLA mismatches at the A locus are also well-known alloimmune risk factors [3]. Alloimmune-independent risk factors can be divided into donor or recipient factors. Studies have shown only weak evidence for ischemia-reperfusion injury (IRI) or primary graft dysfunction (PGD) as risk factors, but there is no evidence for donor age, sex, blood type, or ischemic time [3]. Several recipient factors have also been proposed, such as younger age and transplantation for primary pulmonary hypertension, although these are not yet widely accepted [3]. Patient noncompliance to immunosuppressive treatment may provoke acute rejection and should also be considered a risk factor for chronic lung allograft rejection. Both cytomegalovirus (CMV) infection (without pneumonitis) and CMV pneumonitis are also considered as probable risk factors [3]. As the immunocompromised pulmonary allograft recipient may be particularly susceptible to lung inflammation triggered by exogenous infectious agents, toxins, and irritants, it is no surprise that community respiratory virus infections, bacterial/fungal infections, and airway colonization with gram-negative bacteria (e.g., *P. aeruginosa*) or with fungal species (e.g., *Aspergillus* spp.) as well as exposure to air pollution have been associated with the development of chronic lung allograft rejection [3–5]. Gastroesophageal reflux disease (GERD) with aspiration of gastric contents has also been shown to provoke allograft injury, subsequent activation of the innate and adaptive immune system, airway inflammation, and eventually progression towards chronic lung allograft rejection [6].

This primary allograft insult activates resident airway dendritic cells and/or macrophages and upregulates chemokines and cytokines from the endothelium or epithelium itself, resulting in local attraction and activation of other inflammatory cells (lymphocytes, neutrophils) and production of a broad range of chemokines and cytokines by structural airway cells such as smooth muscle cells. Activated neutrophils may further increase epithelial or interstitial damage—for instance, via the production of reactive oxygen species and matrix metalloproteinases (MMP). It is thought that in a later stage a fibroproliferative phase occurs, which is driven by growth factors and infiltration of fibrocytes, that leads to smooth muscle cell and myofibroblast proliferation and eventually results in collagen deposition and, ultimately, fibrous, obliterative airway lesions (obliterative bronchiolitis, OB) [7]. Moreover, recent evidence also suggests the existence of epithelial-mesenchymal transition (EMT) as a factor in the fibrotic response after initial epithelial damage [8]. Interleukin (IL)-17-producing T-helper cells (T_h17) have recently been shown to participate in chronic lung allograft rejection/BOS [9]. T_h17 may be responsible for driving IL-8 secretion from various cell types in the airways through IL-17. Because IL-8 is the most important neutrophil-attracting chemokine in humans [10], T_h17 may account for the increased BAL neutrophilia seen in some patients with BOS. Histologically, pulmonary allograft lesions are initially characterized by infiltration of mononuclear cells in the lamina propria of the affected airway wall, followed by eosinophilic hyaline fibrosis of the submucosa; a fibrous scarring process affecting non-cartilaginous terminal (membranous or respiratory) bronchioles of the pulmonary allograft ultimately occurs, which may be associated with fibro-intimal changes affecting pulmonary arteries and veins [11].

How Azithromycin May Interact with the Underlying Pathophysiological Mechanisms in Chronic Lung Allograft Rejection/BOS

Macrolides belong to the polyketide group of natural products, originally isolated from *Streptomyces* species [12]. Their characteristic structure consists of a macrocyclic lactone ring to which various deoxy sugars, most commonly cladinose and desosamine, are attached. The most important macrolide antibiotics are 14-, 15-, and 16-membered compounds. The prototype macrolide is erythromycin, a 14-membered macrolide. Drug delivery problems resulting from acid instability prompted the design of newer macrolides. These include (1) clarithromycin, roxithromycin, dirithromycin, and the ketolides and fluoroketolides, all of which have a 14-membered ring structure; (2) the 15-membered azithromycin (AZI; Fig. 15.1),

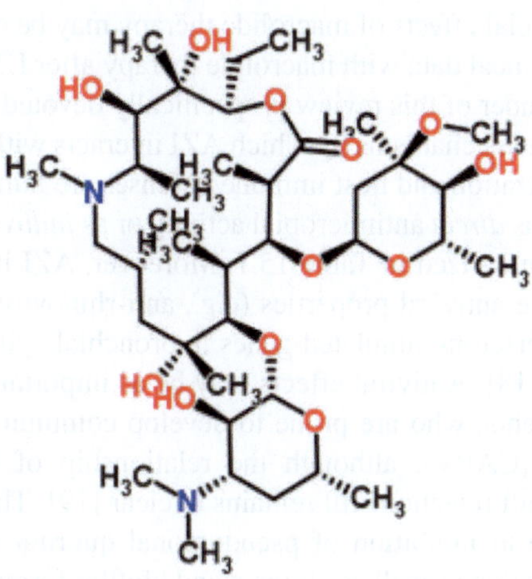

Molecular Formula Azithromycin: $C_{38}H_{72}N_2O_{12}$

Fig. 15.1 Chemical structure of azithromycin

also termed “azalide”; and (3) the 16-membered agents spiramycin, rokitamycin, and josamycin. The more advanced macrolides, AZI and clarithromycin, as well as the (fluoro-) ketolides, have several distinct advantages over erythromycin. These include extended spectrum of activity, improved pharmacokinetics, pharmacodynamics, tolerability, and once-daily administration [12]. For instance, AZI, and to a lesser extent clarithromycin, demonstrate high and prolonged concentrations at sites of infection, reaching tissue levels that are 10- to 100-fold and 2- to 20-fold greater than serum concentrations, respectively [12]. Although predominantly bacteriostatic, the high tissue, macrophage, and polymorphonuclear leukocyte concentrations attained by macrolides and macrolide-like agents may favor bactericidal activity in vivo. Similar to other macrolides, AZI has the ability to reversibly bind to the bacterial 50S ribosome subunit and inhibit protein synthesis, thereby preventing bacterial multiplication. Because AZI demonstrates bacteriostatic activity against gram-positive (e.g., *S. pneumoniae, S. aureus*) and gram-negative pathogens (e.g., *H. influenzae, M. catarrhalis*), as well as atypical respiratory tract pathogens (e.g., *Chlamydia, Mycoplasma, Listeria, Pneumocystis*, and *Legionella* spp.), it is extensively prescribed for the treatment of upper and lower respiratory tract infections [12]. During the 1990s, however, it became clear that the prognosis of patients with diffuse panbronchiolitis, most of whom are chronically colonized with pseudomonas species, dramatically improved after long-term treatment with macrolides was implemented [13]. Additional research showed that macrolides exerted a deleterious effect on the *P. aeruginosa* biofilm formation and epithelial adherence, making individual bacteria more susceptible for more specific antibiotic therapy [13, 14]. Later, long-term, low-dose AZI therapy also proved beneficial in cystic fibrosis (CF) patients with chronic *P. aeruginosa* infection/colonization [14] and in non-CF bronchiectasis [15]. Because airway colonization with pseudomonas, which has a prevalence of 30–40 % after LTx and constitutes an important non-alloimmune risk factor for BOS [4], may induce neutrophilic airway inflammation in a similar way as in the aforementioned neutrophil-driven respiratory disorders [16], comparable beneficial effects of macrolide therapy may be expected after LTx. Because most of the clinical data with macrolide therapy after LTx have been obtained with AZI, the remainder of this review is specifically devoted to AZI therapy.

The mechanisms by which AZI interacts with bacterial (pseudomonal) infection/colonization and host immune defenses are numerous, but generally can be categorized as *direct* antimicrobial activity or as *indirect* immunomodulatory activity [17], as summarized in Table 15.1. Moreover, AZI has recently also been demonstrated to have antiviral properties (e.g., anti-rhinovirus activity and increased production of interferon-stimulated genes in bronchial epithelial cells during rhinovirus infection) [18]. Antiviral effects may be as important as the antibacterial effects in LTx recipients, who are prone to develop community-acquired respiratory viral infections (CARV), although the relationship of CARV with acute and/or chronic allograft rejection still remains unclear [19]. The anti-pseudomonal activity of AZI is due to inhibition of pseudomonal quorum sensing-dependent virulence factor production as well as alginate and biofilm formation, making mucoid bacteria more susceptible to complement- or oxidative stress-mediated killing as well as to

Table 15.1 Cellular mechanisms and proposed sites of action of azithromycin

Effects	Activity	Cellular mechanisms	Site of action [References]
Direct antimicrobial effects	Antibacterial	Binding of 50S ribosome subunit and ↓ protein synthesis	Gram-positive (e.g., *S. pneumoniae, S. aureus*), gram-negative (e.g., *H. influenzae, M. catarrhalis*), and atypical pathogens (e.g., *Chlamydia, Mycoplasma, Listeria, Pneumocystis, Legionella* spp.) [12]
		↓ quorum sensing-dependent virulence factors, ↓ alginate and biofilm formation, ↓ protein synthesis, interaction with outer cellular membrane proteins	*P. aeruginosa* [20–23]
Indirect host immunomodulatory effects	Antiviral	↑ IFN-stimulated genes	Rhinovirus-infected primary human bronchial *epithelial* cells [18]
	Antibacterial	Maintained integrity, ↓ mucin production, ↓ IL-6/8, MMP-1/2/9/10/13, GM-CSF, ↑ phospholipidosis, ↓ mitosis	Pseudomonal infected [24, 25, 27] or LPS-stimulated [26] primary human bronchial *epithelial* cells
		↑ acute degranulation and phagocytosis-associated oxidative burst	Pseudomonal or LPS-stimulated human *polymorphonuclear leucocytes* [43, 45]
	Other in vitro	↑ CD34, E-selectin, ICAM-1	Untreated human *endothelial cells* (EA.hy 926 and primary vascular endothelial cells) [28]
		↓ IL-8, 8-isoprostane and VEGF, direct relaxant effect, antiproliferative and autophagic effect	IL-17 stimulated [31] or FGF stimulated [32] human primary bronchial, precontracted [33] or untreated rabit primary tracheal [34] *smooth muscle cells*
		Reservoir and transfer to other phagocytic cells	Human *fibroblasts* [35]
		↓ IL-1β (beta), CCL-2, TNF-α (alpha), and IL-12p40, ↑ phagocytosis, shift towards M2-phenotype (↑ mannose receptor, CD23 and arginase)	LPS-stimulated [37] or untreated [39] human or murine [38] primary alveolar *macrophages*, LPS- or INF-γ stimulated murine RAW264.7 [40] or J774 [41] macrophage cell line
		↓ IL-8, GRO-α (alpha), MPO and PGE2, ↓ delayed oxidative burst responses, ↑ apoptosis, ↓ chemotactic response	Untreated [42], pseudomonal [44], or LPS-stimulated [46] human *polymorphonuclear leucocytes*
		↓ TNF-*α* (alpha) and GM-CSF, ↑ apoptosis	LPS stimulated PBMCs [48] or anti-CD3/CD28 and IL-2 stimulated human *lymphocytes* [47]
		↑ IL-10 and CD-80, ↓ IL-6, IL-12p40, CXCL10/11, CCL2, CD40, CD86, MHCII and TLR- 4, ↑ regulatory and phagocytic properties	LPS stimulated PBMC-derived human [49] or bone-marrow-derived murine [50, 51] *dendritic cells*
	Other in vivo	↓ leukocyte, lymphocyte and neutrophil numbers, ↓ 8-isoprostane, IL-1β (beta), IL-6, and GRO/KC	Murine lung *ischemia-reperfusion injury* [52]
		↓ BAL IL-1β(beta)/8, MPO, TIMP-1, MMP-8/9, and neutrophils ↓ plasma MIP-1α (alpha), I309, MCP-1, TNF-α (alpha), and IL-8	Human lung transplant recipients with BOS [56–58]

specific antibiotics when in the stationary growth phase [20, 21]. A bactericidal effect through interaction with the outer membrane [22] and inhibition of protein synthesis after intracellular accumulation has also been demonstrated [23].

Modulation of host defenses by AZI during infection/colonization includes effects on the respiratory epithelium that include preserved integrity [24], reduced mucin secretion [25], altered signal transduction (mitogen-activated protein kinase, MAPK) pathways, and gene expression of inflammatory, lipid metabolism, and cell cycle pathways [26, 27]. In untreated endothelial cells, AZI has been shown to upregulate various cell surface markers involved in interactions between endothelial cells and leukocytes [28], yet suppression of adhesion molecule function can be seen with other macrolides in lipopolysaccharide [LPS]-stimulated epithelial cells or neutrophils [29, 30]

AZI not only inhibits interleukin (IL)-17-induced IL-8 and 8-isoprostane release in airway smooth muscle cells [31], but it can also attenuate fibroblast growth factor (FGF)-induced vascular endothelial growth factor (VEGF) production in airway smooth muscle cells via its interactions with MAPK-signaling [32]. AZI also has a direct relaxant effect on precontracted airway smooth muscle cells [33], and it has an antiproliferative and autophagic effect on airway smooth muscle cells [34]. It has also been suggested that fibroblasts may act as a tissue reservoir for AZI and may even be involved in the transfer of AZI to phagocytic cells, such as macrophages and neutrophils [35, 36].

AZI has been shown to inhibit LPS-induced production and expression of pro-inflammatory cytokines by alveolar macrophages via inhibition of nuclear expression of activator protein-1 (AP-1) [37, 38], and it has been shown to increase phagocytosis of apoptotic epithelial cells or neutrophils by upregulation of the macrophage mannose receptor [39]. In LPS or interferon (INF)-γ(gamma)-stimulated macrophages, AZI has also been recently shown to attenuate subsequent T_{h}-1 responses [40], and AZI may also shift macrophage polarization towards the alternatively activated M2-phenotype, which plays a role in directing T_h-2 responses and coordinating repair following an inflammatory reaction [41].

Due to its intracellular accumulation, the concentration of AZI in neutrophils can reach more than 2,000 times that of the plasma concentration [42], which promotes antibiotic delivery to phagocytosed bacteria [43] and may explain the ability of AZI to exert direct effects on neutrophils as it accumulates at the site of inflammation. Uptake of AZI results in acute stimulation of neutrophil degranulation and the phagocytosis-associated oxidative burst, which may contribute towards the acute antibacterial activity of AZI. Acute anti-inflammatory actions include down-regulating effects on chemokine production, and delayed inhibitory effects of AZI on neutrophils include decreased oxidative respiratory burst responses, down-regulating effects on myeloperoxidase (MPO) production, and an increase in neutrophil apoptosis. Additionally, AZI attenuates both chemokine-dependent (e.g., IL-8) and chemokine-independent neutrophil chemotactic responses by having a suppressive effect on the MAPK-signal transduction pathway (inhibition of transcription factors NFκ(kappa)-B and AP-1) [44].

Leukotriene B4 (LTB4), a metabolite of the arachidonic acid cascade that is known to be released from neutrophils and alveolar macrophages in response to various stimuli, is another potent, endogenously formed chemotactic and adhesion-promoting factor for human neutrophils. LTB4-production has been shown to be suppressed by erythromycin and roxithromycin in patients with panbronchiolitis who are colonized with pseudomonas species, which suggests that LTB4 may also be inhibited by AZI [45]. AZI can also inhibit prostaglandin E2-synthesis in LPS-stimulated polymorphonuclear and mononuclear leukocytes by suppressing mRNA-expression for prostaglandin synthetic enzymes (COX-1 and COX-2) [46]. At high concentrations (as can be seen with accumulation of AZI at a site of inflammation), AZI may also promote apoptotic cell death of local lymphocytes via upregulation of Fas/Fas-ligand antigen expression or down-regulation of Bcl-xL expression [47]. AZI has been shown to decrease tumor necrosis factor (TNF)-α(alpha) and granulocyte monocyte-colony-stimulating factor (GM-CSF) production by LPS-stimulated monocytes [48], and AZI also modulates the differentiation and the LPS-induced maturation of dendritic cells (DC) towards a DC phenotype that is associated with regulatory properties and increased phagocytic capacity [49, 50]. Finally, AZI can not only inhibit expression of co-stimulatory molecules (CD40 and CD86) and major histocompatibility complex (MHC) class II in LPS-induced DC, but it can also reduce Toll-like receptor (TLR)-4 expression, IL-12 production, and the allo-stimulatory capacity of DCs, all of which suggests that it has the potential to modulate allogeneic responses [51].

It should be noted that the pleiotropic, anti-inflammatory, and immunomodulatory effects of AZI on the innate immune response described above may occur in the absence of lower respiratory tract colonization or infection by microbes. As an example, in the setting of transplantation, in vivo immunomodulatory effects have been described in a murine model of isolated lung IRI in which AZI pretreatment reduced leukocyte, lymphocyte, and neutrophil numbers and also reduced 8-isoprostane, IL-1β(beta), and, to a lesser extent, IL-6 and GRO/KC levels following ischemia and reperfusion [52]. Additionally, clarithromycin therapy has been shown to attenuate TNF-α(alpha) and IFN-γ(gamma) expression and fibrous obliteration of heterotopic tracheal allografts in a rat model of OB [53]. AZI has also been shown to inhibit the acute phase response of the pentraxin serum amyloid-A (SAA) to a sterile inflammatory stimulus in mice [54]. SAA is synthesized by the liver after IL-1β(beta) or IL-6 stimulation, as is C-reactive protein (CRP); therefore, AZI could also directly (i.e., by inhibiting CRP synthesis in hepatocytes and/or local CRP-producing cells) or indirectly (i.e., by reducing cytokine release at the site of inflammation) reduce circulating or local CRP levels after LTx, and this has been demonstrated in patients with both COPD and CF [39, 55]. Moreover, AZI has not only been shown to reduce local airway inflammation after LTx (e.g., decreased BAL fluid IL-8, MMP-9, and neutrophilia) [56], but it has also been recently shown to attenuate plasma levels of multiple pro-inflammatory chemokines in a cohort of LTx recipients with BOS after 6–12 months of azithromycin treatment [57, 58]. The unique immunomodulatory properties of AZI (as discussed above), combined with its exceptional intrapulmonary pharmacokinetics [59], which promote extensive and sustained lung tissue penetration [60], are not only the likely explanation for its disease-modifying effects in various infectious [55] or noninfectious inflammatory pulmonary conditions [61, 62], but these properties are also likely to be operant in chronic allograft rejection after LTx, as it is clear that many pathophysiological mechanisms involved in airway inflammation and remodeling can be modulated by AZI. One can readily suspect that interaction with or even reversal of ongoing airway inflammation/remodeling by AZI may affect airflow and, thus, FEV_1 measurements in patients with BOS.

Azithromycin in the Treatment of Chronic Lung Allograft Rejection/BOS

Despite the initial use of immunosuppressive protocols that consisted of a triple-drug regimen of prednisolone, cyclosporine A, and azathioprine, recipients remained at risk to develop chronic lung allograft rejection. Although the subsequent introduction of newer immunosupressants such as tacrolimus, mycophenolate mofetil, sirolimus, and everolimus allowed modification of immunosuppressive protocols, these newer agents have also been unable to prevent chronic rejection after LTx [63]. Furthermore, once chronic lung allograft rejection/BOS was diagnosed, conventional treatment with changes to other agents or increased dosages of available immunosuppressives and/or corticosteroids did not seem to significantly improve the typical course of the decreasing FEV_1; at best, such changes could only stabilize FEV_1 [63]. Given these frustrating results of attempts to prevent and treat BOS, it became clear that other therapies were needed. Because of the similarities of BOS with other neutrophilic-driven pulmonary diseases (as discussed above), Gerhardt et al. introduced macrolide therapy to the treatment of BOS and were the first to do so [64]. Maintenance AZI therapy was given (250 mg 3 times a week for a mean of 13.7 weeks) in addition to conventional immunosuppression in this open-label landmark study of six LTx recipients with BOS. Remarkably, five of these six patients demonstrated a significant improvement in FEV_1 of 17.1 % predicted or 0.5 L (as compared with their baseline values at the start of AZI therapy). Two other small studies corroborated these findings shortly thereafter and demonstrated a mean increase in FEV_1 of 18.3 % predicted (0.33 L) and 14 % predicted (0.11 L), respectively [65, 66]. Subsequently, Shitrit et al. were unable to demonstrate similar findings; however, as FEV_1 stabilized after 10 months of AZI treatment (i.e., 40 ± 9 % predicted at initiation vs. 38 ± 10 % predicted at end of follow-up), the authors concluded that AZI may nevertheless slow disease progression [67]. More recently, however, other groups [56, 68–72] were able to demonstrate FEV_1 improvement after initiation of AZI, as summarized in Table 15.2. Comparable results have also been obtained using clarithromycin in BOS [73]. Of note, it has now been reported that AZI treatment could have an effect on structural airway changes in addition to

Table 15.2 Azithromycin for established BOS[a]

Author [Reference]	No. included	No. improved	FEV_1 improvement (responders)	FEV_1 change (mean all patients)
Gerhardt [64]	6	5 (83 %)	+21 %	+17 %
Verleden [65]	8	4 (50 %)	+26 %	+18 %
Yates [66]	20	10 (50 %)	?	+14 %
Shitrit [67]	11	2 (18 %)	?	Stable
Verleden [68]	14	6 (43 %)	At least +10 %	+13 %
Vos [69]	107	43 (40 %)	+12 %	Stable
Porhownik [70]	7	2 (29 %)	At least +10 %	Stable
Gottlieb [71]	81	24 (30 %)	+17 %	Stable
Jain [72]	78	28 (36 %)	At least +10 %	?
Meloni [57]	62	13 (21 %)	+24 %	+7 % (estimate)
Vos [82]	18	11 (61 %)	+15 %	?
Total	412	148 (36 %)	–	+7.6 % (mean estimate)

[a]Note that some patients may have been included in more than one study and that time of evaluation after initiation of azithromycin after transplantation differs between studies and ranges from a mean of 3 months to 3 years

functional improvement, as was seen in a LTx recipient with end-stage chronic rejection (BOS stage 3) who demonstrated a major improvement in bronchiectasis after 5 months of AZI treatment [74]. This was more recently corroborated in a large, retrospective cohort-study that demonstrated radiologic improvement in bronchial dilatation, consolidation, and air trapping in the subgroup of BOS patients responsive to AZI (i.e., those who demonstrated increased airway neutrophilia at initiation of therapy and improvement of FEV_1 while receiving AZI) [75].

How can one explain the observed interactions of AZI on FEV_1 mechanistically? Gottlieb et al. demonstrated that AZI responders at 6 months (i.e., improvement of FEV_1 of at least 10 % predicted or more) demonstrated that higher percentages of neutrophils were present in BAL for responders vs. non-responders [71]. This finding was later confirmed [69] and is corroborated by previous data showing that AZI significantly reduced BAL neutrophilia and IL-8 protein levels in patients with BOS [68]. Moreover, pretreatment BAL neutrophilia had a high positive predictive value for subsequent improvement of FEV1 after initiation of AZI with a cut-off that varied from 15 [68] to 20 % [71]. Thus, modulation of airway inflammation (and associated airway remodeling) by AZI may explain the effect on airflow and improved FEV_1.

Recently, we have obtained additional evidence for modulation of host innate immune responses by AZI. A significant improvement in FEV_1 with AZI therapy was observed in those BOS patients who demonstrated pretreatment upregulation of factors associated with airway inflammation (IL-1β(beta), IL-8), oxidative stress (myloperoxidase), and matrix remodeling (tissue inhibitor of metalloproteinases (TIMP)-1; MMP-8/9) [76]. When various risk factors for BOS were examined, responders seemed to have higher PGD scores and more lymphocytic bronchiolitis (LB) episodes compared to non-responders, and both PGD and LB are associated with airway inflammation and BAL neutrophilia [69]. In addition to its immunomodulatory properties, AZI can enhance esophageal motility and accelerate gastric emptying, and a reduction in airway inflammation caused by aspiration of gastric contents (pepsin and bile acids) after LTx may also partially explain the beneficial effects of AZI in this setting [77]. A remarkable finding by Gottlieb et al., however, was the finding that 23 % of the initial AZI responders eventually developed a progressive decrease in FEV_1 compatible with BOS despite sustained treatment with AZI. This finding was confirmed by our group, and concurrent BAL neutrophilia was absent when relapse occurred [69]. This observation suggests that despite the modulation of some innate pathophysiological mechanisms by AZI, other mechanisms (yet to be unraveled) may nevertheless be unaffected and eventually may lead to recurrence and progression of BOS in initial responders. Despite this finding, however, a significantly better overall survival in responders compared to nonresponders has now been demonstrated by several studies [69, 71, 72]. Additionally, long-term outcome in AZI-treated patients may even be better compared to historical outcomes of untreated patients with BOS (irrespective of their response in FEV_1) [69, 71]. Multivariate analyses have demonstrated that both a response to AZI administration as well as initiation of AZI therapy at an earlier time in the post-transplant course are independent predictors for better allograft outcomes following the onset of BOS [71], which may reflect a better response to AZI if treatment is initiated at an earlier stage of BOS [58, 72].

To summarize the beneficial results of AZI therapy for BOS, we conclude that AZI not only significantly improves allograft function in specific subsets of patients with chronic allograft dysfunction by modulation of host innate immune responses, but, more importantly, it also improves long-term outcome in these patients. From these retrospective, open-label case-series, it became clear that randomized controlled trials (RCT) of AZI, both as preventive or as treatment strategy for established BOS, were required despite the fact that such trials may be of low commercial value to companies marketing AZI [78].

The first RCT of AZI treatment for established BOS was recently completed by the Newcastle group (EudraCT 2006-000485-36) and showed that AZI significantly improves lung function after 12 weeks of therapy as compared to placebo in patients with BOS [79]. Based on these findings of AZI therapy in LTx recipients with BOS, one can conclude that chronic lung allograft rejection/BOS in fact is a heterogeneous condition that likely consists of at least two different BOS phenotypes (Fig. 15.2) that can be distinguished on the basis of a combination of clinical findings, HRCT imaging, BAL neutrophilia, and airway histopathologic changes [80, 81] (Table 15.3). The inflammatory phenotype starts rather early after LTx (often in the first postoperative year), progresses gradually, and is characterized by concurrent neutrophilic airway inflammation and beneficial response to AZI. In contrast, the fibroproliferative phenotype is characterized by later onset after LTx, more rapid progression, absence of overt neutrophilic inflammation, and lack of response to AZI, most often leading to respiratory insufficiency and death in a rather short period of time [80, 81].

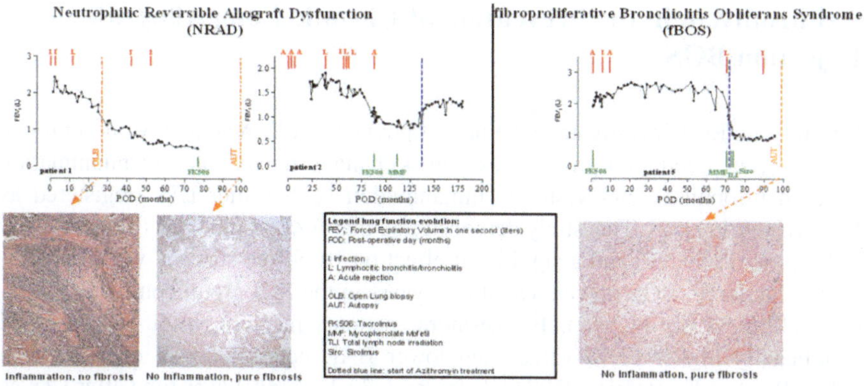

Fig. 15.2 Chronic lung allograft rejection phenotypes based on azithromycin treatment. Adapted from [75, 80, 81]

Table 15.3 Chronic lung allograft rejection phenotypes based on azithromycin treatment[a]

	Neutrophilic reversible allograft dysfunction (NRAD)	Fibroproliferative BOS (fBOS)
Bronchoalveolar lavage	Neutrophilia >15 %	Neutrophilia <15 %
Clinical signs	Coarse crackles, increased sputum production	No crackles, no sputum
Time of onset	Mostly early after transplantation (<1 year)	Mostly later (>1 year)
Progression of FEV_1 decrease	Slow (several years)	Rapid (<6–12 months)
Histology airway wall	Lymphocytic inflammation, ends up in fibrosis	Pure fibrosis
Radiology	Mainly tree-in-bud, airway wall thickening, mucus plugging, bronchiectasis	Mainly air trapping, consolidation
Effect of azithromycin	Decrease in lymphocytic airway wall inflammation and in bronchoalveolar lavage neutrophils	No effects on fibrosis, probably similar effects on possible minor simultaneous airway wall and bronchoalveolar lavage inflammation
	Improvement of FEV_1 (reversible decline)	No improvement of FEV_1 (further decline or temporary stabilization)
	Decrease in severity of tree-in-bud, airway wall thickening, mucus plugging, bronchiectasis, consolidations, ground glass, and airtrapping on chest CT scan	Lesser decrease in severity of possible simultaneous tree-in-bud, airway wall thickening, mucus plugging, and ground glass on chest CT scan, no effect on bronchiectasis, consolidations, and airtrapping

[a]Adapted from [75, 80, 81]

Azithromycin in the Prevention of Chronic Lung Allograft Rejection/BOS

Recently, an RCT investigated whether prophylactic AZI treatment would improve outcome (i.e., freedom from BOS) as well as changes in FEV_1, airway inflammation (BAL neutrophilia), and systemic inflammation (CRP) after LTx (registered as NCT01009619) [82]. This study demonstrated that AZI prophylaxis (initiated prior to hospital discharge) had a significant effect on BOS-free survival with a significant reduction in BOS prevalence after 2 years in the AZI group compared to placebo (12.5 % vs. 44.2 %). Furthermore, patients receiving AZI demonstrated significantly higher FEV_1 values and lower BAL neutrophil cell counts (mean 9.4 ± 1.9 %) and systemic CRP levels (mean 6.7 ± 1.4 mg/L) over time after LTx as compared to patients receiving placebo (19.4 ± 3.7 % and 14.0 ± 3.5 mg/L, respectively) [82]. These data clearly demonstrate the association of prophylactic AZI therapy with better post-transplant outcomes, presumably due to its anti-inflammatory properties and ability to attenuate local airway and systemic inflammation resulting from various alloimmunologic and non-alloimmunologic events that affect the pulmonary allograft. However, a more recent, retrospective analysis of clarithromycin for the prevention of BOS in lung transplant recipients could not confirm a benefit in BOS-free or overall survival in patients receiving clarithromycin, although it remains difficult to explain this discrepancy with AZI [83].

Pitfalls for Long-Term Treatment with Azithromycin

If AZI is used as a prophylactic therapy post-transplant, one should be aware of possible adverse effects related to AZI. However, there are relatively few data that suggest that long-term AZI treatment cannot generally be considered safe. The most common side effects are caused by its effects on the gastrointestinal tract and include nausea, vomiting, diarrhea, or abdominal pain due to stimulation of gut motility. Gastrointestinal intolerance increases in proportion to measured serum concentrations [84], is more common with daily compared to thrice-weekly therapy [85], and may respond to dose reduction or the use of an oral suspension. However, AZI treatment may need to be suspended for some patients. Chronic AZI therapy has a low incidence of laboratory abnormalities, serious adverse events, or drug–drug interactions as compared to other macrolides. Some rare side effects of AZI have been reported, which include aggravation of myasthenia gravis, inappropriate antidiuretic hormone secretion with severe hyponatremia, interstitial nephritis, cholestatic jaundice in case of preexisting liver disease, and reversible tinnitus or hearing loss [86]. Unlike other macrolides, true allergic reactions or anaphylaxis to AZI is highly unlikely. However, a recent study has raised concern that AZI may prolong the QT_c-interval and lead to potentially fatal Torsades de Pointes [87]. Drug–drug interactions are relatively unlikely because AZI does not interact with the hepatic

CYP450 complex (unlike other macrolides), which inhibit the CYP3A4 enzyme and alter metabolism of other drugs (e.g., calcineurin inhibitors, mTOR inhibitors) by the liver [88, 89]. AZI is primarily eliminated unchanged in feces, and urinary excretion is minimal, which makes dosing modifications unnecessary in patients with mild to moderate hepatic or renal impairment, although a transient mild increase in transaminases may be seen shortly after initiation [60]. In patients with subjective intolerance or possible drug interactions with administration or oral AZI, aerosolized administration of AZI represents a potential future strategy to minimize adverse effects while maximizing drug delivery to the target site of disease [90, 91].

Another consideration that should be taken into account with long-term AZI therapy is the potential for selection of antibiotic-resistant bacteria. A recent study in healthy volunteers who received AZI or placebo for 3 days demonstrated that about 50 % of AZI-treated subjects acquired resistant streptococcal flora in the oropharynx after 2 weeks of therapy that decreased to about 35 % after 6 weeks of baseline [92]. Macrolide resistance in streptococci arises from an alteration of the ribosomal drug-binding site by methylation of the 23S bacterial ribosomal RNA, induction of drug-inactivating enzymes (esterases and kinases), or via active drug efflux proteins, which are products of macrolide efflux genes specific for 14- and 15-membered macrolides [93]. However, it should be noted that streptococcal macrolide resistance can significantly vary from one region to another and that in Belgium, for instance, macrolide resistance can be found in up to 30 % of noninvasive *S. pneumoniae* isolates [94]. These data in healthy volunteers were recently corroborated by prospective data in CF patients that associated long-term administration of AZI with an increase in macrolide resistance in *S. aureus* and *Haemophilus* spp. [95, 96]. Also, mutations in multidrug efflux pumps have been described in AZI-resistant *P. aeruginosa* biofilms [97], and this could become more prevalent in *P. aeruginosae* with increased use of AZI.

Conclusion

Chronic lung allograft rejection, which is widely attributed to the onset of BOS, remains the most important hurdle to tackle in improving long-term outcome after LTx. The recent introduction of macrolide therapy in the field of LTx has undeniably changed the current view on chronic rejection after LTx. The promising results regarding pulmonary function and survival benefit obtained with AZI in some patients with BOS, as well as the potential of prophylactic AZI treatment in preventing BOS, will likely change future treatment strategies in LTx. Moreover, numerous other pulmonary disorders, in addition to BOS in LTx, that share many common innate inflammatory mechanisms can potentially benefit from AZI therapy. Additionally, other disorders that present as true bronchiolitis obliterans [98–101] as well as neutrophilic airway disease after non-pulmonary organ transplantation [102] may benefit from such therapy. Indeed, AZI may prove useful for the medical treatment of many chronic pulmonary disorders in the future.

Acknowledgements G.M.V. is holder of the Glaxo Smith Kline (Belgium) chair in respiratory pharmacology at the KULeuven and is supported by the Research Foundation Flanders (FWO): G.0643.08 and G.0723.10 and Onderzoeksfonds KULeuven (OT/10/050). B.M.V., DEVR, and LJD are senior research fellows of the Research Foundation Flanders (FWO G.0518.06, G.0643.08, G.0723.10)

Conflict of Interest Statement: None of the authors has a financial relationship with a commercial entity that has an interest in the subject of the presented manuscript.

References

1. Estenne M, Maurer JR, Boehler A, Egan JJ, Frost A, Hertz M, et al. Bronchiolitis obliterans syndrome 2001: an update of the diagnostic criteria. J Heart Lung Transplant. 2002;21: 297–310.
2. Hagedorn PH, Burton CM, Carlsen J, Steinbrüchel D, Andersen CB, Sahar E, et al. Chronic rejection of a lung transplant is characterized by a profile of specific autoantibodies. Immunology. 2010;130(3):427–35.
3. Sharples LD, McNeil K, Stewart S, Wallwork J. Risk factors for bronchiolitis obliterans: a systematic review of recent publications. J Heart Lung Transplant. 2002;21(2):271–81.
4. Vos R, Vanaudenaerde BM, Geudens N, Dupont LJ, Van Raemdonck DE, Verleden GM. Pseudomonal airway colonisation: risk factor for bronchiolitis obliterans syndrome after lung transplantation? Eur Respir J. 2008;31:1037–45.
5. Nawrot TS, Vos R, Jacobs L, Verleden SE, Wauters S, Mertens V, et al. The impact of traffic air pollution on chronic rejection and mortality after lung transplantation. Thorax. 2011;66(9):748–54.
6. Blondeau K, Mertens V, Vanaudenaerde BA, Verleden GM, Van Raemdonck DE, Sifrim D, et al. Gastro-oesophageal reflux and gastric aspiration in lung transplant patients with or without chronic rejection. Eur Respir J. 2008;31(4):707–13.
7. Boehler A, Kesten S, Weder W, Speich R. Bronchiolitis obliterans after lung transplantation: a review. Chest. 1998;114(5):1411–26.
8. Borthwick LA, McIlroy E, Gorowiec MR, Brodlie M, Johnson GE, Ward C, et al. Inflammation and epithelial to mesenchymal transition in lung transplant recipients: role in dysregulated epithelial wound repair. Am J Transplant. 2010;10(3):498–509.
9. Vanaudenaerde BM, De Vleeschauwer SI, Vos R, Meyts I, Bullens DM, Reynders V, et al. The role of the IL23/IL17 axis in bronchiolitis obliterans syndrome after lung transplantation. Am J Transplant. 2008;8(9):1911–20.
10. DiGiovine B, Lynch 3rd JP, Martinez FJ, Flint A, Whyte RI, Iannettoni MD, et al. Bronchoalveolar lavage neutrophilia is associated with obliterative bronchiolitis after lung transplantation: role of IL-8. J Immunol. 1996;157(9):4194–202.
11. Stewart S, Fishbein MC, Snell GI, Berry GJ, Boehler A, Burke MM, et al. Revision of the 1996 working formulation for the standardization of nomenclature in the diagnosis of lung rejection. J Heart Lung Transplant. 2007;26(12):1229–42.
12. Retsema J, Fu W. Macrolides: structures and microbial targets. Int J Antimicrob Agents. 2001;18(S1):S3–10.
13. Kobayashi H, Ohgaki N, Takeda H. Therapeutic possibilities for diffuse panbronchiolitis. Int J Antimicrob Agents. 1993;3(S1):S81–6.
14. Saiman L, Marshall BC, Mayer-Hamblett N, Burns JL, Quittner AL, Cibene DA, et al. Azithromycin in patients with cystic fibrosis chronically infected with Pseudomonas aeruginosa: a randomized controlled trial. JAMA. 2003;290(13):1749–56.
15. Anwar GA, Bourke SC, Afolabi G, Middleton P, Ward C, Rutherford RM. Effects of long-term low-dose azithromycin in patients with non-CF bronchiectasis. Respir Med. 2008;102(10):1494–6.

16. Vos R, Vanaudenaerde BM, Dupont LJ, Van Raemdonck DE, Verleden GM. Transient airway colonization is associated with airway inflammation after lung transplantation. Am J Transplant. 2007;7:1278–87.
17. Shinkai M, Henke MO, Rubin BK. Macrolide antibiotics as immunomodulatory medications: proposed mechanisms of action. Pharmacol Ther. 2008;117:393–405.
18. Gielen V, Johnston SL, Edwards MR. Azithromycin induces anti-viral responses in bronchial epithelial cells. Eur Respir J. 2010;36(3):646–54.
19. Weinberg A, Lyu DM, Li S, Marquesen J, Zamora MR. Incidence and morbidity of human metapneumovirus and other community-acquired respiratory viruses in lung transplant recipients. Transpl Infect Dis. 2010;12(4):330–5.
20. Kai T, Tateda K, Kimura S, Ishii Y, Ito H, Yoshida H, et al. A low concentration of azithromycin inhibits the mRNA expression of N-acyl homoserine lactone synthesis enzymes, upstream of lasI or rhlI, in Pseudomonas aeruginosa. Pulm Pharmacol Ther. 2009;22(6):483–6.
21. Hoffmann N, Lee B, Hentzer M, Rasmussen TB, Song Z, Johansen HK, et al. Azithromycin blocks quorum sensing and alginate polymer formation and increases the sensitivity to serum and stationary-growth-phase killing of Pseudomonas aeruginosa and attenuates chronic P. aeruginosa lung infection in Cftr(−/−) mice. Antimicrob Agents Chemother. 2007;51(10):3677–87.
22. Sugimura M, Maseda H, Hanaki H, Nakae T. Macrolide antibiotic-mediated downregulation of MexAB-OprM efflux pump expression in Pseudomonas aeruginosa. Antimicrob Agents Chemother. 2008;52(11):4141–4.
23. Kawamura-Sato K, Iinuma Y, Hasegawa T, Horii T, Yamashino T, Ohta M. Effect of subinhibitory concentrations of macrolides on expression of flagellin in Pseudomonas aeruginosa and Proteus mirabilis. Antimicrob Agents Chemother. 2000;44(10):2869–72.
24. Halldorsson S, Gudjonsson T, Gottfredsson M, Singh PK, Gudmundsson GH, Baldursson O. Azithromycin maintains airway epithelial integrity during Pseudomonas aeruginosa infection. Am J Respir Cell Mol Biol. 2010;42(1):62–8.
25. Imamura Y, Yanagihara K, Mizuta Y, Seki M, Ohno H, Higashiyama Y, et al. Azithromycin inhibits MUC5AC production induced by the Pseudomonas aeruginosa autoinducer N-(3-Oxododecanoyl) homoserine lactone in NCI-H292 cells. Antimicrob Agents Chemother. 2004;48(9):3457–61.
26. Murphy DM, Forrest IA, Corris PA, Johnson GE, Small T, Jones D, et al. Azithromycin attenuates effects of lipopolysaccharide on lung allograft bronchial epithelial cells. J Heart Lung Transplant. 2008;27(11):1210–6.
27. Ribeiro CM, Hurd H, Wu Y, Martino ME, Jones L, Brighton B, et al. Azithromycin treatment alters gene expression in inflammatory, lipid metabolism, and cell cycle pathways in well-differentiated human airway epithelia. PLoS One. 2009;4(6):e5806.
28. Millrose M, Kruse M, Flick B, Stahlmann R. Effects of macrolides on proinflammatory epitopes on endothelial cells in vitro. Arch Toxicol. 2009;83(5):469–76.
29. Khair OA, Devalia JL, Abdelaziz MM, Sapsford RJ, Davies RJ. Effect of erythromycin on Haemophilus influenzae endotoxin-induced release of IL-6, IL-8 and sICAM-1 by cultured human bronchial epithelial cells. Eur Respir J. 1995;8(9):1451–7.
30. Lin HC, Wang CH, Liu CY, Yu CT, Kuo HP. Erythromycin inhibits beta2-integrins (CD11b/CD18) expression, interleukin-8 release and intracellular oxidative metabolism in neutrophils. Respir Med. 2000;94(7):654–60.
31. Vanaudenaerde BM, Wuyts WA, Geudens N, Dupont LJ, Schoofs K, Smeets S, et al. Macrolides inhibit IL17-induced IL8 and 8-isoprostane release from human airway smooth muscle cells. Am J Transplant. 2007;7(1):76–82.
32. Willems-Widyastuti A, Vanaudenaerde BM, Vos R, Dilisen E, Verleden SE, De Vleeschauwer SI, et al. Azithromycin attenuates fibroblast growth factors induced vascular endothelial growth factor via p38(MAPK) signaling in human airway smooth muscle cells. Cell Biochem Biophys. 2011 Dec 29. [Epub ahead of print].
33. Daenas C, Hatziefthimiou AA, Gourgoulianis KI, Molyvdas PA. Azithromycin has a direct relaxant effect on precontracted airway smooth muscle. Eur J Pharmacol. 2006;553(1–3):280–7.

34. Stamatiou R, Paraskeva E, Boukas K, Gourgoulianis KI, Molyvdas PA, Hatziefthimiou AA. Azithromycin has an antiproliferative and autophagic effect on airway smooth muscle cells. Eur Respir J. 2009;34(3):721–30.
35. McDonald PJ, Pruul H. Phagocyte uptake and transport of azithromycin. Eur J Clin Microbiol Infect Dis. 1991;10(10):828–33.
36. Idris S, Chilvers E, Haworth C, Mc Keon D, Condliffe A. Azithromycin therapy for neutrophilic airways disease: myth or magic? Thorax. 2009;64:186–9.
37. Meyer M, Huaux F, Gavilanes X, van den Brûle S, Lebecque P, Lo Re S, et al. Azithromycin reduces exagerated cytokine production by M1 alveolar macrophages in cystic fibrosis. Am J Respir Cell Mol Biol. 2009;41(5):590–602.
38. Bosnar M, Cuzic S, Bosnjak B, Nujić K, Ergović G, Marjanović N, et al. Azithromycin inhibits macrophage interleukin-1β production through inhibition of AP-1 in lipopolysaccharide-induced murine pulmonary neutrophilia. Int Immunopharmacol. 2011;11(4):424–34.
39. Hodge S, Hodge G, Jersmann H, Matthews G, Ahern J, Holmes M, et al. Azithromycin improves macrophage phagocytic function and expression of mannose receptor in chronic obstructive pulmonary disease. Am J Respir Crit Care Med. 2008;178(2):139–48.
40. Yamauchi K, Shibata Y, Kimura T, Abe S, Inoue S, Osaka D, et al. Azithromycin suppresses interleukin-12p40 expression in lipopolysaccharide and interferon-gamma stimulated macrophages. Int J Biol Sci. 2009;5(7):667–78.
41. Murphy BS, Sundareshan V, Cory TJ, Hayes Jr D, Anstead MI, Feola DJ. Azithromycin alters macrophage phenotype. J Antimicrob Chemother. 2008;61(3):554–60.
42. Wilms EB, Touw DJ, Heijerman HG. Pharmacokinetics of azithromycin in plasma, blood, polymorphonuclear neutrophils and sputum during long-term therapy in patients with cystic fibrosis. Ther Drug Monit. 2006;28(2):219–25.
43. Miossec-Bartoli C, Pilatre L, Peyron P, N'Diaye EN, Collart-Dutilleul V, Maridonneau-Parini I, et al. The new ketolide HMR3647 accumulates in the azurophil granules of human polymorphonuclear cells. Antimicrob Agents Chemother. 1999;43(10):2457–62.
44. Tsai WC, Standiford TJ. Immunomodulatory effects of macrolides in the lung: lessons from in-vitro and in-vivo models. Curr Pharm Des. 2004;10(25):3081–93.
45. Tamaoki J, Kadota J, Takizawa H. Clinical implications of the immunomodulatory effects of macrolides. Am J Med. 2004;117(9A):5S–11S.
46. Miyazaki M, Zaitsu M, Honjo K, Ishii E, Hamasaki Y. Macrolide antibiotics inhibit prostaglandin E2 synthesis and mRNA expression of prostaglandin synthetic enzymes in human leukocytes. Prostaglandins Leukot Essent Fatty Acids. 2003;69(4):229–35.
47. Mizunoe S, Kadota J, Tokimatsu I, Kishi K, Nagai H, Nasu M. Clarithromycin and azithromycin induce apoptosis of activated lymphocytes via down-regulation of Bcl-xL. Int Immunopharmacol. 2004;4(9):1201–7.
48. Khan AA, Slifer TR, Araujo FG, Remington JS. Effect of clarithromycin and azithromycin on production of cytokines by human monocytes. Int J Antimicrob Agents. 1999;11(2):121–32.
49. Stupin Polancec D, Munic VK, Banjanac M, Vrancic M, Cuzic S, Belamaric D, et al. Azithromycin drives in vitro GM-CSF/IL-4-induced differentiation of human blood monocytes toward dendritic-like cells with regulatory properties. J Leukoc Biol. 2012;91(2):229–43.
50. Sugiyama K, Shirai R, Mukae H, Ishimoto H, Nagata T, Sakamoto N, et al. Differing effects of clarithromycin and azithromycin on cytokine production by murine dendritic cells. Clin Exp Immunol. 2007;147(3):540–6.
51. Iwamoto S, Kumamoto T, Azuma E, Hirayama M, Ito M, Amano K, et al. The effect of azithromycin on the maturation and function of murine bone marrow-derived dendritic cells. Clin Exp Immunol. 2011;166(3):385–92.
52. Geudens N, Timmermans L, Vanhooren H, Vanaudenaerde BM, Vos R, Van De Wauwer C, et al. Azithromycin reduces airway inflammation in a murine model of lung ischaemia reperfusion injury. Transpl Int. 2008;21(7):688–95.
53. Remund K, Rechsteiner T, Guo Z, Rentsch K, Boehler A. The macrolide clarithromycin inhibits experimental post-transplant bronchiolitis obliterans. Exp Lung Res. 2009;35(10):830–40.

54. Glojnaric I, Cuzic S, Erakovic-Haber V, Parnham MJ. The serum amyloid A response to sterile silver nitrate in mice and its inhibition by dexamethasone and macrolide antibiotics. Int Immunopharmacol. 2007;7(12):1544–51.
55. Wolter J, Seeney S, Bell S, Bowler S, Masel P, McCormack J. Effect of long term treatment with azithromycin on disease parameters in cystic fibrosis: a randomised trial. Thorax. 2002;57(3):212–6.
56. Verleden S, Vandooren J, Vos R, Willems S, Dupont LJ, Verleden GM, et al. Azithromycin decreases MMP-9 expression in the airways of lung transplant recipients. Transpl Immunol. 2011;25(2):159–62.
57. Fietta AM, Meloni F. Lung transplantation: the role of azithromycin in the management of patients with bronchiolitis obliterans syndrome. Curr Med Chem. 2008;15(7):716–23.
58. Frederica M, Nadia S, Monica M, Alessandro C, Tiberio O, Francesco B, et al. Clinical and immunological evaluation of 12-month azithromycin therapy in chronic lung allograft rejection. Clin Transplant. 2011;25(4):E381–9.
59. Togami K, Chono S, Morimoto K. Distribution characteristics of clarithromycin and azithromycin, macrolide anti-microbial agents used for treatment of respiratory infections, in lung epithelial lining fluid and alveolar macrophages. Biopharm Drug Dispos. 2011;32(7):389–97.
60. Zuckerman JM, Qamar F, Bono BR. Macrolides, ketolides, and glycylcyclines: azithromycin, clarithromycin, telithromycin, tigecycline. Infect Dis Clin North Am. 2009;23(4):997–1026, ix–x.
61. Beigelman A, Gunsten S, Mikols CL, Vidavsky I, Cannon CL, Brody SL, et al. Azithromycin attenuates airway inflammation in a noninfectious mouse model of allergic asthma. Chest. 2009;136(2):498–506.
62. Martinez FJ, Curtis JL, Albert R. Role of macrolide therapy in chronic obstructive pulmonary disease. Int J Chron Obstruct Pulmon Dis. 2008;3(3):331–50.
63. Sarahrudi K, Carretta A, Wisser W, Senbaklavaci O, Ploner M, Neuhauser P, et al. The value of switching from cyclosporine to tacrolimus in the treatment of refractory acute rejection and obliterative bronchiolitis after lung transplantation. Transpl Int. 2002;15(1):24–8.
64. Gerhardt SG, McDyer JF, Girgis RE, Conte JV, Yang SC, Orens JB. Maintenance azithromycin therapy for bronchiolitis obliterans syndrome: results of a pilot study. Am J Respir Crit Care Med. 2003;168:121–5.
65. Verleden GM, Dupont LJ. Azithromycin therapy for patients with bronchiolitis obliterans syndrome after lung transplantation. Transplantation. 2004;77:1465–7.
66. Yates B, Murphy DM, Forrest IA, Ward C, Rutherford RM, Fisher AJ, et al. Azithromycin reverses airflow obstruction in established bronchiolitis obliterans syndrome. Am J Respir Crit Care Med. 2005;172:772–5.
67. Shitrit D, Bendayan D, Gidon S, Saute M, Bakal I, Kramer MR. Long-term azithromycin use for treatment of bronchiolitis obliterans syndrome in lung transplant recipients. J Heart Lung Transplant. 2005;24:1440–3.
68. Verleden GM, Vanaudenaerde BM, Dupont LJ, Van Raemdonck DE. Azithromycin reduces airway neutrophilia and interleukin-8 in patients with bronchiolitis obliterans syndrome. Am J Respir Crit Care Med. 2006;174:566–70.
69. Vos R, Vanaudenaerde BM, Ottevaere A, Verleden SE, De Vleeschauwer SI, Willems-Widyastuti A, et al. Long-term azithromycin for bronchiolitis obliterans syndrome: divide and conquer? J Heart Lung Transplant. 2010;29(12):1358–68.
70. Porhownik NR, Batobara W, Kepron W, Unruh HW, Bshouty Z. Effect of maintenance azithromycin on established bronchiolitis obliterans syndrome in lung transplant patients. Can Respir J. 2008;15:199–202.
71. Gottlieb J, Szangolies J, Koehnlein T, Golpon H, Simon A, Welte T. Long-term azithromycin for bronchiolitis obliterans syndrome after lung transplantation. Transplantation. 2008;85: 36–41.
72. Jain R, Hachem RR, Morrell MR, Trulock EP, Chakinala MM, Yusen RD, et al. Azithromycin is associated with increased survival in lung transplant recipients with bronchiolitis obliterans syndrome. J Heart Lung Transplant. 2010;29(5):531–7.

73. Benden C, Boehler A. Long-term clarithromycin therapy in the management of lung transplant recipients. Transplantation. 2009;87(10):1538–40.
74. Verleden GM, Dupont LJ, Vanhaecke J, Daenen W, Van Raemdonck DE. Effect of azithromycin on bronchiectasis and pulmonary function in a heart-lung transplant patient with severe chronic allograft dysfunction: a case report. J Heart Lung Transplant. 2005;24(8):1155–8.
75. de Jongh PA, Vos R, Verleden GM, Vanaudenaerde BM, Verschakelen JA. Thin-section computed tomography findings before and after azithromycin treatment of neutrophilic reversible lung allograft dysfunction. Eur Radiol. 2011;21(12):2466–74.
76. Verleden SE, Vos R, Mertens V, Willems-Widyastuti A, De Vleeschauwer SI, Dupont LJ, et al. Airway protein diversity in bronchiolitis obliterans syndrome after lung transplantation. J Heart Lung Transplant. 2011;30(6):667–73.
77. Mertens V, Blondeau K, Pauwels A, Farre R, Vanaudenaerde B, Vos R, et al. Azithromycin reduces gastroesophageal reflux and aspiration in lung transplant recipients. Dig Dis Sci. 2009;54(5):972–9.
78. Williams TJ, Verleden GM. Azithromycin: a plea for multicenter randomized studies in lung transplantation. Am J Respir Crit Care Med. 2005;172(6):657–9.
79. Corris PA, et al. Abstract presented at the 32nd Annual Meeting of the International Society for Heart and Lung Transplantation. Prague; 2012.
80. Vanaudenaerde BM, Vos R, Meyts I, Geudens N, De Wever W, Verbeken EK, et al. A dichotomy in bronchiolitis obliterans syndrome after lung transplantation revealed by azithromycin therapy. Eur Respir J. 2008;32(4):832–43.
81. Vanaudenaerde BM, Vos R, Meyts I, De Vleeschauwer SI, Verleden SE, Widyastuti-Willems A, et al. Macrolide therapy targets a specific phenotype in respiratory medicine: from clinical experience to basic science and back. Inflamm Allergy Drug Targets. 2008;7(4):279–87.
82. Vos R, Vanaudenaerde BM, Verleden SE, De Vleeschauwer SI, Willems-Widyastuti A, Van Raemdonck DE, et al. A randomised controlled trial of azithromycin to prevent chronic rejection after lung transplantation. Eur Respir J. 2011;37(1):164–72.
83. Dhillon GS, Valentine VG, Levitt J, Patel P, Gupta MR, Duncan SR, et al. Clarithromycin for prevention of bronchiolitis obliterans syndrome in lung allograft recipients. Clin Transplant. 2012;26:105–10.
84. Brown BA, Griffith DE, Girard W, Levin J, Wallace Jr RJ. Relationship of adverse events to serum drug levels in patients receiving high-dose azithromycin for mycobacterial lung disease. Clin Infect Dis. 1997;24(5):958–64.
85. Griffith DE, Brown BA, Girard WM, Griffith BE, Couch LA, Wallace Jr RJ. Azithromycin-containing regimens for treatment of Mycobacterium avium complex lung disease. Clin Infect Dis. 2001;32(11):1547–53.
86. Rubinstein E. Comparative safety of the different macrolide. Int J Antimicrob Agents. 2001;18(1):71–6.
87. Ray WA, Murray KT, Hall K, Arbogast PG, Stein CM. Azithromycin and the risk of cardiovascular death. N Engl J Med. 2012;366(20):1881–90.
88. Westphal JF. Macrolide-induced clinically relevant drug interactions with cytochrome P-450A (CYP) 3A4: an update focused on clarithromycin, azithromycin and dirithromycin. Br J Clin Pharmacol. 2000;50(4):285–95.
89. Granowitz EV, Tabor KJ, Kirchhoffer JB. Potentially fatal interaction between azithromycin and disopyramide. Pacing Clin Electrophysiol. 2000;23(9):1433–5.
90. Hickey AJ, Lu D, Ashley ED, Stout J. Inhaled azithromycin therapy. J Aerosol Med. 2006;19(1):54–60.
91. Zhang Y, Wang X, Lin X, Liu X, Tian B, Tang X. High azithromycin loading powders for inhalation and their in vivo evaluation in rats. Int J Pharm. 2010;395(1–2):205–14.
92. Malhotra-Kumar S, Lammens C, Coenen S, Van Herck K, Goossens H. Effect of azithromycin and clarithromycin therapy on pharyngeal carriage of macrolide-resistant streptococci in healthy volunteers: a randomised, double-blind, placebo-controlled study. Lancet. 2007; 369(9560):482–90.

93. Tait-Kamradt A, Clancy J, Cronan M, Dib-Hajj F, Wondrack L, Yuan W, et al. mefE is necessary for the erythromycin-resistant M phenotype in Streptococcus pneumoniae. Antimicrob Agents Chemother. 1997;41(10):2251–5.
94. Vanhoof R, Camps K, Carpentier M, De Craeye S, Frans J, Glupczynski Y, et al. 10th survey of antimicrobial resistance in noninvasive clinical isolates of Streptococcus pneumoniae collected in Belgium during winter 2007–2008. Pathol Biol. 2010;58(2):147–51.
95. Tramper-Stranders GA, Wolfs TF, Fleer A, Kimpen JL, van der Ent CK. Maintenance azithromycin treatment in pediatric patients with cystic fibrosis: long-term outcomes related to macrolide resistance and pulmonary function. Pediatr Infect Dis J. 2007;26(1):8–12.
96. Phaff SJ, Tiddens HA, Verbrugh HA, Ott A. Macrolide resistance of Staphylococcus aureus and Haemophilus species associated with long-term azithromycin use in cystic fibrosis. J Antimicrob Chemother. 2006;57(4):741–6.
97. Gillis RJ, White KG, Choi KH, Wagner VE, Schweizer HP, Iglewski BH. Molecular basis of azithromycin-resistant Pseudomonas aeruginosa biofilms. Antimicrob Agents Chemother. 2005;49(9):3858–67.
98. Stover DE, Mangino D. Macrolides: a treatment alternative for bronchiolitis obliterans organizing pneumonia? Chest. 2005;128(5):3611–7.
99. Mann JM, Sha KK, Kline G, Breuer FU, Miller A. World Trade Center dyspnea: bronchiolitis obliterans with functional improvement: a case report. Am J Ind Med. 2005;48(3):225–9.
100. Khalid M, Al Saghir A, Saleemi S, Al Dammas S, Zeitouni M, Al Mobeireek A, et al. Azithromycin in bronchiolitis obliterans complicating bone marrow transplantation: a preliminary study. Eur Respir J. 2005;25(3):490–3.
101. Wuyts WA, Willems S, Vos R, Vanaudenaerde BM, De Vleeschauwer SI, Rinaldi M, et al. Azithromycin reduces pulmonary fibrosis in a bleomycin mouse model. Exp Lung Res. 2010;36(10):602–14.
102. Verleden GM, Vos R, De Vleeschauwer S, Verleden S, Dupont L, Nevens F, et al. Neutrophilic reversible airways dysfunction after liver transplantation: a case report. Transplant Proc. 2011;43(5):2078–81.

Chapter 16
Other Treatments for Bronchiolitis Obliterans Syndrome

Ramsey Hachem

Abstract Bronchiolitis obliterans syndrome (BOS) remains the leading obstacle to better long-term outcomes after lung transplantation. The incidence of BOS approaches 50 % within 4 years of transplantation, and the median survival after the diagnosis of BOS is approximately 3 years. Because BOS is generally thought to represent chronic alloimmune-mediated rejection, the mainstay of therapy has been intensifying immunosuppression. However, the response to treatment is poor, and the typical clinical course is characterized by progressive allograft dysfunction. Total lymphoid irradiation (TLI) and extracorporeal photopheresis (ECP) are used at some centers, although they are usually reserved as salvage treatments for refractory BOS. Re-transplantation is the ultimate treatment option, but the donor organ shortage and generally marginal outcomes have limited its widespread use.

Keywords Bronchiolitis obliterans syndrome • Total lymphoid irradiation • Extracorporeal photopheresis • Forced expiratory volume in one second (FEV_1) • Survival

Introduction

The clinical course after the diagnosis of bronchiolitis obliterans syndrome (BOS) is often characterized by progressive and relentless loss of lung function. Although the exact pathogenesis of BOS remains unknown, both alloimmune and non-alloimmune insults are recognized as key risk factors in the development and

---

R. Hachem, M.D. (✉)
Washington University School of Medicine/Barnes-Jewish Hospital Pulmonary and Critical Care, 660 S. Euclid Avenue. Campus Box 8052, St. Louis, MO 63110, USA
e-mail: rhachem@dom.wustl.edu

K.C. Meyer and A.R. Glanville (eds.), *Bronchiolitis Obliterans Syndrome in Lung Transplantation*, Respiratory Medicine 8, DOI 10.1007/978-1-4614-7636-8_16,

progression of BOS [1–3]. Furthermore, non-alloimmune insults, such as primary graft dysfunction (PGD), gastroesophageal reflux disease (GERD), and community-acquired respiratory viral (CARV) infections, are thought to mediate the development of BOS by creating an inflammatory milieu that promotes the alloimmune response [4–6]. Therefore, treatment has generally focused on intensifying the immunosuppression, but the response to therapy is often disappointing, with progressive decline in lung function. Indeed, stabilization in the decline in lung function, rather than an improvement in lung function, is usually the goal of treatment. This poor response to intensifying immunosuppression raises the possibility that BOS may be a stereotypic allograft response to injury with an exuberant but disordered repair process, rather than the result of ongoing alloimmune injury. Furthermore, it is possible that BOS may have distinct pathogeneses in different patients; while in some patients, BOS may be directly caused by alloimmune injury, it may be due to a disordered repair process in others. The heterogeneity in presentation and clinical course after the diagnosis supports this paradigm. Nonetheless, accurately phenotyping an individual patient's disease or predicting the clinical course and response to therapy has proven difficult in practice. More importantly, the dearth of clinically available anti-proliferative or anti-fibrotic treatments leaves immunosuppression and immunomodulation as the only viable treatment options.

The conventional immunosuppressive prophylaxis and treatment strategies for BOS are discussed elsewhere in this book. This chapter focuses on other treatments, including total lymphoid irradiation (TLI), extracorporeal photopheresis (ECP), and re-transplantation. In general, there is little consensus on the use of induction immunosuppression and the optimal maintenance immunosuppression regimen, and practices vary widely among centers [7]. This is also true for the management of BOS. TLI and ECP are used at some centers, but both are usually reserved as salvage treatments for refractory BOS.

Total Lymphoid Irradiation

TLI was initially used for the treatment of Hodgkin's disease, and it was recognized that patients treated with radiotherapy had sustained alterations in the number and function of circulating lymphocytes years after treatment [8]. This suggested a potential role in the management of solid organ transplant rejection. TLI was initially used as induction immunosuppression in kidney transplantation, with low-dose steroid monotherapy as maintenance immunosuppression after transplantation [9, 10]. However, although immunological and animal studies suggested that TLI would promote donor organ tolerance [11, 12], its efficacy in clinical practice was marginal [9], and its use became limited to the treatment of refractory rejection after the advent of cyclosporine [13–16].

To target all lymphatic areas, including the spleen, three fields are used. The mantle field includes the cervical, clavicular, axillary, mediastinal, and hilar lymph nodes. The para-aortic field encompasses the para-aortic nodes and the spleen, and the inverted-Y field includes the iliac, inguinal, and femoral lymph nodes. Non-lymphatic structures are shielded with customized blocks. The total dose of radiation used has traditionally been 8 Gy divided into 10 fractions of 0.8 Gy, each administered twice weekly over 5 weeks [17–19]. This dose of radiation is comparatively low, as most regimens used for the treatment of Hodgkin's disease use 30–40 Gy [20]. Leukopenia and thrombocytopenia are common side effects, even with the 8 Gy dose, and treatment is generally delayed when the white blood cell count is less than 2,000–3,000/mm^3 or the platelet count is less than 50,000/mm^3. To mitigate bone marrow suppression, anti-proliferative immunosuppressants, including azathioprine and mycophenolate mofetil, are usually stopped when TLI is initiated and resumed after completion of therapy and resolution of bone marrow suppression.

Critically evaluating the clinical efficacy of TLI in lung transplantation is difficult because the literature is limited to small case series without a concurrent control group. Furthermore, TLI has been reserved clinically as a salvage treatment for patients with refractory or progressive rejection, and this clearly biases survival analyses after treatment. In the first report of the use of TLI in lung transplantation, Valentine and colleagues detailed the outcomes of treating six recipients (two heart–lung and four lung recipients) who had persistent acute rejection that was refractory to high-dose steroids [17]. The mean number of episodes of rejection per 100 patient-days decreased from 3.07 before TLI to 0.12 after TLI, but four of the five recipients who survived more than year after completing TLI developed obliterative bronchiolitis, (OB) and the median time from transplantation to the development of OB was 353 days [17]. In addition, four of the six patients died a median 568 days after completing TLI. While the high incidence of BOS may be related to the patients' underlying refractory acute rejection, it is noteworthy that TLI did not uncouple the association between acute rejection and BOS and did not prevent BOS in this high-risk cohort.

In the earliest publication of the use of TLI for progressive BOS, Diamond and colleagues reported their experience among 11 patients [18]. In the 3 months before initiating TLI, the mean FEV_1 was 1.2 L, the mean decrease in FEV_1 was 34 %, and the patients had a median of three augmentations in immunosuppression, including treatment with methylprednisolone, anti-thymocyte globulin, and OKT3. Only 4 of the 11 patients completed all 10 treatments; TLI was discontinued in 4 patients because of progressive allograft dysfunction, in 2 patients because of infection, and in 1 patient because of persistent thrombocytopenia [18]. TLI failed in 7 of the 11 patients within 8 weeks of completion; 6 patients died, and 1 was re-transplanted. Four deaths were due to progressive BOS, and two deaths were due to preexisting infection. Four patients had a positive response to TLI; this was characterized by a change in FEV_1 from an average 40 % decline in the 3 months before TLI to an average 1 % improvement in the 3 months following TLI [18]. In this cohort, factors predictive of a positive response included initiating TLI at a later time point after transplantation, a higher FEV_1 at the initiation of TLI, and the absence of preexisting pulmonary infection. The authors concluded that a subset of patients with refractory and progressive BOS responded favorably to TLI and opined that better results might be achieved if TLI is initiated earlier in the course of BOS [18].

In a more recent publication, Fisher and colleagues reported the results of TLI for progressive BOS in 37 patients treated over a 12-year period at their center [19]. Seven patients had BOS stage 1, 14 had BOS stage 2, and 16 had BOS stage 3, and the mean FEV_1 before initiating TLI was 1.35 L. Twenty-seven of the 37 patients completed 8 of the planned 10 treatments; 2 died of progressive BOS before completion of the 10 treatments, 6 developed myelosuppression, and 2 developed serious infections. Efficacy was evaluated among the 27 who completed eight treatments, and the mean FEV_1 increased from 1.35 L before TLI to 1.60 L after TLI, with some patients having a remarkable improvement in lung function [19]. Similarly, the rate of decline in FEV_1 decreased from 122 mL/month before TLI to 25 mL/month after TLI [19]. Nine of the 27 were alive at the end of follow-up, with a median survival of 27 months after TLI.

In the most recent publication regarding the efficacy of TLI, Verleden and colleagues reported the results of treating six patients with refractory BOS [21]. Three patients had BOS stage 2, three patients had BOS stage 3, and all patients completed all 10 fractions (8 Gy). Overall, there was a significant reduction in the rate of decline in FEV_1 from a mean 221 mL/month to 94 mL/month, but the FEV_1 did not improve in any of the patients, and three patients died, two patients were re-transplanted, and one patient was stable at BOS stage 3 [21]. The authors compared the rate of decline in FEV_1 among those treated with TLI to a historical control group, and the historical control group had an ongoing decline in FEV_1 of 193 mL/month compared to 209 mL/month.

It is difficult to determine the efficacy of TLI from the published data. In all studies, TLI was used as a salvage treatment for patients with progressive BOS refractory to first- and second-line therapy. This patient population is generally unlikely to have a favorable response to any treatment and is at increased risk of death. Furthermore, while the individual patients served as their own controls in before-and-after analyses, the natural history of BOS and the rate of decline in FEV_1 are unknown. It is possible that the rate of decline in FEV_1 is nonlinear and may plateau at some low measurement where a large proportion of respiratory and membranous bronchioles have been obliterated. However, a minority of patients responded well to TLI and actually had an improvement in lung function, although the number of patients is too small to develop reliable predictors of a favorable response. Obviously, a randomized controlled trial would be ideal to assess the efficacy and safety of any treatment, but it is extremely difficult and challenging to conduct a clinical trial in this setting.

Extracorporeal Photopheresis

ECP was originally used for the treatment of the skin manifestations of cutaneous T-cell lymphoma [22, 23]. The treatment consists of three steps. In the first step, peripheral blood mononuclear cells are separated from whole blood via apheresis. Next, the mononuclear cells are incubated with a photo-activating substance (8-methoxypsoralen) then irradiated with ultraviolet A (UVA) light. This results in cell membrane damage, DNA crosslinking, apoptosis, and antigen-presenting cell activation [24, 25]. In the last step, the treated cells are reinfused into the patient. Because of its immunomodulating effects, ECP has been used in a variety of inflammatory disorders, including rheumatoid arthritis, systemic sclerosis, systemic lupus erythematosus, and pemphigus vulgaris [26–29]. It is currently most frequently used for the management of graft-versus-host disease (GVHD) after allogeneic hematopoietic stem-cell transplantation [30, 31]. The use of ECP in the management of solid organ rejection dates back to the early 1990s, and it is currently approved in the United States for refractory heart transplant rejection [32, 33], but its exact mechanism of action in allograft rejection remains unknown.

During each ECP procedure, 2–5 % of the total peripheral blood mononuclear cells are exposed to 8-methoxypsoralen. This crosslinks and damages cellular DNA upon exposure to UVA. The majority of treated cells undergo apoptosis via the Fas/FasL and Bcl-2 protein family pathways [34, 35]. Macrophages and dendritic cells then phagocytose apoptotic lymphocytes. The presentation of apoptotic cell antigens on antigen-presenting cells appears to promote peripheral tolerance in the absence of inflammation and "danger" signals [36, 37]. Furthermore, ECP stimulates the proliferation of CD4+CD25+ regulatory T cells [37–39]. In fact, one study demonstrated that patients with refractory BOS who responded favorably to ECP had an increase or stabilization in the number of peripheral blood CD4+CD25+ regulatory T cells, while those who had a progressive decline in lung function had a decline in their peripheral regulatory T-cell numbers [40]. This also demonstrates that the immunological and clinical responses to ECP are heterogeneous. ECP also appears to promote a favorable cytokine profile. One study of patients with GVHD treated with ECP demonstrated a shift in the cytokine profile of cultured T cells from IL-2 and IFN-γ (gamma)-producing Th1 cells to IL-4 and IL-10-producing Th2 cells [41]. Similarly, co-culturing ECP-treated mononuclear cells with dendritic cells in vitro increased the production of IL-10 and reduced the expression of co-stimulatory molecules on dendritic cells after stimulation with lipopolysaccharide (LPS), suggesting a potential mechanism for the immunomodulation induced by ECP [42].

In the first publication describing the use of ECP in BOS, Slovis and colleagues reported their experience with three patients who developed progressive BOS refractory to anti-thymocyte globulin and high-dose steroids in 1995 [43]. One patient had an improvement in FEV_1 from 0.94 to 1.3 L, and two patients had stabilization in their lung function, although the measurements were not reported [43]. None of the patients had any adverse effects, and the response was durable, although at least one patient continued ECP for 23 months. In a similar publication, Salerno and colleagues reported their experience in eight patients [44]. Seven patients had refractory BOS and were in BOS stage 3, and one patient had undergone re-transplantation for BOS without improvement in lung function; the patients received 3–13 treatments, and there was a statistically significant decrease in the median rate of decline in FEV_1 after ECP compared to before ECP [44]. During the study period, one patient died, three required re-transplantation (15, 21, and 25 months after ECP), and four were alive and clinically stable. The authors compared patient survival in this cohort with a concurrent group of patients with BOS stage 3 who were not treated with ECP and found a trend to improved survival associated with ECP, although this was not statistically significant [44]. Importantly, it is not clear why the control group was not treated with ECP and whether this may have influenced the survival results. Nevertheless, there were no adverse events associated with ECP. In a larger report of 14 patients with BOS (including 3 with stage 0'b', 5 with stage 1, 3 with stage 2, and 3 with stage 3), Villanueva and colleagues divided the cohort into those with early BOS (stage 0'b' and stage 1) and those with advanced BOS (stage 2 and stage 3) [45]. All patients received six ECP treatments. Among those with early BOS, four remained in the same BOS stage, one improved from stage 1 to stage 0, and three progressed to a higher stage; the mean survival after ECP was 43 months in this subgroup. Among the six patients with advanced BOS, five died and one was re-transplanted a mean 14 months after ECP [45]. Two patients had catheter-associated sepsis that responded to antibiotic treatment and removal of the catheter. These findings suggest a potential benefit for ECP primarily when used in the early stages of BOS.

In a more recent publication, Benden and colleagues reported their experience with ECP for BOS and recurrent acute rejection over a 10-year period [46]. Twelve patients were treated with ECP for progressive BOS, and all received 24 treatments. Five had BOS stage 1, two had stage 2, and five had stage 3. The rate of decline in FEV_1 before ECP initiation was calculated based on serial measurements from the best post-transplant measurement to the last measurement before ECP initiation; similarly, the rate of decline in FEV_1 after ECP was calculated based on serial measurements from the completion of ECP until the end of follow-up. The rate of decline in FEV_1 improved significantly from 112 mL/month before ECP to 12 mL/month after ECP [46]. There were no complications related to ECP. During the study period, two patients required re-transplantation and four patients died because of progressive BOS [46]. The authors conclude that the use of ECP at earlier stages of BOS would be ideal to prevent further loss of lung function and suggest that there may be a role for ongoing therapy beyond 24 treatments for sustained stabilization in lung function.

In the largest published series, Morrell and colleagues reported their experience with 60 patients treated with ECP for progressive BOS over a 7-year period [47]. Five patients had BOS stage 1, 20 had stage 2, and 35 had stage 3. All patients had refractory BOS; 58 had been treated with anti-thymocyte globulin, and 54 had been treated with azithromycin but had a progressive decline in lung function. Four patients died of progressive BOS shortly after initiating ECP and were excluded from the primary lung function analysis. Among the remaining 56 patients, the mean rate of decline in FEV_1 over the 6-month period before ECP initiation was 116 mL/month, and there was a significant decrease in the rate of decline in the 6-month period after the initiation of ECP to 28.9 mL/month [47]. In addition, the four patients who died early after the initiation of ECP were included in a separate analysis and were assigned an FEV_1 of 0 at the time of their death; the rate of decline in FEV_1 after the initiation of ECP increased to 57.2 mL/month after this group was included, but this was still a significant change compared to the rate of decline in FEV_1 before the initiation of ECP [47]. It is noteworthy that 14 patients

(25 % of the cohort) had an improvement in FEV_1 during the 6 months after ECP initiation. Ten patients had ECP-related complications; eight had catheter-associated bacteremia, one of whom died, one had catheter-related thrombosis, and one had transient hypotension. Twenty-seven patients died during the study period, and the median survival after the initiation of ECP was 2.6 years; BOS was the leading cause of death [47]. The authors constructed regression models to identify clinical factors that might predict a favorable response but could not find any demographic or disease-specific variable that predicted the response to ECP.

Collectively, these results suggest that ECP slows the decline in lung function in many patients and may improve lung function in a minority of patients. However, all of these reports have important methodological limitations. The most important limitation is the absence of a control group. While individual patients may serve as their own control by analyzing the change in lung function before and after ECP, this may be biased if the rate of decline in FEV_1 is different at different stages of BOS. Indeed, one study demonstrated that FEV_1 varied over time after the diagnosis of BOS, and the steepest decline was seen in the first 6 months [48]. However, the temporal association between the initiation of ECP and the change in the rate of decline in FEV_1 implies a treatment effect. Nevertheless, a control group is necessary to critically evaluate the effect of ECP on lung function. Furthermore, all studies evaluated efficacy as the effect of ECP on FEV_1. While FEV_1 is an important clinical variable, none of the studies have evaluated quality of life. In addition, although most studies reported survival after ECP, it is impossible to assess the impact of ECP on survival without a control group. An additional limitation of most studies is that the rate of change in FEV_1 is not usually linear and a regression line is drawn through the data points to calculate a slope of FEV_1. Nonetheless, it is important to note that ECP has been used as a salvage treatment for patients with refractory BOS, as TLI has been used. By definition, this group of patients is unlikely to respond to treatment and is at increased risk of death. Lastly, although ECP may slow the rate of decline in lung function, many patients may still become severely impaired from a respiratory standpoint, since ECP is often used as a salvage treatment. Clearly, a randomized controlled trial in this group of high-risk patients would be difficult, but developing sound clinical evidence is necessary to improve outcomes.

Re-transplantation

Re-transplantation is the ultimate treatment option for carefully selected patients with refractory BOS. However, only a small minority of patients with BOS has undergone re-transplantation. In fact, among 30,673 lung transplant recipients reported to the latest ISHLT Registry Report, only 472 (1.5 %) had undergone re-transplantation for BOS [7]. The annual number of re-transplants has increased in recent years; 21 re-transplants were reported to the ISHLT Registry in 2000, and this increased to 69 in 2005 and 107 in 2009 [7]. In part, this is related to the change in the lung organ allocation system in the United States that was implemented in 2005 [49]. Under this system, organ allocation is based on medical urgency and expected survival after transplantation, and waiting time has become irrelevant. Clearly, this favors candidates with unpredictable or rapidly deteriorating clinical courses and makes re-transplantation feasible for patients with end-stage BOS. In addition to the change in the organ allocation system, outcomes after re-transplantation have improved over time, and this probably accounts for some of the increasing activity in recent years. Nevertheless, many patients with end-stage BOS are not candidates for re-transplantation because of multiple comorbidities and complications related to the immunosuppressive regimen that accumulate over time. In addition, re-transplantation raises difficult ethical questions because of the donor organ shortage and the resultant mortality on the waiting list for primary transplantation.

In 1991, an international registry of lung re-transplantation was established to determine outcomes and predictors of survival in a large cohort of patients. In the initial report of the first 61 patients enrolled in the registry, 32 underwent re-transplantation for BOS, 14 for graft failure, 8 for airway problems, 5 for severe acute rejection, and 4 for other indications [50]. Survival 1 year after re-transplantation was 35 %; the indication for re-transplantation and the operation performed did not affect survival, but there was a trend to improved survival among patients who were ambulatory before re-transplantation. Importantly, survival after re-transplantation was significantly worse than after primary transplantation [50]. A follow-up report was published in 1995 describing the experience with 139 re-transplant recipients at 34 centers in the United States and Europe [51]. Eighty patients underwent re-transplantation for BOS, 34 for acute graft failure, 13 for airway complications, 8 for acute rejection, and 4 for other indications. Survival was 65 % one month after re-transplantation and 45 % at 1 year. Fifty-six percent of deaths were due to infection, and 22 % were due to acute graft failure [51]. In this analysis, ambulatory status was the most important predictor of survival, although only 29 % of patients were ambulatory (defined as being able to walk 50 m). Importantly, survival in the more recent era (1992–1994) was significantly better than in the earlier era (1985–1991). Although re-transplant recipients as a group had a similar incidence of BOS as primary transplant recipients, patients who underwent re-transplantation for BOS had a more rapid decline in FEV_1 than those who underwent re-transplantation for other indications [51]. This suggests that they had a higher risk of recurrent BOS than those re-transplanted for other indications. The last report of the registry was published in 1998, and this detailed the outcomes of 230 re-transplant recipients from 47 international centers [52]. In this report, survival was 47 % at 1 year and 33 % at 3 years after re-transplantation. Ambulatory status and re-transplantation after 1991 were again associated with better survival, whereas the need for mechanical ventilation was associated with increased mortality. Indeed, ambulatory patients who did not require mechanical ventilation and were re-transplanted after 1991 had a 1-year survival of 64 %. Another important predictor of survival that emerged was the time interval between primary transplantation and re-transplantation. Patients who underwent re-transplantation within 2 years of primary transplantation had a significantly worse survival than those who underwent re-transplantation more than 2 years after primary transplantation. The leading cause of death after re-transplantation was infection, which accounted for 42 % of deaths; acute graft failure accounted for 29 % of deaths, and BOS accounted for 21 % of deaths [52]. Of note, 62 % of patients were free from BOS 3 years after re-transplantation [52]. The authors concluded that re-transplantation was a reasonable treatment option among carefully selected patients.

In addition to the multi-center pulmonary re-transplantation registry, single-center series have been published, and these can provide outcomes and complications data with greater detail. Brugiere and colleagues reported their experience with 15 patients who were re-transplanted for BOS between 1988 and 2002 [53]. All patients had a single lung re-transplant; 4 had ipsilateral transplants, 9 had contralateral transplants, and 2 had single lung re-transplants after a bilateral primary transplant. One-year survival was 60 % and 5-year survival was 45 %; infection was the leading cause of death, accounting for 60 % of deaths [53]. It is noteworthy that the retained primary allograft was the initial site of the fatal infection in four of the six patients who died because of infection, and two other patients who had a retained allograft had chronic and disabling pulmonary infection [53]. This demonstrates that a chronically rejected and damaged lung can become a nidus for serious infection after re-transplantation and suggests that replacing the rejected lung or lungs at re-transplantation has an important impact on outcomes. However, pleural adhesions as a result of the primary transplant, pneumonia, or the chronic lung inflammation associated with BOS can make this approach technically difficult in some cases. Finally, among the 10 patients who survived beyond 6 months, freedom from BOS was 72 % at 3 years and 66 % at 5 years after re-transplantation [53].

In a larger single-center series, Strueber and colleagues reported the outcomes of 54 re-transplant recipients at their center [54]. Thirty-seven of the 54 were re-transplanted for BOS, 10 for primary graft failure, and 7 for airway complications. Those re-transplanted for primary graft failure and airway complications had significantly worse survival than those re-transplanted for BOS and those who underwent primary transplantation. In fact, those re-transplanted for primary graft failure had a 50 % 1-year survival, and those re-transplanted for airway complications had a 33 % 2-year survival. In contrast, those re-transplanted for BOS had a 62 % 5-year survival, which was comparable to primary transplant recipients who had a 63 % 5-year survival [54]. The authors analyzed causes of death among re-transplant recipients, but there were no clear trends other than infection accounting for four of the six deaths among those re-transplanted for primary graft failure. Finally, there was a trend to an increased incidence of BOS among those re-transplanted for BOS compared to those who had a primary transplant, but this was not statistically significant [54].

Osaki and colleagues reported their results among 15 patients who underwent re-transplantation and 2 who underwent a third transplant procedure [55]. Five of the 17 patients underwent re-transplantation for acute graft failure, and 12 underwent re-transplantation for BOS. Overall, re-transplant recipients had a 59 % 1-year survival and a 42 % 5-year survival; these results were significantly worse than primary transplant recipients at this center, which had an 88 % 1-year survival and a 65 % 5-year survival for primary lung transplant recipients [55]. Importantly, those re-transplanted for acute graft failure had a 40 % 1-year survival compared to those re-transplanted for BOS who had a 67 % 1-year survival and a 44 % 5-year survival. Both third transplant recipients died within 1 year of transplantation. Again, infection was the leading cause of death, accounting for 45 % of deaths, and the retained primary graft was the source of fatal infection in 40 % [55]. Aigner and colleagues reported the results of 46 patients who underwent re-transplantation at their center; 23 had primary graft failure, 19 had BOS, and 4 had airway complications [56]. Those re-transplanted for primary graft failure had a significantly worse survival than those who had BOS. The 1-year and 5-year survival rates were 35 % and 29 % for the primary graft failure group compared to 73 % and 61 % for the BOS group, respectively [56]. All patients re-transplanted for airway complications were alive at the end of follow-up. It is noteworthy that 8 of the 23 patients re-transplanted for primary graft failure were on extracorporeal membrane oxygenation (ECMO) before transplantation, while none of those who had BOS or airway complications were on ECMO. Again, infection was the leading cause of death in all groups, accounting for 14 of the 24 deaths [56].

Kawut and colleagues performed a large retrospective analysis of re-transplantation in the United States using United Network for Organ Sharing (UNOS) data [57]. Patients who underwent re-transplantation were divided into those re-transplanted between 1990 and 2000 ($n=184$) and those re-transplanted between 2001 and 2006 ($n=205$), and outcomes were compared to patients who underwent primary transplantation between 2001 and 2006 ($n=5,657$). In both re-transplant groups, over 50 % of patients underwent re-transplantation for BOS, 10–15 % underwent re-transplantation for primary graft failure, and the indication for re-transplantation was unknown in approximately 30 % of patients. One-year survival among re-transplant recipients in the modern era was 62 %, and 5-year survival was 45 %; however, this was significantly better than survival among re-transplant recipients in the earlier era [57]. Nonetheless, re-transplant recipients in the modern era had a 30 % higher risk of death than primary transplant recipients transplanted during the same time period. In addition, patients re-transplanted in the modern era for BOS had a twofold higher risk of BOS than primary transplant recipients. In fact, the incidence of BOS among re-transplant recipients was 22 % at 2 years and 46 % at 4 years compared to 12 % at 2 years and 30 % at 4 years among primary transplant recipients [57].

Taken together, the published data demonstrate that survival after re-transplantation is generally worse than after primary transplantation, although outcomes after re-transplantation have improved over time. Furthermore, survival after re-transplantation for primary graft failure is particularly limited and is worse than survival after re-transplantation for BOS. Infection appears to be the leading cause of death after re-transplantation, and a retained graft is often the source of fatal infection. This suggests that removing chronically rejected and failed allografts at the time of re-transplantation might mitigate the risk of infection and improve survival. However, this is sometimes not feasible because of pleural adhesions. Nevertheless, survival among ambulatory patients with BOS and few comorbidities after re-transplantation approaches that of survival after primary transplantation. However, patients re-transplanted for BOS appear to have an increased risk of recurrent BOS compared to primary transplant recipients in the largest series [57]. This association has not been demonstrated consistently in earlier registry studies or in small single-center studies because survival was severely limited by infection, and many small series may have been underpowered to detect this association.

Re-transplantation raises serious ethical questions that are difficult to answer by the medical community alone. Utilitarianism supports the allocation of organs to those who are most likely to derive the most benefit from transplantation. On the other hand, egalitarianism supports equal access to donor organs for patients in need. In addition, the ethical considerations of re-transplantation vary between different societies and cultures, and donor organs are generally considered resources of society as a whole. Therefore, the community and its citizenry would address these questions best with input from the medical profession regarding outcomes data. Nevertheless, re-transplantation is not an ideal treatment for patients with BOS. Few patients are good candidates for re-transplantation, and the donor organ shortage means that some candidates will die on the waiting list.

Other Novel Potential Approaches

Traditional treatments for BOS have consisted primarily of conventional immunosuppressive drugs, such as tacrolimus, sirolimus, and anti-thymocyte globulin. While the use of conventional immunosuppression has made lung transplantation clinically feasible and has been reasonably effective preventing and treating acute rejection, its efficacy in the treatment of BOS has been disappointing. There is preliminary evidence suggesting a potential role for novel immunomodulating agents, including 3-hydroxy-3-methylglutaryl coenzyme A (HMG CoA) reductase inhibitors (or statins) and angiotensin converting enzyme (ACE) inhibitors [58, 59]. Johnson and colleagues performed a retrospective study comparing the outcomes of 39 patients treated with statins for hypercholesterolemia to 161 contemporary control patients [58]. Patients treated with statins were less likely to develop acute rejection, and none of the 15 patients who were initiated on statins within 1 year of transplantation developed BOS [58]. In addition, those treated with statins had lower total cell counts, neutrophil counts, and lymphocyte counts in their bronchoalveolar lavage fluid than control patients. Most importantly, survival 6 years after transplantation among those treated with statins was 91 % compared to 54 % in the control group [58]. Iuppa and colleagues analyzed the effect of statins on the development of BOS and survival in a retrospective cohort study at their center [60]. Fifty-one patients were treated with statins for hypercholesterolemia and 101 were not; there was no difference in freedom from BOS and no difference in survival between the two groups [60]. Reasons for the discrepant results between these two studies are unknown, but the inability to replicate the favorable results reported in the original study suggests that the effect of statins on BOS development may be heterogeneous. Of note, there are no reports of the effect of statins as a treatment for BOS. A randomized controlled trial is necessary before statin use can be recommended for BOS prevention or treatment.

In general, immunosuppressive and immunomodulating therapies do not directly impact the fibroproliferation that is characteristic of OB. Thus, anti-fibrotic and anti-proliferative agents are appealing choices. Data suggesting a therapeutic role for ACE inhibitors, endothelin receptor antagonists, and pirfenidone in BOS are limited to animal studies [59, 61–63]. Clearly, human studies are needed to evaluate these approaches further.

Conclusion

BOS remains the leading obstacle to better long-term outcomes after lung transplantation. The response to treatment is generally disappointing, and the goal is usually to stabilize the decline in lung function, although this is often difficult to achieve over time. ECP and TLI have been used at some centers for refractory BOS, but a critical evaluation of the efficacy of both treatments is difficult because of inherent limitations in the study design of all published series. Nonetheless, both treatments appear to stabilize the decline in lung function in some patients and improve lung function in a minority of patients. Randomized controlled trials are needed to evaluate the efficacy and safety of ECP and TLI in BOS. Re-transplantation is the ultimate treatment for refractory BOS, but only a minority of patients are candidates, and long-term outcomes remain inferior to those after primary transplantation. In addition, the donor organ shortage limits the access to re-transplantation as a treatment for BOS.

References

1. Estenne M, Hertz MI. Bronchiolitis obliterans after human lung transplantation. Am J Respir Crit Care Med. 2002;166:440–4.
2. Belperio JA, Weigt SS, Fishbein MC, Lynch JP. Chronic lung allograft rejection. Mechanisms and therapy. Proc Am Thorac Soc. 2009;6:108–21.
3. Weigt SS, Wallace WD, Derhovanessian A, Saggar R, Saggar R, Lynch JP, et al. Chronic allograft rejection: epidemiology, diagnosis, pathogenesis, and treatment. Semin Respir Crit Care Med. 2010;31:189–207.
4. Daud SA, Yusen RD, Meyers BF, Chakinala MM, Walter MJ, Aloush AA, et al. Impact of immediate primary lung allograft dysfunction on bronchiolitis obliterans syndrome. Am J Respir Crit Care Med. 2007;175:507–13.
5. Davis RD, Lau CL, Eubanks S, Messier RH, Hadjiliadis D, Steele MP, et al. Improved lung allograft function in patients with gastroesophageal reflux disease undergoing lung transplantation. J Thorac Cardiovasc Surg. 2003;125:533–42.
6. Khalifah AP, Hachem RR, Chakinala MM, Schechtman KB, Patterson GA, Schuster DP, et al. Respiratory viral infections are a distinct risk for bronchiolitis obliterans syndrome and death. Am J Respir Crit Care Med. 2004;170:181–7.
7. Christie JD, Edwards LB, Kucheryavaya AY, Benden C, Dobbels F, Kirk R, et al. The registry of the International Society for Heart and Lung Transplantation: Twenty-eighth adult lung and heart-lung transplant report—2011. J Heart Lung Transplant. 2011;30:1104–22.

8. Fuks Z, Strober S, Bobrove AM, Sasazuki T, McMichael A, Kaplan HS. Long term effects of radiation on T and B lymphocytes in peripheral blood of patients with Hodgkin's disease. J Clin Invest. 1976;58:803–14.
9. Waer M, Vanrenterghem Y, Roels L, Verberckmoes R, Hauglustaine D, van der Schueren E, et al. Renal cadaveric transplantation in diabetics using total lymphoid irradiation or cyclosporine A. A controlled randomized study. Leuven Collaborative Transplantation Group. Transpl Int. 1988;1:64–8.
10. Saper V, Chow D, Engleman ED, Hoppe RT, Levin B, Collins G, et al. Clinical and immunological studies of cadaveric renal transplant recipients given total lymphoid irradiation and maintained on low-dose prednisone. Transplantation. 1988;45:540–6.
11. Strober S, Slavin S, Gottlieb M, Zan-Bar I, King DP, Hoppe RT, et al. Allograft tolerance after total lymphoid irradiation (TLI). Immunol Rev. 1979;46:87–112.
12. Strober S, Modry DL, Hoppe RT, Pennock JL, Bieber CP, Holm BI, et al. Induction of specific unresponsiveness to heart allografts in mongrel dogs treated with total lymphoid irradiation and antithymocyte globulin. J Immunol. 1984;132:1013–8.
13. Evans MA, Schomberg PJ, Rodeheffer RJ, Katzmann JA, Schnell Jr WA, Tazelaar HD, et al. Total lymphoid irradiation: a novel and successful therapy for resistant cardiac allograft rejection. Mayo Clin Proc. 1992;67:785–90.
14. Salter SP, Salter MM, Kirklin JK, Bourge RC, Naftel DC. Total lymphoid irradiation in the treatment of early or recurrent heart transplant rejection. Int J Radiat Oncol Biol Phys. 1995;33:83–8.
15. Ross HJ, Gullestad L, Pak J, Slausaon S, Valantine HA, Hunt SA. Methotrexate or total lymphoid radiation for treatment of persistent or recurrent allograft cellular rejection: a comparative study. J Heart Lung Transplant. 1997;16:179–89.
16. Lim TS, O'Driscoll G, Freund J, Peterson V, Hayes H, Heywood J. Short-course total lymphoid irradiation for refractory cardiac transplantation rejection. J Heart Lung Transplant. 2007;26:1249–54.
17. Valentine VG, Robbins RC, Wehner JH, Patel HR, Berry GJ, Theodore J. Total lymphoid irradiation for refractory acute rejection in heart-lung and lung allografts. Chest. 1996;109:1184–9.
18. Diamond DA, Michalski JM, Lynch JP, Trulock EP. Efficacy of total lymphoid irradiation for chronic allograft rejection following bilateral lung transplantation. Int J Radiat Oncol Biol Phys. 1998;41:795–800.
19. Fisher AJ, Rutherford RM, Bozzino J, Parry G, Dark JH, Corris PA. The safety and efficacy of total lymphoid irradiation in progressive bronchiolitis obliterans syndrome after lung transplantation. Am J Transplant. 2005;5:537–43.
20. Yeoh K, Mikhaeel NG. Role of radiotherapy in modern treatment of Hodgkin's lymphoma. Advances in Hematology 2011; 2011: Article ID: 258797.
21. Verleden GM, Lievens Y, Dupont LJ, Van Raemdonck DE, De Vleeschauwer SI, Vos R, et al. Efficacy of total lymphoid irradiation in azithromycin nonresponsive chronic allograft rejection after lung transplantation. Transplant Proc. 2009;41:1816–20.
22. Edelson R, Berger C, Gasparro F, Jegasothy B, Heald P, Wintroub B, et al. Treatment of cutaneous T-cell lymphoma by extracorporeal photochemotherapy. N Engl J Med. 1987;316: 297–303.
23. Heald P, Rook A, Perez M, Wintroub B, Knobler R, Jegasothy B, et al. Treatment of erythrodermic cutaneous T-cell lymphoma with extracorporeal photochemotherapy. J Am Acad Dermatol. 1993;28:1023–4.
24. Yoo EK, Rook AH, Elenitsas R, Gasparro FP, Vewels BR. Apoptosis induction of ultraviolet A and photochemotherapy in cutaneous T-cell lymphoma; relevance to mechanism of therapeutic action. J Invest Dermatol. 1996;107:235–42.
25. Berger CL, Hanlon D, Kanada D, Girardi M, Edelson RL. Transimmunization, a novel approach for tumor immunotherapy. Transfus Apher Sci. 2002;26:205–16.
26. Menkes CJ, Andreu J, Heshmati f, Hillikquin P. Treatment of refractory rheumatoid arthritis by extracorporeal photochemotherapy. Br J Rheumatol. 1992;31:789–90.

27. Rook AH, Freundich B, Jegasothy BV, Perez MI, Barr WG, Jimenez SA, et al. Treatment of systemic sclerosis with extracorporeal photochemotherapy. Results of a multicenter trial. Arch Dermatol. 1992;128:337–46.
28. Knobler RM. Extracorporeal photochemotherapy for the treatment of lupus erythematosus: preliminary observations. Springer Semin Immunopathol. 1994;16:323–5.
29. Rook AH, Jgasothy BV, Heald P, Nahass GT, Ditre C, Witmer WK, et al. Extracorporeal photochemotherapy for drug resistant pemphigus vulgaris. Ann Intern Med. 1990;112:303–5.
30. Dall'Amico R, Messina C. Extracorporeal photochemotherapy for the treatment of graft-versus-host disease. Ther Apher. 2002;6:296–304.
31. Foss FM, Divenuti GM, Chin K, Sprague K, Grodman H, Klein A, et al. Prospective study of extracorporeal photopheresis in steroid-refractory or steroid-resistant extensive chronic graft-versus-host disease: analysis of response and survival incorporating prognostic factors. Bone Marrow Transplant. 2005;45:1187–93.
32. Costanzo-Nordin MR, Hubbell EA, O'Sullivan EJ, Johnson MR, Mullen GM, Heroux AL, et al. Photopheresis versus corticosteroids in the therapy of heart transplant rejection: preliminary clinical report. Circulation. 1992;86(5 suppl):II242–50.
33. Barr ML, Meiser BM, Eisen HJ, Roberts RF, Livi U, Dall'Amico R, et al. Photopheresis for the prevention of rejection in cardiac transplantation. Photopheresis Transplantation Study Group. N Engl J Med. 1998;339:1744–51.
34. Di Renzo M, Rubegni P, Sbano P, Cuccia A, Castagnini C, Pompella G, et al. ECP-treated lymphocytes of chronic graft-versus-host disease patients undergo apoptosis which involves both the Fas/FasL system and the Bcl-2 protein family. Arch Dermatol Res. 2003;295:175–82.
35. Bladon J, Taylor PC. Extracorporeal photopheresis: a focus on apoptosis and cytokines. J Dermatol Sci. 2006;43:85–94.
36. Enk AH. Dendritic cells in tolerance induction. Immunol Lett. 2005;99:8–11.
37. Lamioni A, Parisi F, Isacchi G, Giorda E, Di Cesare S, Landolfo A, et al. The immunological effects of extracorporeal photopheresis unraveled: induction of tolerogenic dendritic cells in vitro and regulatory T cells in vivo. Transplantation. 2005;79(7):846–50.
38. Biagi E, Di Biaso I, Leoni V, Gaipa G, Rossi V, Bugarin C, et al. Extracorporeal photochemotherapy is accompanied by increasing levels of circulating CD4+ CD25+ GITR+Foxp3+CD62L+ functional regulatory T-cells in patients with graft- versus-host disease. Transplantation. 2007;84:31–9.
39. Bladon J, Taylor P. Extracorporeal photopheresis normalizes some lymphocyte subsets (including T regulatory cells) in chronic graft-versus-host-disease. Ther Apher Dial. 2008;12:311–8.
40. Meloni F, Cascina A, Miserere S, Perotti C, Vitulo P, Fietta AM. Peripheral CD4+CD25+ TREG cell counts and the response to extracorporeal photopheresis in lung transplant recipients. Transplant Proc. 2007;39:213–7.
41. Gorgun G, Miller KB, Foss FM. Immunologic mechanisms of extracorporeal photochemotherapy in chronic graft-versus-host disease. Blood. 2002;100:941–7.
42. Di Renzo M, Sbano P, De Aloe G, Pasqui AL, Rubegni P, Ghezzi A, et al. Extracorporeal photopheresis affects co-stimulatory molecule expression and interleukin-10 production by dendritic cells in graft-versus-host disease patients. Clin Exp Immunol. 2008;151:407–13.
43. Slovis BS, Loyd JE, King LE. Photopheresis for chronic rejection of lung allografts. N Engl J Med. 1995;332:962–3.
44. Salerno CT, Park SJ, Kreykes NS, Kulick DM, Savik K, Hertz MI, et al. Adjuvant treatment of refractory lung transplant rejection with extracorporeal photopheresis. J Thorac Cardiovasc Surg. 1999;117:1063–9.
45. Villanueva J, Bhorade SM, Robinson JA, Husain AN, Garrity ER. Extracorporeal photopheresis for the treatment of lung allograft rejection. Ann Transplant. 2000;5:44–7.
46. Benden C, Speich R, Hofbauer GF, Irani S, Eich-Wanger C, Russi EW, et al. Extracorporeal photopheresis after lung transplantation: a 10-year single-center experience. Transplantation. 2008;86:1625–7.

47. Morrell MR, Despotis GJ, Lublin DM, Patterson GA, Trulock EP, Hachem RR. The efficacy of photopheresis for bronchiolitis obliterans syndrome after lung transplantation. J Heart Lung Transplant. 2010;29:424–31.
48. Lama VN, Murray S, Lonigro RJ, Toews GB, Chang A, Lau C, et al. Course of FEV_1 after onset of bronchiolitis obliterans syndrome in lung transplant recipients. Am J Respir Crit Care Med. 2007;175:1192–8.
49. Yusen RD, Shearon TH, Quian Y, Kotloff R, Barr ML, Sweet S, et al. Lung transplantation in the United States, 1999–2008. Am J Transplant. 2010;10:1047–68.
50. Novick RJ, Kaye MP, Patterson GA, Andreassian B, Klepetko W, Menkis AH, et al. Redo lung transplantation: A North American-European experience. J Heart Lung Transplant. 1993;12:5–15.
51. Novick RJ, Schafers HJ, Stitt L, Andreassian B, Duchatelle JP, Klepetko W, et al. Recurrence of obliterative bronchiolitis and determinants of outcome in 139 pulmonary retransplant recipients. J Thorac Cardiovasc Surg. 1995;110:1402–14.
52. Novick RJ, Stitt LW, Al-Kattan K, Klepetko W, Schafers HJ, Duchatelle JP, et al. Pulmonary retransplantation: predictors of graft function and survival in 230 patients. Ann Thorac Surg. 1998;65:227–34.
53. Brugiere O, Thabut G, Castier Y, Mal H, Dauriat G, Marceau A, et al. Lung retransplantation for bronchiolitis obliterans syndrome. Long-term follow-up in a series of 15 recipients. Chest. 2003;123:1832–7.
54. Strueber M, Fischer S, Gottleib J, Simon AR, Goerler H, Gohrbandt B, et al. Long-term outcome after pulmonary retransplantation. J Thorac Cardiovasc Surg. 2006;132:407–12.
55. Osaki S, Maloney JD, Meyer KC, Cornwell RD, Edwards NM, De Oliveira NC. Redo lung transplantation for acute and chronic lung allograft failure: long-term follow-up in a single center. Eur J Cardiothorac Surg. 2008;34:1191–7.
56. Aigner C, Jaksch P, Taghavi S, Lang G, Reza-Hoda MA, Wisser W, Klepetko W. Pulmonary retransplantation: is it worth the effort? A long-term analysis of 46 cases. J Heart Lung Transplant. 2008;27:60–5.
57. Kawut SM, Lederer DJ, Keshavjee S, Wilt JS, Daly T, D'Ovidio F, et al. Outcomes after lung retransplantation in the modern era. Am J Respir Crit Care Med. 2008;177:114–20.
58. Johnson BA, Iacono AT, Zeevi A, McCurry KR, Duncan SR. Statin use is associated with improved function and survival of lung allografts. Am J Respir Crit Care Med. 2003;167:1271–8.
59. Weber J, Tiriveedhi V, Takenaka M, Lu W, Hachem R, Trulock E, et al. Inhibition of rennin angiotensin aldosterone system causes abrogation of obliterative airway disease through inhibition of tumor necrosis factor-α-dependent interleukin-17. J Heart Lung Transplant. 2012;31:419–26.
60. Iuppa JA, Wills AR, Bowman LJ, Patterson GA, Trulock EP, Hachem RR. An evaluation of the impact of statin use on the progression to bronchiolitis obliterans in lung allografts [abstract]. J Heart Lung Transplant. 2011;30(Suppl):S150–1.
61. Antus B, Sebe A, Fillinger J, Jeney C, Horvath I. Effects of blockade of the renin-angiotensin and endothelin systems on experimental bronchiolitis obliterans. J Heart Lung Transplant. 2006;25:1324–9.
62. Antus B, Fillinger J, Sebe A, Jeney C, Horvath I. Late treatment with angiotensin-converting enzyme inhibitors plus endothelin receptor antagonists ameliorates rat tracheal allograft rejection. Transpl Int. 2008;21:801–7.
63. McKane BW, Fernandez F, Narayanan K, Marshbank S, Margolin S, Jendrisak M, et al. Pirfenidone inhibits obliterative airway disease in a murine heterotopic tracheal transplant model. Transplantation. 2004;77:664–9.

Index

K.C. Meyer and A.R. Glanville (eds.), *Bronchiolitis Obliterans Syndrome in Lung Transplantation*, Respiratory Medicine 8, DOI 10.1007/978-1-4614-7636-8,

D

MIX
Papier aus verantwortungsvollen Quellen
Paper from responsible sources
FSC® C105338

If you have any concerns about our products,
you can contact us on
ProductSafety@springernature.com

In case Publisher is established outside the EU,
the EU authorized representative is:
Springer Nature Customer Service Center GmbH
Europaplatz 3, 69115 Heidelberg, Germany

Printed by Libri Plureos GmbH
in Hamburg, Germany